Kenneth R. Valpey

Cow Care in Hindu Animal Ethics

palgrave
macmillan

Kenneth R. Valpey
Oxford Centre for Hindu Studies
Oxford, UK

The Palgrave Macmillan Animal Ethics Series
ISBN 978-3-030-28407-7   ISBN 978-3-030-28408-4   (eBook)
https://doi.org/10.1007/978-3-030-28408-4

This Palgrave Macmillan imprint is published by the registered company Springer Nature Switzerland AG
The registered company address is: Gewerbestrasse 11, 6330 Cham, Switzerland

For all who would care more for our kin, including kine

In the memory of my preceptor, Swami Prabhupada, whose care begins to sprout within me

Series Editors' Preface

This is a new book series for a new field of inquiry: Animal Ethics.

In recent years, there has been a growing interest in the ethics of our treatment of animals. Philosophers have led the way, and now a range of other scholars have followed from historians to social scientists. From being a marginal issue, animals have become an emerging issue in ethics and in multidisciplinary inquiry.

In addition, a rethink of the status of animals has been fueled by a range of scientific investigations which have revealed the complexity of animal sentiency, cognition, and awareness. The ethical implications of this new knowledge have yet to be properly evaluated, but it is becoming clear that the old view that animals are mere things, tools, machines, or commodities cannot be sustained ethically.

But it is not only philosophy and science that are putting animals on the agenda. Increasingly, in Europe and the United States, animals are becoming a political issue as political parties vie for the "green" and "animal" vote. In turn, political scientists are beginning to look again at the history of political thought in relation to animals, and historians are beginning to revisit the political history of animal protection.

As animals grow as an issue of importance, so there have been more collaborative academic ventures leading to conference volumes, special journal issues, indeed new academic animal journals as well. Moreover, we have witnessed the growth of academic courses, as well as university posts, in Animal Ethics, Animal Welfare, Animal Rights, Animal Law, Animals and Philosophy, Human-Animal Studies, Critical Animal Studies, Animals and Society, Animals in Literature, Animals and Religion—tangible signs that a new academic discipline is emerging.

"Animal Ethics" is the new term for the academic exploration of the moral status of the non-human—an exploration that explicitly involves a focus on what we owe animals morally, and which also helps us to understand the influences—social, legal, cultural, religious, and political—that legitimate animal abuse. This series explores the challenges that Animal Ethics poses, both conceptually and practically, to traditional understandings of human–animal relations.

The series is needed for three reasons: (i) to provide the texts that will service the new university courses on animals; (ii) to support the increasing number of students studying and academics researching in animal-related fields, and (iii) because there is currently no book series that is a focus for multidisciplinary research in the field.

Specifically, the series will:

- provide a range of key introductory and advanced texts that map out ethical positions on animals;
- publish pioneering work written by new, as well as accomplished, scholars, and
- produce texts from a variety of disciplines that are multidisciplinary in character or have multidisciplinary relevance.

The new Palgrave Macmillan Series on Animal Ethics is the result of a unique partnership between Palgrave Macmillan and the Ferrater Mora Oxford Centre for Animal Ethics. The series is an integral part of the mission of the Centre to put animals on the intellectual agenda by facilitating academic research and publication. The series is also a natural complement to one of the Centre's other major projects, the *Journal of Animal Ethics*. The Centre is an independent "think tank" for the advancement of progressive thought about animals and is the first Centre of its kind in the world. It aims to demonstrate rigorous intellectual enquiry and the highest standards of scholarship. It strives to be a world-class center of academic excellence in its field.

We invite academics to visit the Centre's Web site www.oxfordanimalethics.com and to contact us with new book proposals for the series.

Oxford, UK   Andrew Linzey
Villanova, USA   Priscilla N. Cohn
                                                          General Editors

Foreword

As human populations have increased, so also the need for food has increased. With the global introduction of mechanized agriculture, the demand for and consumption of meat have grown, in both total and per person. Today, it is estimated that 56 billion land animals are killed for food every year, including 800,000 cows every day around the world (www.sentientmedia.org). Because so few people have direct contact with the process of food production, it can be all too easy to ignore the tremendous amount of suffering inflicted on animals for the sake of human sustenance and, in many instances, human vanity, luxury, and status.

This book offers important insight into what might be done in terms of awareness of this problem and describes possible small-scale solutions. As Margaret Mead once commented, "Never doubt that a small group of thoughtful, committed, organized citizens can change the world; indeed, it's the only thing that ever has." For many centuries, the cow has been deemed sacred in India and advocates for vegetarianism have been quite effective in developing a healthy cuisine that does not include meat, fish, or eggs. In terms of harm reduction to both the animals and the human body itself, plant-based diets have grown in popularity throughout the world.

Vegetarianism can be a complex undertaking. Important leaders of modern India, including Dayananda Saraswati, M. K. Gandhi, and B. R. Ambedkar advocated adoption of a meat-free diet, each for different reasons. However, Gandhi asserted that one should allow oneself to be killed for the protection of the cow, but must not kill in order to defend a cow. Some would argue that even the gifts of the cow such as milk and ghee and by-products such as cheese and yogurt must be abandoned because of the inevitable maltreatment of the cow and the possible ill effects to human health of a dairy-heavy diet.

This book employs the ethical decision-making processes of three contemporary thinkers in outlining the case for cow protection. Philosopher Vrinda Dalmiya expands the ethics of care developed by Carol Gilligan to include the non-human realm. Political scientist Jonathan Haidt posits that loyalty and sanctity must be included with care, along with reliance on reliable data. Theologian Larry Rasmussen advocates the formation of anticipatory communities that demonstrate the possibility of enhanced goodness.

Valpey provides direct accounts of four intentional communities inspired by A. C. Bhaktivedanta Swami Prabhupada dedicated to the well-being of the cow: Mayapur Chandrolaya Mandir in West Bengal, New Vraja Dhama in Hungary, Bhaktivedanta Manor in London, and Govardhan Eco Village in Maharashtra. And even in these idyllic small-scale communities, complexities arise. With the widespread use of the tractor, the employ of oxen (castrated bulls) for ploughing has diminished worldwide, causing an increase in the killing of young male cattle for veal, who otherwise would serve no economic function. Artificial insemination further decreases the demand for the services of adult male bulls. Govardhan has opted for castration of bulls, while some of the other communities listed above do not castrate.

At the core of all these conversations can be found a common concern: how might harm to animals and the consequent suffering be mitigated in the world? Awareness of the problem is a first step toward the development of conscience. As Margaret Mead has reminded us, change and movement toward goodness lies in the hands of the citizenry. By describing in detail the commitments made by individuals to eschew meat consumption and actively work for the protection of cattle, Valpey reminds us of what is possible, while noting multiple political and biological complexities that inevitably arise.

Christopher K. Chapple
Doshi Professor of Indic and Comparative Theology
Loyola Marymount University, Los Angeles
Author, *Nonviolence to Animals, Earth, and Self in Asian Traditions*

Preface

Growing up in suburban America, my connection with cows was almost exclusively through drinking their milk—delivered to our door in glass bottles—and in eating their meat at supper. Not until several years later, when I became a "Hare Krishna" monk (and thereby, a vegetarian) and eventually was stationed at the mission's small farm in Bavaria, southeast Germany, did I begin to have growing awareness of cows as beings with lives of their own. Those twenty-odd cows were to be cared for their entire natural lives—a practice introduced in a few nascent Western Krishna farm communities by their founder, my spiritual guide, A. C. Bhaktivedanta Swami Prabhupada. Cows became, therefore, part of our lives, an important reason why we lived as we did, pursuing an ideal of "plain living and high thinking," as Prabhupada urged us to do.

As I began visiting India (first in 1978, then almost every year since then), I saw how cows are part of the everyday landscape in most places there, whether country, village, town, or city. As different as this was from my experience of cows in America and Germany, it strangely made sense: humans and cows somehow belong together. But gradually I learned more about cows in India. On the one hand, they are treated as special, even worshipped. On the other hand, many cows are neglected, and increasing numbers (millions) are victims of a burgeoning beef and leather industry. I also learned that years of political and legal action on behalf of cows had done relatively little for them. How to understand these anomalies?

This book has come about as a result of my attempt to understand more about cows in Indian tradition and current practice, and my wish to help others to understand cow care, whether or not in connection with India. Much has been written on this subject, but obviously I find there is more to be said, hopefully prompting more serious discussion and then action to reverse what needs to be recognized as a deep anomaly and a great shame on our human species.

I write from a position of liminality: Western in background and culture, as a young man adopting ways and ideas generally labeled "Hindu" and, more specifically, "Vaishnava," later (re-)entering the academy to study my adopted tradition from scholarly perspectives. Out of this mix, I present my own comprehension of a complex subject, and my own "constructive" approach to the ethics of what I call "cow care" (the practice of keeping and caring for cows throughout their natural lives, translating the Sanskrit and Hindi term *go-seva*). Truth be told, I don't speak from direct experience of cow care. Observing cows (and occasionally brushing them or offering them snacks), observing and listening to those with experience caring for cows, conversing with cow care activists and colleagues, reading and thinking a lot—these have been my ways of learning about, being moved by, caring about, my subject.

Oxford, UK   Kenneth R. Valpey

Acknowledgements

I'm ever grateful to those who have shared their knowledge and wisdom with me and who have helped me in numerous other ways. I can mention only some of them.

Professor Andrew Linzey, Director of the Oxford Centre for Animal Ethics, has so kindly invited me to publish this work in the Palgrave Macmillan Animal Ethics book series, which he co-edits. Initially, I was resistant to the idea, but I'm grateful for his gentle persistence. Andrew's lovely daughter, Clair Linzey, has also been a big help and encouragement, as has Anna King.

Many friends and colleagues have helped in various ways, including some Vaishnavas (Vaishnava Hindus). Typically, Vaishnavas address each other by their initiation names, and many prefer to be known by these (names ending in "Das" or "Dasi" as you will see below). My thanks to Allan Andersson and his wife Petra for their careful reading and suggestions on early drafts; similarly, Hrvoje Cargonja and Ravi Gupta have helped illumine the way, as has Graham Schweig. Barbara Holdredge, Tony Stewart, Jessica Frazier, Rembert Lutjeharms, Brian Hatcher, and Tattvavit Das gave useful suggestions for sources, as did Rasamandala Das, Hari Parshad Das, Brijabhasi Das, and Brahma Muhurta Das.

Chirayu Thakkar and Sugopi Sadhu alerted me to relevant news items; and Jonathan Banks helped numerous times accessing online materials. Acyuta Das, at Bhaktivedanta Research Centre, Kolkata, was very helpful, and Akrura Das gave helpful advice on project strategizing.

My heartfelt thanks go to several patient interviewees, including Shivarama Swami, Swami B. V. Tripurari, Satya Narayan Das Babaji, Radha Krishna Das, Revatiraman Das, Akhandanand Das, Hrimati Dasi, Sitaram Das, Indraneelamani Das, Arca-murti Dasi and Raju, Dayal Mukunda Das, Damodar Dulal Das, Janmastami Das, Saci Kumar Das, Vishnu Nama Das, Keshi Nisudana Das, Prahlada Bhakta Das, Sanak-Sanatan Das, Datta Saranananda Swami and his assistants, Arvind and Prabhav, Gopal Sutariya, Satya Narayan Das Babaji, Shrivatsa Goswami, Uttam Maheshwari, Brig. S. S. Chohan, and Maneka Gandhi.

I'm particularly grateful to my colleagues at the Oxford Centre for Hindu Studies for their constant encouragement and support, especially Shaunaka Rishi Das, Anuradha Dooney, and Rembert Lutjeharms. For research funding through the OCHS, I am grateful for receiving the Ramlal B. Patel and Harish I. K. Patel Bursaries.

Hearty thanks to Narottamadas Thakur Das, his wife Manjari Dasi, and son Kartamisha, who hosted me with great warmth and the best imaginable devotional cuisine for several weeks in their Mumbai home and facilitated my travel in Maharashtra and Gujarat, with their expert and careful driver, Ram-ji. Thank you Madhu Gauranga Das, for enthusiastically arranging to meet *go-raksha* activists, and to Kalakantha Das for thoughtful discussions on cow care and its many challenges and rewards.

While back in Europe I've been assisted by several friends keeping me peacefully sheltered and well-fed, allowing me to concentrate on writing: My thanks to Radharaman Das, Mukunda-mala Dasi and family, Madhai Jivan Nitai Das, Malati-mala Dasi and Nadiya Nimai Das, Vira Gopal Das (who also helped sourcing materials and with Hindi translation), and Indulekha Dasi. I was also assisted in Hindi translation by Madhavi Kishori Dasi, her mother Nandimukhi Dasi, Sunil and Sunita, and Vrishabhanu Kumari Dasi, and Pulkit Gupta. I also appreciate the help of Gaura Mitra Das and Uddhava Mitra Das, who scanned materials in my library, enabling me—an itinerant monk—to reference them while traveling. Many thanks to you all. Then, there are Suzanne and Ludwig Jacob, who have caringly kept me physically fit and mentally cheerful, for which I'm ever deeply grateful.

It has been a pleasure working with the folks at Palgrave Macmillan, including April James and Lauriane Piette. Also I thank the anonymous reviewers for their helpful suggestions.

With the generous donations of several persons it has become possible to bring this book to the public through open access under Palgrave Macmillan's auspices. I am grateful to the publisher for this opportunity, and to several donors who have made this option possible for this book. In particular, I wish to thank Prema-rasarnava Das and Sita Dasi, Purushottama Kshetra Das, Mitra Balaram Das, Dino and Adisa Muhović, Harry Kwok, Wilhelm Kinn, Beate Düringer, Jacek Brycki, Julia Brycka, Anna Johansson, and Rolf Peters. I am grateful to Mandali Mendrila, Madhu van Paare, and Gopal Lila Patel for encouraging and guiding me in this fundraising venture.

Professor Christopher Key Chapple, thank you for kindly taking the time to write your thoughtful Foreword for the book.

Praise for *Cow Care in Hindu Animal Ethics*

"A thoroughly researched and most timely book analyzing the place-
ment of the cow throughout Hindu culture, and its potential role in
human well-being more broadly. While the growing Western animal
rights movement is primarily based in human-centric concerns, and
the protection of animals objectified and valued in terms of benefits to
human health, diet, ecology and environment, Valpey introduces us to
the notion of the cow as subject and as citizen in its own right. Using
traditional as well as modern theoretical frames of references, Valpey
leads us to the inexorable conclusion that the welfare of human civilization and cow protection are inextricably linked."
 —Edwin Bryant, *Professor of Hinduism, Rutgers University, USA*

"There has been growing academic interest in the more-than-human
these days, and this certainly includes nonhuman animals. The cow
within Hinduism has been either regarded as the most special of animals, or even as the representative of all animals. Kenneth Valpey has
produced a wonderful book that invites us to look at cows as "subjects,"
and explores the special nature of them from a wide variety of sources
within India. In so doing, he offers a very thoughtful ethical perspective

for our consideration. Those interested in the larger field of animal ethics will find much of value in this book."
—David L. Haberman, *Professor of Religious Studies, Indiana University, author of* People Trees: Worship of Trees in Northern India

"An extensive and nuanced meditation on the relationship between human and animal kingdoms in India and the world at large: this volume examines the philosophical underpinnings of the ethics of cow care and protection in India and goes on to make a credible environmental case for their contemporary implementation. It offers a very rich blend of cultural studies, intellectual history, and environmental awareness and will clearly develop and deepen the discourse on inter-species dharma."
—E. H. Rick Jarow, *Associate Professor of Religion and Asian Studies, Vassar College*

"The cow is integral to the economic, cultural and spiritual well being of Hindus and is central to the natural, human and divine spheres of life, which interrelate for mutual benefit. Kenneth Valpey's book 'Cow Care in Hindu Animal Ethics' discusses the historical and current issues that surround the cow as a sacred animal in Indian culture. It highlights how both dharma and bhakti are balanced in the daily care of cows, requiring the long term well-being of all animals, with the human—cow relationship as a starting point. The book is well researched on Hindu animal ethics from the Vedic to the contemporary and is an important contribution to our knowledge of the co-operation between human beings and the animal world."
—Dr. Nanditha Krishna, *President, C. P. Ramaswami Aiyar Foundation, Chennai, India*

"This is a path-breaking book that deserves to be widely read. Valpey expands our understanding of animal ethics and complexifies our notion of devotion. Original and thought-provoking, this book will open up new venues for discussion and reflection regarding cow care."
—Mary Evelyn Tucker, *Yale Forum on Religion and Ecology, Yale University, USA*

Contents

Abbreviations

Bg, Gita	Bhagavad Gita
BhP	Bhagavata Purana
CC	Chaitanya Charitamrita
CMNG	Community of the Many Names of God
GEV	Govardhan Eco Village
ISKCON	International Society for Krishna Consciousness
MBh	Mahabharata
NVD	New Vraja Dhama
TB	Taittiriya Brahmana
TOVP	Temple of the Vedic Planetarium
YS	Yoga Sutras of Patanjali

List of Figures

1

Introduction

Cows—certain types of *bovinae*—can evoke strong emotions among people, different emotions rooted in different worldviews. One worldview, which is arguably a galaxy of worldviews emerging over centuries in India, has come to be called "Hindu." Some people who identify themselves as Hindus have strong feelings about cows—feelings that tie into their sense of conviction that cows are not just different from, but are *more than* animals, that they are in an important sense sacred, set apart, worthy of reverence, and therefore worthy of special care and protection. With a slight wordplay echoing the term *divinity*, we can speak in this context of *bovinity* as a descriptor for cows as more than animals.

For persons with other worldviews, cows may also evoke strong emotions. For some, the emotion evoked may be rooted in a strong sense of possessiveness. Oddly, such possessiveness has affinity with affects of Hindus who see cows as more than animal. Both regard cows as valuable. The difference is that the (*possibly* non-Hindu) persons in the second group find value in cows' bodies more for what they provide once dead than what they provide while living.

© The Author(s) 2020
K. R. Valpey, *Cow Care in Hindu Animal Ethics*,
The Palgrave Macmillan Animal Ethics Series,
https://doi.org/10.1007/978-3-030-28408-4_1

I say *possibly* non-Hindu because some who might identify themselves as at least nominally Hindus, whether or not they would admit it, share this latter sense of cows' value.

Again, cows—bovines—can evoke strong emotions among people; conversely, cows can also be objects of indifference. Surprisingly, this is—or has become—especially true in India, a land typically associated with Hindu worldviews that include high regard for cows. A strange state of cultural cognitive dissonance appears to affect many people throughout the entire country of India, from top government officials to simple farmers.

Again, strangely, whether objects of strong emotions (either as bovinity or as commodity) or objects of indifference, all three of these sorts of persons tend to regard cows as *objects*. As objects, cows serve humans, or not. If they serve humans, it is either by divine arrangement that they do so, or by welcome accident that they can be used by humans, as sources of commodities. If they do not serve humans, cows are expendable, perhaps to be left to become either rewilded or extinct.

To consider cows as *subjects* is the starting point of this book, as it is the starting point for an ethical consideration of cows and, with cows, other nonhuman animals, in particular "farm animals." Also, since positive regard for cows (more or less as bovinity) is strongly associated with Hindu traditions, this book is concerned with what has come to be called Hinduism, although the Hindu landscape may be better described in the plural, as "Hinduisms." For many (both Hindus and non-Hindus), concern for cows beyond their utility is, or has come to be, a defining feature of Hinduism.[1]

However, the process of defining Hinduism can lead to objectification, or rather, to *misplaced* objectification, by which I mean a misunderstanding or failure to recognize what is regarded in Hindu philosophical traditions as objective metaphysical truth. Some—perhaps many—Hindus objectify themselves with the label *Hindu*, such that they may forget or ignore basic teachings of sacred texts they would readily identify as Hindu. Yet, somewhat ironically, to these texts the term "Hindu" is unknown.

More specifically, this term is foreign to the Bhagavad Gita, widely regarded as a key text of several Hindu traditions. The Gita (for short)

---

[1] For a book-length discussion on issues involved in defining Hinduism, see Llewellyn (2005).

does, however, mention cows, including them in a brief list of living beings: "A learned brahmin, a cow, an elephant, a dog, or a 'dog-eater'—a wise person sees [them all] with equal vision" (Gita 5.18). The equation of wisdom (or a well-educated person—*pandita*) with "equal vision" toward living beings points to subjectivity, rooted in an essential understanding of Hindu metaphysics, namely that consciousness is foundational to existence, being prior to, and indeed the source of, matter. In turn, arguably for most Hindus, consciousness indicates *personhood* as a fundamental category of reality; in contrast, designations such as "Hindu" and "cow" are of a secondary order, of identities that do not endure. Seeing equally means seeing all creatures as conscious beings who, depending on the particular bodies they occupy, exhibit varying degrees of the potential for full, enduring personhood. The implications of this worldview for animal ethics are considerable.

But if equal vision is so highly valued, why are cows singled out for special attention by Hindus, and why are they selected as the focus of this book? Why indeed. Much of this book will be concerned with answering this question, and in the attempt, the book will function largely as an extended commentary to the Gita stanza just quoted. I will argue that there are good reasons that cows are to be privileged (insofar as subjectivity of cows and other nonhuman animals is recognized or valued, at least in principle), and there are also less than ideal reasons that cows are privileged (insofar as objectification—of cows, nonhuman animals, and humans) is the result. The "less than ideal" reasons are nonetheless reasons for privileging cows: living cows do provide substances that humans benefit from, and this fact cannot and need not be ignored.

One reason for singling out cows for special attention has little to do with Hinduism as such, and more to do with soil. Healthy, well-cared-for cows (and ruminants more generally) and healthy soil go together; the opposite is also true, and the misuse and abuse of cows have accelerated degradation of soil throughout our planet, leading to expanding—indeed runaway—desertification.[2] Another important sacred text of Hindus, the

---

[2]According to Prof. Sir Bob Watson, chair of the Intergovernmental Science-Policy Platform on Biodiversity and Ecosystem Services, currently some 3.2 billion people worldwide are effected by degraded soils. https://www.bbc.com/news/science-environment-48043134. Accessed 29 April 2019.

Bhagavata Purana, seems to acknowledge this relationship when it identifies earth with cow and, in other texts, the dung of cows—which is extremely nourishing to soil—with Lakshmi, the goddess of fortune.

Considering the bio-zoological relationship of earth and cows, and considering the environmental damage from cattle farming for meat, leather, and other by-products—all for nonessential human uses, the sheer numbers of cows slaughtered annually give pause for thought: Worldwide, the lives of some 300 million cows annually, or roughly 34,000 cows per hour, are cut short by human intervention. Surprisingly, cow slaughter in India accounts for a substantial percentage of these numbers. In 2016, nearly nine million cows were slaughtered, putting India fifth among nations with the greatest numbers of cows slaughtered.[3] It seems that despite India's legacy of special regard for cows, counter-forces have increased and accelerated, such that high regard for cows as beings to be cared for throughout their natural lives competes with disregard and purely instrumental regard that condemns them to commodification's relentless ways of disposal.

In this book, I sketch a sphere of Hindu ethical concern for animals that has as its locus the care and protection of cows. My aim is to (1) set out prominent features of the historical and current complexity of issues surrounding cows as animals of special concern in India; (2) suggest ways that some aspects of Hindu thought may contribute to and enrich present-day animal ethics discussion; (3) highlight limits on the value of Hindu animal ethics thought and practice, insofar as the priority of values is located in being Hindu rather than in respecting animals; and (4) illustrate practical ways that nascent "anticipatory communities"— communities with Hindu roots but reaching beyond this designation—are demonstrating alternative ways of living—both in and outside India—in which what I will be calling *cow care* is an integral feature. With the phrase

---

[3] https://faunalytics.org/global-animal-slaughter-statistics-and-charts/. Accessed 1 April 2019; page dated 10 October 2018), based on data from the United Nations Food and Agriculture Organization. China ranks highest, with almost 50 million cows slaughtered in 2016, Brazil is next, at over 37 million, then United States, at 31 million, followed by Argentina at 11.7 million. Taking into account population, the per capita number of cows slaughtered in India is relatively small. Still, these numbers are vastly greater than would have to be assumed in pre- or early modern India. I should note that another source consulted gave a much higher number for cows slaughtered annually in India, but I suspect that this higher number (some 38 million) includes water buffaloes.

"cow care" I generally mean the practice, or set of practices, centered on keeping and caring for cows (which will mainly, though not always, be referring to both male and female bovines) throughout their natural lives.

As a wide-ranging overview focused on cows, my aim is to make a case for cow care in particular and to set this case within a viable animal ethics discourse framework. I will be attentive to the practical challenges involved in cow care practice while questioning the current dominant instrumentalist and extractive economics of agribusiness that blinds us to the possibility of a different vision, a vision we may loosely call *traditional*. What I offer here are some rudiments of a vision of balance, as suggested by the Indic word *dharma*, and of interspecies care, as suggested by the Indic word *bhakti*.

Present-day Hindus who champion cow care are likely to invoke the tradition of sacred texts as evidence for cows' special regard from ancient times. In Chapter 2, I offer a diachronic literary overview of relevant texts, beginning with the earliest known work, the collection of hymns known as Rigveda. Continuing with relevant references in later Vedic, post-Vedic, and classical Sanskrit works—the philosophically reflective Upanishads, the epic narrative Mahabharata, and the preeminent work of the Purana (ancient lore) genre, the Bhagavata Purana—we then touch on vernacular pre-modern and present-day literature. What emerges from this survey are two sorts of polarity—one of values, ranging between the Indic terms dharma and bhakti, and the second polarity one of meaning, ranging between literal and figurative understanding. These two polarities converge in the Sanskrit term *artha,* which indicates both *value* and *meaning*. Thus, cows as living beings and "cow" as a concept converge as a central locus of thought and action that strives for ethical integrity in all aspects of human life.

The textual survey of Chapter 2 listens mainly to the voices of brahmanical Hinduism, that of the literati and priesthood through the ages. This bias continues in Chapter 3, but with a significant shift in the face of modern critical thought. Since ancient times, the pursuit of ethical integrity has taken ritual form, centrally in performance of *yajna* (Sanskrit: *yajña*), usually translated as "sacrifice." Controversy in modern times for some Hindus has revolved around whether or to what extent animals—especially cows—have been immolated in ancient sacrificial rites. In Chapter 3,

I examine this controversy, after surveying the modern emergence of a Cow Protection movement in India out of which the controversy emerged. I introduce four prominent makers of this history—Dayanand Sarasvati, M. K. Gandhi, B. R. Ambedkar, and Bhaktivedanta Swami Prabhupada. Here, in calling attention to cow protectionism's Hindu identity politics within a growing nationalist movement toward independence from British rule, the semantic field of bovine meaning reaches well into the sphere of modern state governance. Consequently, a rhetoric of dharma— especially *sanatana-dharma* (unchanging dharma) takes a pivotal role, but in the process, I suggest, the dharma concept becomes impoverished as it is privileged over dharma's important counterpart, bhakti. The interest of actual cows is served when both principles are held in balance, the one dynamically complementing the other.

As modernization and globalization extend their reach throughout India, one response of cow carers wishing to preserve bovine sanctity has been to establish cow shelters or sanctuaries (*goshalas*). Throughout present-day India, there are several thousand goshalas of widely varying size and quality. Attempts to demonstrate the importance and viability of cow care can be seen in these goshalas, where one can also see sincere and determined people doing their best to realize a balance of dharma and bhakti in their daily care for cows. In Chapter 4, I offer snapshots of a few such current projects, hearing from their managers or owners about the challenges involved in pursuing an ideal amidst adverse conditions. I also survey economies of cow care in terms of charity and of (living) bovine products, ranging from tangible goods (especially milk and dung, and oxen traction) to less tangible or intangible goods (such as positive influence of cows on the environment and on people). The aim is to examine the inherent tension between utility and care, seeing how this tension is perceived, negotiated, resolved, or unresolved, within the ideological framework of the dharma and bhakti paradigms. Again, I suggest, if dharma is divorced from bhakti, the impulse toward self-centeredness persists, a tendency that plays out in the broadest sense as anthropocentrism, the root of human alienation from nature and hence from nonhuman animals.

Chapters 2 through 4 provide a setting for what follows in Chapter 5. Having viewed the literary, historical, and present-day complexities surrounding cow care, we step back to consider Hindu ethics with respect to animals more broadly, drawing largely from the Indic classical literature to see how the dharma-bhakti polarity of values might be constructively applied. Here, I point to three aspects of dharma—as settled duty, deliberation, and cultivation of virtue, each with positive aspects and limitations. I then introduce *yoga*, an important Hindu tradition of intentional self-cultivation toward spiritual freedom, as a link between dharma and bhakti paradigms. Turning then to bhakti, the key point is to suggest a complementarity between bhakti and the contemporary (Western) "ethics of care" thought stream applied to animal ethics. To appreciate how the bhakti paradigm can enrich the ethics of care approach, I consider the theistic character of bhakti in terms of what I call *divine preference ethics*, which holds human choice to be crucial in realizing the full depth of loving relationship that leads to the good—the aim of ethical deliberation and action. Further, the practical application of ethics of care in bhakti calls for a consideration of an expanded understanding of *citizenship*, as proposed by Sue Donaldson and Will Kymlicka (2013). The citizenship ideal honors nonhuman animals that are in direct relationship with humans ("domestic" or "farm" animals) while acknowledging their varied contributions to human well-being in non-exploitative conditions, always in the pursuit of ahimsa—nonviolence—as ideal toward which human society must purposefully aim. To illustrate how nonhuman animal citizenship might be applied in relation to cows, I consider four of the nine "specific areas of presupposition for citizenship" discussed by Donaldson and Kymlicka, namely (1) mobility and the sharing of public space; (2) use of animal products; (3) use of animal labor; and (4) sex and reproduction. Yet it is further necessary to consider the broader political framework in which such citizenship might function. The proposed framework is *dharma-based communitarian* in character, which is currently being implemented (in very small scale) in "anticipatory communities" in which cow care is a key element.

In Chapter 6, the focus returns to cow care, and the aim is to imagine a possible positive future for cows whereby the principles outlined in Chapter 5 are applied, at least initially in anticipatory communities. Here, I point to two existing such communities, one in India (West Bengal) and one in Central Europe (Hungary), both affiliated with the institution established by Swami Prabhupada (introduced in Chapter 3). As young as both these communities are, only time will tell how successful they will be; yet they point in a direction and strive to realize the sort of dharma- and bhakti-centered cultures in which the ideals of cow care can be practiced in contemporary life. Inevitably, one of the challenges these communities face is end-of-life care for cows. Keeping with the theme of futures for cows, I therefore briefly consider this, referring to two specific cases seen as wrongly treated and one case seen as a good and indeed glorious cow (bull) death leading to what his carers regarded as a bright future in this animal's expected afterlife. I then move to another register of future-thinking, namely, that of activism in the public sphere, to suggest lesser and greater effectiveness of such efforts in terms of the Indic thought system of Samkhya, with its threefold typology of qualities (*gunas*). This brings us back to the theme of objectification. In this context, objectification happens when cows are championed more as symbols than as actual living beings with needs for extensive care. Such "fallacy of misplaced concreteness" (as A. N. Whitehead might put it) displays characteristics of the two lower, or denser, *gunas* (*rajas* and *tamas*—passion and darkness). By way of contrast, I offer a sixfold series of *affirmations on the dharma of cow care* to illustrate what a luminous (*sattva-guna*) future for cows could look like.

These six affirmations may give the impression of a hopelessly utopian vision—a wishful but impossible dream. Yet Hindu traditions, reaching back at least three thousand years, suggest that a longing to find a meaningful and mutually enriching relationship of humans with nonhumans has persisted. In Chapter 7—Concluding Ruminations—we consider this book's utopian/dystopian binary through two further visions presented in Vaishnava Hindu texts, raising the question whether "human nature" is changeable for the better, and if so, how. The bhakti paradigm offers a way forward toward deep transformation, specifically, transformation of *taste*. Through such transformation, *care-full* engagement with our environment—our world—becomes possible and feasible. Today, there is a pressing need to find a way forward toward long-term well-being for animals—both nonhuman and human—in relation to the whole of being. A good starting point may be the very meaningful and mutually enriching relationship of humans with cows, a relationship that can be well nourished by the inclusive, devotional spirit of bhakti.

Terminology and Spelling

As we are discussing Indian (generally Hindu, but more broadly Indic) texts and thought, this book will make considerable use of terms, phrases, and book titles from Sanskrit and Hindi traditions. I have generally removed standard transliteration diacritic marks, in the interest of accessibility to a wide readership. I have, however, retained original diacritic marks in quotations and in bibliographical references. On occasion, I have also retained diacritic marks of a few in-text Sanskrit and Hindi terms and phrases.

As I am discussing *cows* throughout the book, I take the liberty to occasionally change terms. As in common English usage, the word "cow" often refers to both male and female bovines, so also in contemporary Hindi (*gāi/gau*). I sometimes refer to "bovines," as a gender-inclusive term, and when referring to male bovines specifically I will use the word "bull" or "ox."

References

Donaldson, Sue, and Will Kymlicka. 2013. *Zoopolis: A Political Theory of Animal Rights*. Oxford: Oxford University Press.
Llewellyn, J.E. (ed.). 2005. *Defining Hinduism: A Reader*. London: Routledge.

2

The Release of Cosmic Cows

In the Rigveda (Sanskrit: Ṛgveda), the earliest extant sacred text of India, we find this passage in a celebrated hymn dedicated to the storm-god Indra. The poet tells of Indra's victory over Vritra, a serpent monster, and of the cosmic waters' subsequent release from the serpent's grip. As his victory award, Indra then claims the prized *soma* drink:

> … Like bellowing milk-cows, streaming out, the waters went straight down to the sea. Acting the bull, (Indra) chose for his own the soma. He drank of the pressed soma among the Trikadrukas …

Later in the same hymn, the poet describes the waters' condition prior to their release by Indra, whom he then addresses:

> The waters stood still—their husband was the Dāsa; their herdsman, the serpent [Vṛtra]—hemmed in like the cows by the Paṇi. What was the hidden opening for the water—that Indra uncovered after he smashed Vṛtra. You, Indra, then became the tail of a horse when he struck his fangs at you—you,

© The Author(s) 2020
K. R. Valpey, *Cow Care in Hindu Animal Ethics*,
The Palgrave Macmillan Animal Ethics Series,
https://doi.org/10.1007/978-3-030-28408-4_2

the god alone. You conquered the cows, and, o champion, you conquered the soma. You set loose the seven rivers to flow.[1]

Within this short sampling of Rigvedic poetry is a web of names, images, concepts, and narrative that, with all its obscurity for us modern readers, will serve well as a starting point for our journey through literature—ancient to modern—to sketch the main contours of a Hindu imaginaire of cows, what we might venture to call *bovinity*. What we want to note initially from this hymn is simply how it is an indicator that cows are very much a presence in Hindu literature, beginning already from this early text.[2] Over at least three millennia, people of South Asia have engaged with domesticated bovines as integral to their economic livelihood and their cultural and spiritual well-being, and this is richly reflected in their literature. In our survey of this corpus, we will focus mainly on the texts most prominent and revered in the tradition, especially of the brahmanical, or priestly, classes who have produced and preserved them. For the most part we are concerned with texts composed in Sanskrit, though we will also look briefly at later works in modern Hindi.

What the Rigveda and the post-Vedic corpus (including the Sanskrit epics and Puranas[3]) as a whole shows is a constellation of associations in which *cow*—whether referred to literally or figuratively—holds an important, often key, place in articulating notions of cosmic order and regularity, fecundity and abundance, auspiciousness of circumstances, human possession of wealth, general well-being, life as it is meant to be lived, and related notions of desirability. When bulls are mentioned in distinction

---

[1] Rigveda translation—Jamison and Brereton (2014, p. 135; vv. i.32.2, 11–12). All subsequent Rigveda quotations translated by Jamison and Brereton.

[2] As I have noted in the Introduction, the term "Hindu" can be problematic. I use it largely as an inclusive term of convenience, recognizing that, while historically it is an anachronism to refer to early texts such as Rigveda as Hindu, the much later and present-day identification of a broad corpus of literature as Hindu by persons regarding themselves as Hindus justifies this usage. Srinivasan (1979, p. 1) notes that collectively, among the Rigveda's more than one thousand hymns, the seven or eight terms for "cow" appear almost 700 times, more than any other animal. Of these terms, *gó* is the most inclusive.

[3] "Epics" refers to the two classical Sanskrit epic poems, the Valmīki Ramayana and the Mahabharata, both of which are generally given several centuries of developmental time, typically from the 5th c. BCE to the 4th c. CE (Brockington 2003, p. 116). "Puranas" ("ancient lore") are several texts of varying length and focus, with the earliest extant Puranas usually dated to the 4th to 5th c. CE, and later Puranas dating up to the 16th c. or even later.

from cows, further notions of righteous virility and power are added to this constellation of meaning. But as we might expect, over such a vast time period there are shifts and reshapings of this semantic field. From one perspective—typically that of Hindus—these are not so much *changes* in understanding as they are reiterations and amplifications of persistent concerns, attitudes, and truths in relation to cows. In any case, what we find in later literature is elaboration, especially through narratives, of what may be in only germinal form in the earliest literature.

Of particular interest to us will be narratives in the Bhagavata Purana (usually dated 4th–9th c. CE), a text of enduring pan-Indian popularity due especially to its detailed account of the irresistably charming cowherd divinity Krishna in the ideal and idyllic land of cows, Vraja. What will be important to consider here will be how the notion of cow care is interwoven with the major current of Indic religiosity known as *bhakti*—devotion to a particular divinity, especially to Krishna or Shiva, or possibly to the divine feminine in a form such as Parvati. Also, because it is Krishna in particular who is associated with cows, we find a wealth of post-Bhagavata literature focused on Krishna-*bhakti* that will concern us with its portrayals of a pastoral world that enhances and sustains divine play (Sanskrit: *līlā*). Looking back in time from the later to the earliest literature, what we will find as a consistent thread, I will argue, is a notion of divine-human-animal cooperation that is sustained in a matrix of ritual and *bhakti*. Yet this interconnected triangle is at times threatened by adverse forces such that the very possibility of stable worldly well-being is perpetually questioned. This questioning, in turn, brings forth and nurtures renunciant ideologies, which will be crucial for development of the Indic concept and practices of *ahimsa*—nonviolence. The development of ahimsa ideology will be treated in the next chapter.

The Rigveda—Cows Ranging in Meaning

The Rigveda, generally considered the earliest of four collections of sacred utterances, assembled probably well before 1000 BCE, enjoys a position of highest regard and authority by most, if not all, persons who would identify themselves as Hindu (Smith 1998, pp. 13–14).[4] By modern scholarly estimation, it is "the oldest literary monument of the Indo-European languages" and, indeed, "one of the oldest and most precious documents of man" (Myers 1995, p. 25, quoting Macdonell 1917, p. xi; Maurer 1986, p. 1). And although but a tiny number of Hindus have any idea of its specific content; their reverence for the work is evident in its continued application in ritual practices to the present day. Pundits (scholars or priests learned in Hindu sacred texts) are similarly revered as custodians of Vedic writ, and it is likely they who will be most ready to affirm with Rigveda excerpts the sanctity of cows. Thus, we do well to examine Rigvedic bovine references to gain a sense of the value system in which cows are so important and within which the term "cow" plays a significant role in a dynamic web of meanings.

In the Rigveda hymn quoted above, the poet employs cows and a bull figuratively in connection with water and Indra, respectively; also, the poet alludes, within the main narrative of Indra's victory, to another Rigvedic narrative about cow confinement that we will discuss later. The motif of confined cows released, often identified with their milk-giving capacity, points to a broad Vedic symbol for flourishing life: freely roaming and grazing milk-producing cows seek and find their watering place (Myers 1995, p. 40). In direct opposition to flourishing life is constriction or obstruction (*vritra*, Sanskrit *vṛtra*, means "obstacle") which is, or brings about, decay, destruction, chaos, and death. Here, the waters' freedom is constrained by their "husband," identified as the Dasa (Sanskrit: Dāsa) people—essentially "outsiders" to the Rigvedic community, which designated itself as Aryan peoples, roughly "the civilized ones" (Jamison and Brereton 2014, p. 54).

Indra, the hero in this narrative, is the powerful storm-god, often regarded as the king of the heavenly realm. He is repeatedly praised in the Rigveda for his indomitable bull-like valor, often in the context of

---

[4]Smith writes, "Hinduism is the religion of those humans who create, perpetuate, and transform traditions with legitimizing reference to the authority of the Veda." This definition that looks back in time may be augmented by Frazier (2017, p. 21), who notes, "The Vedic tradition … is a bricolage that developed over two millennia into a complex culture that turned again and again to its source in order to renew its identity."

recalling his having slain the serpent monster Vritra. In this and numerous other Rigveda hymns, the implication is that as he prevailed in the past he shall prevail again, this time on behalf of the petitioner(s). And it is Indra, in particular, who is regarded as the rightful claimant of the prized juice of the *soma* plant, an invigorating, apparently intoxicating, probably psychotropic drink that was ritually prepared and offered in major sacrificial rites. Significantly, the ritual preparation of the soma drink involved mixing it with water and milk prior to offering it.[5] As an essential ingredient of this crucial offering, milk is frequently identified metonymically with cows, or simply referred to as cows. Finally, in reference to the passage quoted above, Indra's valor is underlined in the affirmation that he "conquered the cows" at the same time that he "conquered the soma." Indra is an aggressive and confrontational divinity (Glucklich 2008, p. 96), but he thereby accomplishes the needful: "You set loose the seven rivers to flow."

As a predominantly pastoral people, the Vedic Aryans were naturally concerned to acquire, retain, and protect their cattle from predators and rustlers. To do so successfully was largely a function of generously sponsored, well-executed ritual performance, broadly referred to as *yajna*, roughly translated as "sacrifice" but also meaning "act of worship or devotion, offering, oblation." Efficacious ritual required, in turn, the engagement of expert priests, brahmins who, like their sponsors, would likely be keepers of cattle. Many of the Rigvedic hymns reflect these considerations, such that much poetic attention is given to inspiring a ritual's divine dedicand to be generous in his (or in some cases her) rewards to the sponsors and priests. One example showing this concern is Rigveda 2.11. Again, the dedication is to Indra:

Drink and drink the soma, o Indra, our champion! Let the exhilarating soma-pressings exhilarate you. As they fill your cheeks, let them strengthen you. When properly pressed among the Paura, (the soma) has helped Indra.

We inspired poets have abided by you, Indra. Serving according to the truth, we would gain insight. Seeking your help, we would create for ourselves a proclamation of your praise. On this very day, we would be those to be given wealth by you.

---

[5]For a detailed description of a contemporary *agni-shtoma* sacrifice including the preparation and offering of *soma*, see Knipe (2015, pp. 212–214).

Then, in the same hymn, Indra is again urged to drink the soma "among the Trikadrukas" (possibly referring to the Maruts, a group of divinities associated with the wind). Again, Indra is reminded that he has slain Vritra, by which, this time, he "uncovered the light for the Arya"; and there is again allusion to the second cow-confinement narrative involving Indra, whereby cows had been hidden in "the Vala cave." The hymn concludes:

> Now should the generous priestly gift yield your boon for the singer as its milk, Indra. Exert yourself for the praise singers. Let fortune not pass us by. May we speak loftily at the ritual distribution, in possession of good heroes.[6]

Here "milk" is the reward rendered presumably to the poet who has composed the hymn, through the (obligatory) "gift" (*dakshina*) given to the priests who have performed the rite in which this hymn would have been recited.

We begin to see the contours of a Vedic cosmic economy, in which three interrelated spheres of life—natural, human, and divine—interact for mutual benefit.[7] In this economy, cows and their products—especially milk—are indispensable. While providing milk and its derivatives that give nourishment for the cows' young and for humans, they also contribute, by their milk, in the preparation of the crucial ritual offering, soma.

We also see contours of Vedic Aryan self-perception as a people threatened by outsiders. Thus, at times Aryans are engaged in battles with their enemies—various sorts of beings (human or nonhuman) associated with darkness. Between the darkness and the light, serving to end darkness and bring on the light, is the dawn. Connecting the cosmic light versus darkness opposition with the Aryans' experience of themselves versus their enemies, some Rigvedic hymns celebrate the dawn as the great Distinguisher which, as an essential, life-giving and sustaining aspect of nature

---

[6] Rigveda 2.11.11–12, 17a, 18, 21 and Jamison and Brereton (2014, pp. 414–415).

[7] Having registered such conceptualization, we do well to also heed A. T. de Nicolás' caution in reading the Rigveda (1976, p. 11): "It is … essential … that we get ourselves ready to move, in one swift jump, from the prosaic, discursive, lengthy and conceptual ground on which we are accustomed to stand, into the moving, shifting, resounding, evanescent, vibrating and always sounding silence of the *musical* world on which the Ṛg Veda stands" (emphasis in original). See de Nicolás, pp. 13–15, for a succinct overview of Eastern and Western Rigveda exegetical approaches.

like water, is also identified as "cows."[8] In turn, the cows = dawns signification serves also the linkage between cows and the soma *yajna*, for it is at the time of the morning pressing of the soma juice (which, we recall, is mixed with cows' milk) that priestly gifts are distributed, among which may be cows.

In such a culture wherein ritual plays such a major role, it may be no surprise that the gifting of cows to priests at the conclusion of their ritual services in the *yajna* has itself ritual aspects. And so, there is a charming Rigvedic hymn (6.28) dedicated to cows which, it is surmised, may have originally been sung "to bless the cows given as a *dakshina* (priestly gift) as they enter the home of their new owner" (Jamison and Brereton 2014, p. 812). We may note the sorts of dangers to cows that are being warded off by the blessing:

> These [cows] will not be lost, and no thief will take them by deception. No enemy will venture against their meandering course. Those (cows) with which he [the cow owner] sacrifices and gives to the gods, he keeps company with them as their cowherd for a very long time.
>
> No dusty-necked steed gets to them (in a cattle raid), nor do they go to the place for dressing [=slaughterhouse]. The cows of the mortal who sacrifices wander far across wide-ranging (space) free of fear.

Continuing in the same hymn, the receiver of the gift of cows rejoices, counting the several benefits bestowed by them while identifying them with soma and Indra:

> Fortune has appeared to me as cows; Indra as cows. The draught of the first soma is cows. These cows here—they, o peoples, are Indra. I am just searching, with my heart and mind, for Indra.
>
> You fatten even the thin man, o cows. You make even one without beauty to have a lovely face. You make the house blessed, o you of blessed speech. Your vigor is declared loftily in the assemblies.[9]

---

[8] For example, see RV 3.31.4: "The victorious (clans [=Aṅgirases?]) escorted the contender [=Indra?]. They distinguished the great light from the darkness. Recognizing him, the dawns rose up in response. He became the lone lord [/husband] of the cows—Indra" (Jamison and Brereton 2014, p. 509; bracketed terms in original).

[9] Rgveda 6.28.3–6; Jamison and Brereton (2014, pp. 812–813).

There is assuredness of well-being in this hymn, based on the presence of cows which—it is hoped and expected by the owner—themselves will experience well-being and indeed "enjoyment" (Rigveda 6.28.1).[10] Cows are regarded as ever givers, and as such they are identified with creation and sustenance, motherhood, fertility, and liberality. They are therefore associated or identified with cosmic waters, which are like the lowing cows that flow with milk. Further, "rain is shed as milk from cows; poetic vision is like a cow flowing with a thousand streams of milk; the breasts of a goddess are like the cow's udder" (Srinivasan 1979, p. 4).

Especially from the last two verses quoted, we get a deeper sense of how cows were highly valued by Rigvedic Aryans. Now we are in a position to appreciate the significance of the story of cows' confinement in the second narrative alluded to in our initial Rigveda excerpt (in 1.32), where it was mentioned that the waters were "hemmed in like the cows by the Pani." In the story of the Panis, cows, horses, and other treasures are stolen by a group of opposers to the Vedic sacrifice—the demonic Panis—who keep the booty hidden in a cave, or within a great rock. To recover these valuables, Indra dispatches his messenger Sarama (in the form of a female dog); the latter, confronting the Panis with threats, tries but fails to persuade the Panis to relinquish the goods. Finally, by force of sacred utterances (*mantra*) Brihaspati, the chief divine priestly assistant to Indra, smashes asunder the enclosure and reclaims the treasures, including, of course, the cows.[11]

This story is important for its celebration of the Vedic sacrificial way of life, whereby cosmic order, rooted in the mysterious ordering principle *rita* (Sanskrit: *ṛta*), positions human beings as intermediaries between the tangible world of nature and the invisible world of the gods—the divine. Vedic *yajna* is an act of generosity, a display of largess. The Panis (*paṇi*

---

[10]One Atharvaveda hymn addresses a cow, in the context of donating a bull to a brahmin (priest): "This young male we set toward you here; with him go you (fem.) playing according to your wills..." (Whitney, 2009, p. 240). Playing (*krīḍantī*) according to their wills (*vaśaṁ anu*) indicates a sense of bovine's subjectivity.

[11]Tales involving bovines are present in several mythological traditions of the world, some of which show interesting parallels with Vedic or post-Vedic accounts of bovines. For example, in south and southeast Asia, several versions of the epic Ramayana tell of a buffalo demon who is encountered and killed by the monkey king Vali in a cave—in some versions enabling Vali to get free from the cave. See Kam (2000, pp. 85–89).

elsewhere in the Rigveda means "miserly") are the opposite of the Aryan sacrificers, and their formidable effort to prevent the sacrifice must be overcome. But this is possible only with the same technology as constitutes the sacrifice, namely well-composed and properly uttered hymns and mantras.

The web of bovine signification in the Rigveda (and in related ritual texts) expands considerably, as cows become associated with speech itself, especially the poetic speech of Vedic hymns, also referred to as mantras. As cows are embodiments of wealth and well-being, rightly pronounced speech facilitates successful sacrificial rites by which, in turn, cattle may be awarded.[12] Indeed, the most basic component of speech, the syllable (*akshara*, meaning unbreakable, irreducible, inexhaustible) is identified with "cow" (Jamison and Brereton 2014, p. 882; Rigveda 7.1.14).[13]

We can make a few generalizations about cows in the Rigveda before moving on to the Upanishads. First, we can see the text as a whole as *modeling* the proper (right) way of living for human beings. As a means of sensitizing humans to cosmic order, cows are living signs of such order with all their characteristics of giving and nurturing. Second, in the sphere of material well-being, possession and care of cows is integral to right living, and such well-being is embodied and sustained in ritual acts of

---

[12]Indeed, in a later reflection on Vedic ritual, in the Brihadaranyaka Upanishad (5.5.8; Olivelle 1998, p. 135), the equivalence of speech and the cow extends to an equation of her four teats with four important syllable pairs pronounced in fire rites: "One should venerate speech as a cow. It has four teats—*Svāhā, Vaṣaṭ, Hanta,* and *Svadhā.* The gods live on two of those teats—Svāhā and Vaṣaṭ. Humans live on Hantā, and the ancestors on Svadhā. The bull of this cow is the breath, and her calf is the mind." Beyond the award of cattle for correctly performed ritual and correctly pronounced speech in the ritual was the award of freedom from death. This will be elaborated in later texts, especially the Brihadaranyaka Upanishad and the Shatapatha Brahmana (Calasso 2015, p. 34). This is also alluded to within the Rigveda, for example I.154.6: "We wish to go to the dwelling places belonging to you two [=Viṣnu and Indra], where there are ample-horned, unbridled cows" (Jamison and Brereton 2014, p. 331).

[13]We have barely scratched the surface of cow associations in the Rigveda and other Vedic texts, especially the Atharvaveda. For a quite thorough referencing and analysis of these associations, see Gonda (1985, pp. 39–53). The web of bovine signification extends yet further when words indicating parts of a cow's body are included. So, for example, the word *padá* means "cow's hoofprint"; and it also means track, sojourn, region, (metrical) foot, radius, (single) word, and speech. Calasso (2015, p. 19) notes, "If we are talking about the 'hidden *padá*', [Louis] Renou says it is 'the mystery par excellence, which the poet tries to reveal'. Already we are a long way from the cow's hoof print, which itself is mysterious and venerable, since a special 'libation on the hoof print,' *padāhuti,* is dedicated to it."

sacrifice. As a consequence, third, literal, actual cows are sought after, as wealth and—of equal or greater importance—prestige, which is regarded as a requirement for achieving human dignity. Fourth, metaphorical cows expand meaning by linking natural phenomena and elements to human existence, especially embodied in the feminine maternal principle. Again, related to the fourth point, value in the paradigmatic human activity of *yajna* is underscored with the correct recitation of appropriate hymns. In their expansion of meaning, cows tend to wander, and in their wandering, they embody the human pursuit of the unknown (Srinivasan 1979, p. 7), which is a central theme in the next important genre of early Sanskrit texts associated with Hindu traditions, the Upanishads.

The Upanishads—Cows and the Acquisition of Higher Knowledge

We step forward in time from the Rigveda to the early formation of a new genre of texts, appearing by the sixth century BCE, a genre that comes to be known as Upanishad (Sanskrit: *upaniṣad*), "to sit down near" (the spiritual teacher earnestly) (Grimes 1996, p. 330). The Upanishads are known for their philosophically reflective character, with discussions conducted mainly in the form of dialogues between teacher and student. In their general pursuit of higher knowledge prompted by fundamental, existential questions (especially, What is the nature of the self? What is the basis of all existence?), they offer engaging interlocutions in which occur occasional, tangential yet telling references to cows. As noted with regard to Rigvedic bovinity, where emerges a sense of association between cows and pursuit of the unknown, cows and concerns about cows in the Upanishads hint strongly of this connection. Also related to our theme of Hindu animal ethics as a whole, the Upanishads are important as a record of a developing renunciant ideology, for which the concept and practice of nonviolence—ahimsa—becomes important, to be discussed in Chapter 3.

Here we look briefly at two cow-related Upanishadic narratives. The first, found in the early Chandogya Upanishad, concerns a certain young boy, Satyakama Jabala, whose strong urge to receive higher knowledge from sage Haridrumata Gautama is eventually rewarded. First, however,

2 The Release of Cosmic Cows   21

the lad must prove his resolve and sincerity by service. The service task assigned is to tend (*anusamvraja*) four hundred of the sage's leanest and feeblest (*nirakritya*) cows. Satyakama promises that he will not only do this, but that he "will not return without a thousand" (cows). Some years later, this number of cattle is reached, at which time "the bull" (*rishabha*) speaks to the lad, informing him that this number has been reached and requesting him to bring them all back to the master. "Take us back to the teacher's house, and I will tell you one quarter of *brahman*."

Brahman, the mysteriously ineffable ultimate reality that is such a major subject of the Upanishads, will now be revealed to Satyakama in four phases, first by the bull, then by fire, third by a gander, and finally by a water bird. When, after four days of travel herding the cattle, Satyakama arrives before Gautama, the latter calls out, "Son, you have the glow of a man who knows *brahman*! Tell me—who taught you?" Satyakama (*satya* means "truth": he who desires truth) tells all of what has happened and then requests the teacher to give him the same teaching "for I have heard from people of your eminence that knowledge leads one most securely to the goal only when it is learnt from a teacher." Gautama is apparently pleased, such that he gives Satyakama the teaching "without leaving anything out" (Chandogya Upanishad 4.4–9; Olivelle 1998, pp. 219–223).[14]

Here the connection between service to a teacher and knowledge received from the teacher is clearly underlined; yet we may note that the service rendered is caring for cows.[15] Moreover, that the first teaching (in this account) about *brahman* comes from the mouth of a bull is worth noting. Here we find a direct connection made between cows (here used

---

[14]The satisfaction of the teacher by tending his cows finds expression in a somewhat similar story of Upamanyu in the Mahabharata. Feller notes that it may be significant that in both these accounts, the students' tending cows may be signaling the boys' isolation in the forest, as a preliminary preparation for initiation. That they are also tending cows during this time suggests additional auspiciousness and purity accruing to the candidates for higher knowledge. Incidentally, the Upamanyu story also finds resonances in the Rigveda (Mahabharata 1.3.19–31; see Feller 2004, pp. 208–211, 216, 227; also see 242–245, on a different, significant account of Upamanyu, later in the Mahabharata).

[15]In a contemporary popular book of stories about cow protection (*go-raksa*), the author urges his readers to understand that Satyakama's service is *for* the cows, and that it is because he serves the cows that he is rewarded with knowledge of *brahman* (Das 2013, pp. 35–37).

as a gender-inclusive term) and higher knowledge that would seem to be only obliquely pursued in Rigvedic hymns.[16]

The other cow-related passage from the Upanishads to concern us is in the Katha Upanishad, a somewhat later work than the Chandogya. The Upanishad opens with this curious scene: A certain young man, Nachiketas, watches while his father, Ushan, gives away all his possessions in charity, or as sacrificial gifts. Among his possessions were old, barren cows. As the cows are being led away, the boy thinks,

> They've drunk all their water, eaten all their fodder, they have been milked dry, they are totally barren—'Joyless' are those worlds called, to which a man goes who gives them as gifts.

Testily Nachiketas asks his father, "Father, to whom will you give me?" Annoyed and impatient with his son (who repeats the same question thrice), Ushan blurts out "I'll give you to Death!"—so that Nachiketas proceeds immediately to the abode of Yama, the lord of death. As it happens, Yama is absent from home for three days while Nachiketas waits for him. Upon his return, Yama anxiously offers to fulfill three wishes, in recompense for the three nights that the young man, a brahmin (who should by no means be neglected), had been kept waiting. Nachiketas obliges, first with two simple wishes that Yama happily and immediately grants; but at his third wish—to receive instruction from Yama on whether or not a person who dies continues to exist or not—Yama balks, unwilling to reveal this great secret.

Initially Yama tries to offer substitutions for Nachiketas' wish, in the form of long life, beautiful women, a vast kingdom, and "much livestock." The point for us to note here is that what was so much sought after in the Rigveda, including wealth in the form of cattle (which Nachiketas

---

[16]An intriguing connection between the bull-like god of fire, Agni, the hidden track of the cow, and poetic speech can be found in ṚV 4.5.3: "A great melody (he [the fire god Agni] gave)—the doubly lofty, sharp-pointed, thousand-spurting, powerful bull--/having found the word hidden like the track of the cow. Agni has proclaimed the inspired thought to me" (Jamison and Brereton 2014, p. 566). The ways in which higher knowledge is expressed in the Upanishads—especially through homologies—can be traced through the language of the post-Vedic Brahmana texts back to Rigvedic poetic expressions (see Witzel 2003, p. 83).

perceives his father as giving begrudgingly), is of no interest to this Upanishadic seeker of enduring truth beyond the apparent truths of temporal life.[17] Times have changed. The Vedic pastoral way of life fades as towns have grown and sociopolitical order has become more complex. And with these new circumstances comes, for many, a resolve to head for the forest to embrace austerities and aloofness from worldly cares, taking the way of disengagement (*nivritti*) and spurning the way of engagement in the world (*pravritti*). With this opposition in mind, we can proceed to bovine representations in the great Sanskrit epic of India, the Mahabharata, wherein the relative value of worldly engagement and disengagement is extensively debated, and cows can prove to have important roles in a human being's destiny.[18]

The Mahabharata—Pursuing Dharma with Cows

As with the Upanishads, the vast-ranging story of fratricidal war that is the Mahabharata can be seen as a work propelled by fundamental questioning. But whereas the Upanishads are more concerned with knowledge of ultimate being, *brahman*, in the Mahabharata the central concern is to know what is right behavior—*dharma*.[19] The desire to comprehend this elusive term, dharma, is not new with the Mahabharata; the Rigveda also refers to dharma in enigmatic ways—but with the Mahabharata there is a sense of increasingly pressing need to establish unequivocally the principles and practices for human well-being, due to a felt acceleration of time's degrading influence. The vortex of such degradation is seen in the massively destructive war between the five Pandava brothers and their

---

[17]Katha Upanishad 1.1–29 (Olivelle 1998, pp. 375–381).

[18]Discussion of the Bhagavad-gīta in relation to cows, and in relation to the issue of violence versus nonviolence toward animals, is relevant in the Mahabharata context, and we take up this subject in Chapter 3.

[19]The word *dharma* is hugely important in Indic texts (including Jain, Buddhist, and Sikh traditions). With both prescriptive and descriptive uses, in its broadest sense it may simply be rendered as "ethics." It can also carry the sense of "justice," as suggested in some texts that refer to the "dharma bull" (Hiltebeitel 2011, p. 213). More on this subject in later chapters. For an extensive analysis of the development of the notion and use of the term *dharma* in Indic literature, see Hiltebeital (2011).

cousins, the Kauravas, over the rule of their contested kingdom. In two didactic interludes to the epic's main story—one in the account of preliminary events leading to this war, and another in the account of the war's aftermath—the subject of cows becomes the focus. It is these moments that will occupy us, as indicators of further development of the bovine imaginaire in the early Hindu literary corpus. This development is such as will develop into an explicit link between cows, the care of cows, and human right action, dharma.

The first passage has the prima facie purpose of teaching that the power of brahmins—priests, teachers, or sages—is superior to that of kshatriyas (Sanskrit: *kṣatriyas*)—members of the martial order.[20] Vasishtha, a brahmin ascetic forest resident, is approached by Vishvamitra, the king of Kushika, while the latter has been hunting deer and boar with his large retinue. The sage warmly welcomes the king to his hermitage, hosting him and his entourage generously with refreshments. The refreshments are of such a fine quality and quantity that the king's curiosity is piqued. How is it possible for Vasishtha, living in such simplicity, without any previous warning, to suddenly supply such goods—not only fruits of the forest, but also grains, milk, clarified butter, and plentiful other comforts, and in such quantities? The explanation is forthcoming: Vasishtha has a special cow named Nandini that—or who—when requested, instantly yields whatever the sage desires.

Seeing the handsome cow, Vishvamitra resolves that he must possess her. But Vasishtha declines the king's offer of ten thousand cows and his entire kingdom in exchange. A battle ensues when Vishvamitra fails to drag Nandini away and Vasishtha calls her to remain with him. The sage's call

---

[20]Although this distinction of brahmins and kshatriyas in terms of a power differential is important in the Mahabharata, also emphasized is the interdependence of the two positions. Biardeau (1997, p. 78 and n. 8) notes that brahmins are generally dependent on the gifts of kshatriyas, typically in the form of gold, cows, and (later) land. They are also (generally) dependent on kshatriyas for protection. Their interdependence is highlighted in the Vedic sacrificial rite, a continuing practice in the Mahabharata (Biardeau 1989, p. 36), at which such gifts will be given by the kshatriya sponsor of the rite as reward to the brahmin for executing the rites. Biardeau also notes, incidentally, that "[Hindu] [m]yths always symbolize the Brahman's [brahmin's] sacerdotal function by means of a cow, and the latter eventually symbolizes the Brahman himself, since a Brahman without a cow is less than a complete Brahman." Because of the brahmin/cow identification, "To kill a cow is almost as abominable as to kill a Brahman, although the revealed texts are categorical: certain rites included a cow as sacrificial victim. But 'to sacrifice is not to kill'" (Biardeau 1989, p. 36).

(following a verbal exchange with the cow) prompts her to manifest from her body hordes of soldiers—tribal peoples who quickly rout, unharmed, Vishvamitra's soldiers. Vishvamitra now understands: kshatriya power is insignificant; brahmin power (*tejas*) is true power. Resolving to become a brahmin, he abandons his kingdom, takes up extreme ascetic practices, and after years of determined ordeal, is granted recognition as a brahmin.[21]

One implication from this story is that cows show their largesse when cared for by brahmins, and they provide all necessities for them. Brahmins, in turn, possessing the superior power of austerity, are the guardians of a society's higher values. Their strength is in their self-restraint, the basic principle of disengagement from the world (*nivritti*), a principle that complements and supports the sheltering of bovine animals, which in turn come to embody the observance of dharma—ethical rightness and realization of individual and collective good (Ranganathan 2017, pp. 5–6).[22]

Unlike the Rigveda, which extols the gifting of cows to priests (brahmins) specifically in sacrificial rituals, the Mahabharata emphasizes a more general principle of cow-gifting as charity, especially to brahmins but not necessarily in relation to their ritual acts. Following the Pandava-Kaurava war (a Pyrrhic victory for the dharmic Pandavas), the dying warrior-grandsire Bhishma prepares the chief Pandava, Yudhishthira, for ruling his kingdom by instructing him in all aspects of dharma. Set in this context are several chapters extolling the virtues and benefits of gifting cows, along with explanations about cows' particular virtues.

In one such passage (13.69), Bhishma speaks with unrestrained enthusiasm on this subject. First, he notes that (because the word *go* can mean "cow," "earth," or "speech") to give cows, earth, or knowledge are of "equal

---

[21]MBh 1.164–165. A fuller account of this episode is to be found in the Valmīki Ramayana (1.50.20–1.64), the other of the two great Sanskrit epics (Sathaye 2011). For brevity, I have discussed the shorter version in the MBh. However, one point to note from the Ramayana version is that Vishvamitra's initial offer in trade for the cow (in that text referred to as Shabala) is one hundred thousand of his own cows. He then asserts, "[Shabala] is truly a gem, and all gems belong to the king. Therefore, brahman, you must give me Śabala. By rights she is mine" (Goldman 2005, p. 279).
[22]Here I draw on Shyam Ranganathan's general consideration of both ethics and dharma being about the same concerns, namely the right or the good. More on this in Chapter 5.

26 K. R. Valpey

merit."[23] Further, the merit received by one who gifts cows accrues immediately. Indeed, cows are "the mothers of all creatures," able to "bestow
every kind of happiness," for they are "goddesses and homes of auspiciousness" which therefore "always deserve worship."[24] And yet, although
giving cows in charity is strongly encouraged, Bhishma also warns that
they should be given only to "deserving" persons. Who are deserving?
Bhishma's standard is high: "A cow should never be given unto one that is
not righteous in behaviour, or one that is sinful, or one that is covetous or
one that is untruthful in speech, or one that does not make offerings unto
the Pitris [ancestors] and deities." Bhishma later quotes the lord of death
and justice, Yama, speaking to Nachiketas, on positive qualifications for a
recipient of cows[25]:

> He is regarded as a proper person for receiving a cow in gift who is known to
> be mild towards kine [cows], who takes kine for his refuge, who is grateful,
> and who has no means of subsistence assigned unto him. (Ganguli 1991,
> vol. 11, p. 94; Mahabharata 13.71)

Simply by giving cows in charity to a proper recipient and in the proper
way one can anticipate the full rewards of eternal transcendence following one's present life. As Yama informs Nachiketas (as told by Bhishma),
beyond the heavenly realm, which itself is a place of stunning beauty and
exalted pleasure, there are "other eternal worlds" that are "reserved for
those persons that are engaged in making gifts of kine" (Ganguli 1991,
vol. 11, p. 93; Mahabharata 13.71).

---

[23]The passage is 13.69 in Mohan Ganguli's English translation (Ganguli 1991 [1970], vol. 11,
pp. 88–89), 13.68 in the Mahabharata Critical Edition (Dandekar 1966, vol. 17, pp. 380–382).
Here and elsewhere I reference Ganguli's edition, as the "vulgate" version that would be known to
many Hindus.

[24]We will consider details of current cow care and veneration practices in Chapter 4. Here we may
note three examples of careful treatment of cows (including bulls) mentioned by Bhishma, namely
(1) at no time, except when tilling the ground in preparation for a sacrificial rite, may bullocks
struck with a goad or whip; (2) when cows are grazing or lying down, no one should disturb them
in any way; and (3) no one should ever deny cows access to any source of water, for them to drink.

[25]Here the MBh gives its own version of the Nachiketas-Yama story from that of the Katha Upanishad. In the Mahabharata version, Yama allows Nachiketas to visit the heavenly realm where,
stunned by its beauty, he hears from Yama of the exalted destiny for givers of cows. Yama also prescribes the procedure for donating cows, including consideration of the proper time, the condition
of the cows to be donated, and whether the recipient will properly care for them.

Such are the rewards that one may anticipate for giving away cows. Yet there are also potential dangers, for even an unintentional mistake in bovine charity could bring about a quite opposite result from what is expected.[26] To illustrate how this is so, Bhishma narrates the story of a certain King Nriga. Nriga was a generous and conscientious giver of cows to brahmins. However, once he unwittingly gave a brahmin a cow that had wandered into his herd from that of another brahmin. The latter brahmin, the proper owner, noticing that his cow was missing, eventually found it with the other brahmin, who had received it as a gift from the king. After some altercation both brahmins approached the king. To rectify the mistake, Nriga begged the recipient brahmin to accept hundreds of other cows in exchange for this one; but the man declined, giving several reasons why this would not be possible. Nriga then offered a hundred thousand cows (!) to the brahmin whose cow had wandered away and which the king had then mistakenly given away in charity, but to no avail: the brahmin refused, saying that he accepts no gifts from the royal order. And so, explains Bhishma, as punishment, after his death the king had to live for countless years as a large lizard before being finally rescued and sent to heaven (for his many pious acts) by the highest divinity in his form as Krishna.[27]

This last story hints strongly at the Mahabharata's struggle to reconcile seeming contradictory principles within one vision of rightness and goodness that would be codified as dharma. And somehow, in the persistent pursuit of this vision as one of integrity among nature, humanity, and divinity, it appears that cows take an increasingly significant place. To be sure, their place is not regarded as that of subjective agency as we might understand it; rather, cows are in large part passive objects of possession,

---

[26]Another noteworthy unintentional mistake involving a cow in the Mahabharata relates to the epic's main story. Karna, the great warrior and arch-rival of Arjuna, while practicing archery in the forest, accidentally kills a brahmin's cow—one that had been supplying milk for the brahmin's sacrificial rites. The brahmin curses Karna that, while fighting in the impending war, his chariot wheel will become stuck in the mud, at which time his enemy will remove his head. Incidentally, we may note the connection between cow and earth in this curse (Bowles 2008, pp. xxxiii–xxxiv).

[27]The Bhagavata Purana 10.64 has an almost identical version of this story, adding that when the king dies, he is given a choice by Yama to either first enjoy results of his pious acts or to first suffer the results of his impious acts. Nriga chooses the latter, and thus he suffers life in the body of a large lizard, until Krishna saves him. Thereafter, Krishna delivers a speech warning of the great dangers of taking the property of brahmins.

symbols and generators of wealth and well-being. And yet as embodiments of power—particularly as embodiments of maternal nurturing and, in the case of bullocks, embodiments of steadfast righteousness—cows become something substantially more than "just animals" in the Hindu imaginaire. As we continue this survey of literary cows, this trend extends further, with a considerable shift in the religious currents to a dominance of what may be called the "bhakti paradigm" or bhakti spirit, the spirit of devotion to a supreme deity for whom cows are integral to his identity and his ways of engagement in the world.

The Bhagavata Purana—Cows in the World of Bhakti

One of the most popular among classical Sanskrit texts in India remains to the present day the Bhagavata Purana. Doubtless the reason for its popularity is its extensive account of Krishna's life, especially of his early life as a charming and mischievous cowherd in the pastoral land of Vraja. While Krishna's winsome ways with his friends, relatives, and cows are captive to the imagination, there is also a persistent and coherently developed message throughout the text—that bhakti, devotion, is the most felicitous way to human perfection and the sublime. To get a sense of this vision and to relate it to what we have encountered thus far with regard to "bovinity," we look at some details of two key passages from the text's early portions before turning to relevant episodes in Krishna's life in a later portion of the text. Both early stories are allegorical in structure and both involve kings whose concern is the well-being of the earth, personified as a cow.

The first episode serves an etiological function, explaining the origin of the current cosmic age, *kali-yuga*—the fourth and last in a cycle of increasing discord and decreasing human capacities, especially for spiritual culture.[28] In a prelude to the main story, a dialogue takes place

---

[28] Previously, while introducing the Mahabharata, I noted its concern with the sense of "time's degrading influence." That text locates its events at the end of the previous cosmic age, *dvapara-yuga*. The understanding is that the full force of degradation unfolds in the present age, the *kali-yuga*. The Puranic calculation of the Kali age's inception places it at ca. 3000 BCE, see Holdrege (2015, p. 319, n. 2, and Ch. 1).

between Dharma, in the form of a bull, and Earth, in the form of a cow (BhP 1.16.18–35). Dharma has lost three of his legs (indicating humanity's morally disabled condition) and, seeing that Earth is grieving, he asks her to identify the cause of her grief, suggesting several possible reasons— exploitation by unprincipled persons; neglect of prescribed sacrificial rites; drought and famine; unprotected women and children; neglect of the goddess of learning by lapsed brahmins; disturbed and unqualified kshatriyas; or the unregulated habits of the human population. Earth replies to Dharma initially by listing some forty virtues and qualities that, having their basis in the supreme Lord (*bhagavan*), have largely disappeared from the world due to the departure from the earth of Krishna (identified throughout the text as *bhagavan*).[29]

To explain briefly: This prelude dialogue is within the first of twelve "books" of the Bhagavata Purana, and the entire first book serves as a prelude to the remainder, the high point of which is Book 10, which tells specifically of Krishna's descent (*avatara*) to the earth. However, in this introductory Book 1, readers are introduced to the story by, in effect, telling its conclusion. Thus, after Krishna has come to the world and then, some 125 years later, has departed, the world languishes in this degenerated state.

---

[29]The concept of divinity as *bhagavan* is of great importance in Vaishnava Hindu traditions. Particularly because Krishna, the divine cowherd, is identified as *bhagavan*, it is worth noting a detailed definition of the term, given by the sixteenth-century theologian of the Caitanya Vaishnava tradition, Jīva Gosvāmī: "He who is the very form of existence, consciousness, and bliss; who possesses inconceivable, multifarious, and unlimited energies that are of his own nature; who is the ocean of unlimited, mutually contradictory qualities, such that in him both the attribute and the possessor of attributes, the lack of differences and varieties of differences, formlessness and form, pervasiveness and centrality [*madhyamatva*]—all are true; whose beautiful form is distinct from both gross and subtle entities, self-luminous, and consisting entirely of his own nature; who has unlimited such forms that are manifested by his chief form called Bhagavan; whose left side is beautified by Lakṣmī—the manifestation of his personal energy, suitable to his own form; who resides in his own abode, along with his associates, who are furnished with a form that is a special manifestation of his own splendor; who astonishes the hosts of *atmaramas* (those who take pleasure in the self) by his wonderful qualities, pastimes, etc., which are characterized by the play of his personal energy; whose own generic brilliance is manifested in the form of the reality of Brahman; who is the sole shelter and life of his marginal energy, called the living entities [*jīvas*]; whose mere reflected energy are the modes of nature [*guṇas*], visible in the unlimited phenomenal world—he is Bhagavan" (Gupta 2007, p. 33, quoting Jīva's *Bhagavat-sandarbha* 100).

To continue the story, the earth-cow (*dharani*—"she who sustains") bemoans the pervasive influence of the current Kali age and its deleterious effect on herself, on the divinities, sages, ancestors, ascetics, and pious upholders of social traditions. She fondly remembers the time of Krishna's presence, when she was relieved from the burden of military hordes (alluding to the annihilation of armies in the Mahabharata war), a time when Dharma was relieved of his distress as well. It was a time of such joy that Earth's "hair" (suggesting grass) would "stand on end," suggesting an abundance of grass available for cows (BhP 1.16.35).

We next read that King Parikshit (sole surviving grandson of Arjuna, the Pandava warrior-king hero prominent in the Mahabharata epic), having become alerted to Kali's increasing influence in his kingdom, sets out from his palace to rectify the situation by reestablishing his authority throughout the realm (BhP 1.17). Eventually he comes upon an uncultured man dressed as a king, cruelly beating a cow and bull, which are trembling, crying, and urinating in their helpless state. Parikshit accosts the man, noting the contradiction between his dress and his behavior and, enraged, thunders, "For harming innocent beings, you deserve to be killed!"

Then, addressing the bull and cow, the king reassures them that he, upholding his duty as king, will protect them. He urges the bull to name the perpetrator of its mutilations—the loss of three of its legs. The bull replies thoughtfully, saying that it is difficult to identify the culprit, for there are so many theories of causation: One's own self, destiny, or one's disposition could be the cause; or else the cause may be impossible to determine by any means. King Parikshit congratulates the bull, identifying him as the embodiment of dharma and affirming his reply as fitting to the correct understanding of dharma.[30] Further, he identifies the four

---

[30]Parīkṣit's affirmation of the bull's reply includes a reference to divine arrangement (1.17.23): Behind all possible causes is the Lord, whose energies are *agocara*, literally "absent of (or beyond) [human] range." The word alludes to cows (*go*) and their movement (*cara*) or the range for their grazing.

"legs" of dharma, three of which are now destroyed, as four principles sustaining human well-being, namely austerity (or "ardor"—*tapas*),[31] cleanliness (*shaucha*), mercy (*daya*), and truthfulness (*satya*). The first three of these have been destroyed respectively by indulgence in intoxication, unrestrained sexual activity, and pride. But now, explains the king, quarrel personified—the personage of the current age, Kali—tries to destroy even truthfulness, the last leg of the dharma bull (BhP 1.17.8–25).

The episode concludes with the king preparing to slay Kali (who had been impersonating a king while torturing the cow and bull); but when Kali abandons his disguise and throws himself in submission before the king, Parikshit relents. Sparing his life, Parikshit initially banishes the troublemaker; but upon Kali's plea for some place to remain within his kingdom (since his kingdom extends throughout the world), the king allows him to remain in five types of places. Wherever there is gambling, drinking, prostitution, animal slaughter, and accumulated gold, Kali would henceforth reside and exercise his pernicious influence. Nonetheless, the narrator reports on a hopeful note, in the end the king restores the bull's three lost legs and restores the cow's (the earth's) health by his responsible rule (BhP 1.17.28–42).

As mentioned, this episode can be read as an etiological story for the origin of the current age (*kali-yuga*), seen as a time of widespread cultural and environmental degradation. Significantly, prior to this episode, the Bhagavata extolls recitation of the Bhagavata as the best antidote to this condition.[32] Within such recitation would be reminders of this cosmic time frame in which the debilitations of Kali are understood to be in effect, and this effect is understood to play out both for human beings and for animals. In particular, although the story just recounted concerns allegorical bovines, the implication is that while, as a whole, the principles of dharma and welfare of the earth suffer, real bovines in particular are

---

[31] Calasso (2015, p. 99) notes that "austerity" as a translation of *tapas* is a product of a Christianizing tendency, whereas *ardor* (or fervor) highlights its original meaning indicating the production of heat, as in the Latin *tepor*, a cognate of *tapas*. As will be discussed in Chapter 5, in considering Hindu ethics as an expression of virtue ethics, these four principles may appropriately be considered as basic elements for the cultivation of virtue.

[32] To the present day, formal Bhagavata Purana recitation is practiced widely, especially in India but now increasingly elsewhere, wherever the Indian Hindu diaspora resides.

victims of the present age (even as, in this account, hope is held out in the restoration to wholeness of the earth-cow and dharma-bull).

We move on to the Bhagavata Purana's Book 4 to consider a second episode involving a king and the earth personified as a cow—in this case an account recalled from an age of relatively greater well-being, long before the present age of Kali. The king is Prithu, considered to be a "portion" of the supreme divinity Vishnu, and his queen, Archi, is counted as a portion of Lakshmi, Vishnu's divine consort. Sage Maitreya narrates how, at the time of Prithu's coronation, there had been famine in the land due to Prithu's predecessor's ill-motivated and wrongheaded governance. Taking his subjects' plight to heart, in a move that seems initially quite the opposite of Parikshit's behavior, Prithu resolves to force the earth to yield its bounty: Taking bow and arrow, he aims it at the earth which, out of fear, assumes the form of a cow and begins to flee from the king's presence. He gives chase, following her into outer space and back to earth, where she pleads with him (BhP 4.17.18), "O knower of dharma, to whom unfortunate creatures are dear, who are established as the protector of living beings, deliver me!"

Here, unlike in the Parikshit-Kali confrontation of Book 1, the earth-cow is represented as having a voice of resistance. She protests to the king: Why is he attacking her who is innocent, who is a woman, who is the earth upon which all beings depend? Prithu defends his behavior: The earth has not been yielding grains, despite proper execution of sacrificial rites; she does not yield seeds of herbs and grains; and despite eating sufficient grass, the earth-cow is not yielding milk; hence, she is not at all innocent. And then the king brashly threatens the earth-cow: "With my arrows I shall pacify the hungry, distressed people with your sliced flesh" (BhP 4.17.25). Indeed, he even accuses the earth-cow of being a "false cow" (*maya-gam*; BhP 4.17.27) that he is justified in killing as the cause of suffering to living beings, which he will henceforth maintain without the earth's help, by the strength of his own mystic power of yoga (concentrated discipline of physical and mental self-restraint).

At this point, the earth humbles herself before Prithu, addressing him as the supreme, fully independent divinity Vishnu, the Lord who is beyond reproach. Although she asks him again why he, for whom dharma is of primary importance, desires to kill her, she recognizes him as the source of creation and cause of all conditions in creation. Hence his behavior is at once contradictory and wondrous. Then the earth-cow explains why she has been withholding her bounty: Until now her yields of grain, herbs, and seeds have been enjoyed by contemptible people, persons who have no spiritual vision or understanding. In consequence, she has been neglected and victimized by thieves, and her gifts have been misused for selfish ends rather than being offered in sacrifice. However, because Prithu, an expansion of Vishnu, is now the king, she wishes to cooperate with him, and she will do so if he arranges to bring a "calf" suitable for "milking" the earth.

Then follows a list of beings who, each with an appropriate "calf" and "milk container," are able to "milk" the earth for the particular substance of her or his desire. First, Prithu demonstrates the milking process by transforming the cosmic progenitor Manu into a calf, enabling Prithu to milk into his cupped hands all grains and herbs from the earth. Similarly, the world's sages make the celestial priest Brihaspati into a calf and milk the Vedic hymns into the senses; Indra, king of the heavens, becomes a calf for the gods, who milk the ritual soma drink into a golden pot. Cosmic demons draw liquor and beer into an iron pot, their calf being the devoted demon-born hero, Prahlada. Thus, all the various sorts of beings of this world and beyond—predator and prey animals, yogis, trees, and even mountains—receive their desired "milk" prizes, each with the help of appropriate "calves" (BhP 4.18.12–26).

Consistent with earlier texts, this story continues the association of cows with abundance. In addition, in this and in the Parikshit-Kali encounter, the Bhagavata Purana makes an explicit identification of cows and earth. In both instances, violence or the threat of violence to the earth-cow is featured, and in both there is verbal communication between a human and the (allegorical) bovine. As with almost all the narratives we have thus far considered, kings or divinities are involved, as protectors of a threatened world-as-bovine. But in the case of Prithu's encounter with the earth-cow, there is the surprising initial threat by the king against her. Also, in this case, unlike in the Mahabharata, there is a sense that dharma—closely linked to brahmins and cows—can be properly upheld when the supreme divinity Vishnu (albeit initially with the threat of violence) intervenes.

The Bhagavata Purana certainly regards Vishnu as the supreme divinity, consistent with a long tradition that regards him as superior to all other gods of the Rigveda. Yet the Bhagavata aims to establish Krishna, the cowherd boy of Vraja, as the original form of *bhagavan*, of whom Vishnu, in countless forms, is a primary manifestation. This distinction is made briefly early in the text, but the entire Book 10 (approximately one third of the entire text) celebrates Krishna as the actual supreme, primordial divine being. Without digressing into the theological details by which this argument is made, for us to note is the notion sustained in the text that, being—or despite being—the supreme God himself, Krishna enjoys the pleasure of acting and being regarded as an ordinary cowherd boy. Thus, the sequence of his adventures from birth to childhood and to youth urges readers/listeners to imagine themselves participating in these events, experiencing Krishna much as Krishna's friends and family in Vraja experience him. He is an ordinary cowherd boy, but then again, he is supraordinary in so many ways, including his stunning beauty and handsomeness, his charming, joking speech and mischievous smiles, and his irresistible dallying with Vraja's young cowherd maidens.

Here we can consider three Book 10 episodes relevant to our topic. To keep well in mind is the text's foregrounding of the *bhakti* principle, or what may be called the "bhakti paradigm." Bhakti is typically translated as "devotion" or "devotionalism," yet the rich import of the term for the tradition in which bhakti is foregrounded is best understood through such literature as the Bhagavata Purana. Important for us to be alert to in appreciating the spirit of bhakti is a sense of cultivated emotive, reciprocal relationality between human and nonhuman devotees and the divinity—in this case Krishna. Such relationality operates within a "spatio-temporal 'neighborhood' of both mortal and non-human persons" (Frazier 2017, p. 177) that is inclusive of nonhuman animals and even of plants and trees. Further, it is in the Vraja neighborhood of bhakti that the sense of *lila*—divine play, pastime, or sport—comes to its full significance.[33] *Lila* is contrasted with *karma*, action which invariably implicates the actor in

---

[33] Vraja (Hindi: Braj) is identified as an area in present-day northern India that straddles three states—Hariyana, Uttar Pradesh, and Rajasthan. More importantly for the tradition, Vraja is Krishna's ever-existing transcendent abode which Krishna manifests on the earthly plane when he exhibits his earthly childhood life. For a detailed explanation, see Holdrege (2013).

the bound, embodied life of enjoyment and suffering, framed by birth, death, and rebirth, each time in a physical aggregation of previous actions, a mortal body. By contrast, divine *lila* carries no residue of karmic selfishness, and thus there is no impedance to the steady flow and swelling of selfless love, leading ultimately to a state of freedom said to be realized in a nonphysical, yet richly multifarious, counterpart to the land of Vraja on earth. In that nontemporal realm called Goloka—the realm (*loka*) of cows (*go*)—the same *lila* that Krishna and his associates enact in the temporal, physical realm is said to go on perpetually, with ever-expanding variation and selfless joy.

Krishna and His Cows in Vraja

Krishna is seven years old when his foster father, Nanda, chieftain of the Vraja cowherd district, begins preparations for the community's annual Indra worship ritual. When Nanda explains to his curious son the reasons why this ritual is performed, Krishna is unconvinced. "Why we don't worship Mount Govardhana instead, since this lush green mountain supplies everything needed for our cows, the direct source of our well-being?" Because Krishna is so lovably charming to Nanda and the other village elders, they are happily inclined to follow his proposal this year and see how it goes.

When Indra, the great storm-god of the heavens, sees that the Vraja villagers are irreverently neglecting his worship, instead dedicating all ingredients and rituals to a nearby mountain, in furious retaliation he sends world-inundating storm clouds over the town. A terrible tempest ensues, enveloping Vraja in torrential rain, hailstones, and blasting winds. The villagers, as well as the cows and other domestic animals, trembling with cold, all rush to Krishna, begging him (who had convinced them to neglect Indra's worship) to save them from the deluge.

Bent on teaching Indra a lesson while fulfilling his vow to protect his devotees, Krishna miraculously places his left arm under Mount Govardhana and raises it into the air, effortlessly balancing it on his hand "just as a child holds aloft a mushroom" (BhP 10.25.19). With the mountain now serving as a vast umbrella, smiling Krishna invites his family and all villagers, with their cows, to come take shelter under the mountain. Doing so, all are comfortably accommodated and, the text reports, for seven days Krishna stands, left hand keeping the mountain above them, unmoving from this position while all gaze upon him, none disturbed by hunger or thirst. After seven days, Indra withdraws the storm clouds, the villagers step out from underneath the mountain, and Krishna carefully sets it down in its previous position. The villagers are beside themselves with gratitude and praises for Krishna, who then unaffectedly returns to his "routine" *lila* of tending the cows.

Indra, now remorseful, comes personally before Krishna, bows before him, and offers him praises as cosmic father, primordial teacher, supreme Lord, and master of time. Acknowledging that Krishna has rightly humbled him, Indra regards Krishna's way of dealing with him as divine mercy and therefore begs Krishna for pardon and refuge. Krishna then blesses Indra to resume his duties as lord of the heavens, warning him not to again succumb to pride.

At this point in the narrative, the celestial cow Surabhi, together with her progeny, approaches and speaks to Krishna (here referred to as *gopa-rūpi*—he who has the form of a cowherd): "You are our supreme divinity; lord of the world, please become our Indra—lord of cows, brahmins, gods, and saints!"[34] Then she, with the help of the heavenly Indra and other divinities, performs a ritual royal consecration, concluding with Indra addressing Krishna as "Govinda" (Indra of Cows). The episode ends with a display of natural abundance and harmony: The cows, out of joyfulness, drench the earth with their milk, rivers flow with various liquids, the trees flow with sweet sap, vegetables thrive without cultivation, and mountains yield jewels on their surfaces. Even predator animals are said to shed their vicious natures (BhP 10.27.18–27).[35]

[34]There are several stories about the celestial Surabhi cow in various Sanskrit texts, including the Mahabharata and as early as the Taittiriya Brahmana, a portion of the very early text, the Yajurveda. The BhP (8.8) mentions Surabhi (referred to as Havirdhani—she who provides ingredients for sacrificial rites) as the first of the beings that emerge from the Churning of the Cosmic Ocean by the gods and anti-gods, a story widely known throughout South and Southeast Asia.

[35]One can easily recognize in the BhP Govardhana episode the message of Vedic orthodox brahmanical *yajna* replacement with the bhakti paradigm, whereby the bhakti spirit and practices are contrasted with the ritualism of Vedic practices. Also, Indra's humiliation in this account contrasts

In our second Book 10 narrative, a noteworthy similar testing of Krishna's divinity in which cows are involved is ventured by the cosmic demiurge, Brahma. There are sufficient features of this episode differing from the encounter with Indra to merit our attention, particularly its echoing of the Rigvedic story of bovine theft by the Panis.

In days prior to the encounter with Indra, when Krishna is just old enough to herd the calves, he roams the Vraja forest with the calves and with his young cowherd friends. Eventually the friends sit together to enjoy the lunch they have brought with them from their homes. While eating, after some time the boys notice that the calves have wandered off, and Krishna sets off alone to fetch them while the boys continue with their picnic. During Krishna's absence from both the boys and the calves, Brahma invisibly takes them all—all the boys and all the calves—and hides them away. Krishna, now alone, understands that this is the work of Brahma to test him, for Brahma had been observing Krishna's previous wonderful deeds, and he hoped to ascertain the limits to Krishna's power.

Krishna's simple solution to the problem of missing friends and their calves is to instantly replicate them all. By his unlimited divine powers, Krishna creates a perfect copy of each boy and each calf, each one exactly like its prototype, in both appearance and character. That afternoon, in these many forms, Krishna returns to each appropriate home and cowshed, where both human and bovine mothers joyfully welcome their would-be offspring. Because it is actually Krishna, the supremely attractive *bhagavan*, whom the mothers meet, their feelings of love for whom they think are their offspring redoubles. And with all their devotionally imbued attentions upon these boys and calves, these respective "mothers" unknowingly render devotional services to Krishna in a particular emotional mode of bhakti called *vatsalya*—the caring and protecting mood of parents and elders for children and dependents. The charade continues for an entire year, with the affection of the cowherd men and women for their sons intensifying from day to day, and that of the cows for their calves similarly increasing.

---

with his exalted identity in the Rigveda to highlight the more exalted position of Krishna as "Indra of the cows."

Meanwhile, after only a moment by his own experience of time, Brahma returns to see how Krishna has reacted to his trick. To his surprise and astonishment, he finds Krishna playing with his friends and surrounded by calves just as before. Looking back to the boys and calves he has kept hidden, he is now confused: Which of them are the real ones? In this state of bewilderment, Krishna gives him a divine vision, in which all of Krishna's expanded calves and boys assume forms of Vishnu, with Vishnu's four arms and other insignia. Finally, Krishna reveals to the ever more astonished Brahma a vision of Vraja in which hunger, thirst, and anger are dissolved, and where naturally inimical animals and humans reside like friends.

We may recall that in the Rigveda is a story of cattle theft by the Panis, who hide the cows in a cave (or in/behind a rock). In this account of Brahma's cattle and cowherd theft, the specific location of their captivity is not indicated; only it is mentioned that they are kept "sleeping in the bed of *maya*," that is, they are kept under a sleep-like spell for one year's duration. In any case, the more important contrast to note here is between the Rigvedic sacrificial world and the Bhagavata's devotional world. The Rigvedic world is one in which the danger of scarcity is always to be overcome by keeping the sacrificial process—in which cows play an integral role—intact at all cost. The devotional world of Vraja in the Bhagavata Purana echoes to some extent the Rigvedic sacrificial world, but in contrast, this is a world of assured abundance, where threats of deprivation are always overcome by the object of devotion, Krishna. And this is assured because, after all, Krishna is an "ordinary" cowherd boy *and* he is the Indra of cows, Govinda, making him superior even to Indra, the lord of the heavens (BhP 10.13).

Our final episode from the Bhagavata's Book 10 takes us still further back in the life of Krishna, to his time as a toddler as he is doted upon by his foster mother, Yashoda. Here again, the theme is the power of devotion, again highlighting the *vatsalya* mood of parental affection, but now child Krishna displays his mischievous nature while showing how the products of cows—milk and its derivatives—become uniquely apt media for exchange in the "economy of love" (Hawley 1983, p. 283). And here again, the naughty thievery of Krishna is an echo of ancient dangers related to cows, now replayed on the register of divine pranks and the passion for fresh butter.

It is early morning, and Yashoda, wife of Nanda (the Vraja cowherd chieftain), is in the home courtyard churning yogurt. Yashoda's beloved child Krishna interrupts her work to suckle her breast milk; but then their exchange is interrupted when Yashoda must dash to the kitchen to save some cooking milk from boiling over. While Yashoda is thus preoccupied, Krishna, now upset by this interruption, shows his spite by smashing the pot in which yogurt was being churned, and makes off to a side room with part of the pot to enjoy its contents. When his mother finds him, little Krishna is sharing the contents with some monkeys. Seeing Yashoda approaching him with a stick in hand, Krishna flees "as if afraid," but she soon apprehends him. Seeing the child's fear and his tears, Yashoda discards the stick. But then she resolves to bind Krishna with a rope to something immovable, to teach him a lesson and to prevent further mischief.

The Bhagavata's main narrator, Shuka, points out that Krishna, as *bhagavan*, has neither beginning nor end, neither interior nor exterior. Hence, it is impossible for anyone to capture and bind him. Nonetheless, Yashoda is resolved to do so. Since the first rope she wraps around Krishna's small belly is slightly too short, she ties a second rope to the first. Yet, strangely, the combined ropes are still too short, as are three ropes and any number more that she adds to the previous ones. When Krishna sees that Yashoda now perspires with her determined effort, he finally accedes to her wish and allows himself to be bound by her, to a large wooden grinding mortar.[36] The narrative concludes with an explicit lesson to be learned: The supreme Lord, the butter thief Krishna, cannot be attained by anyone who would try by one's own power; yet he allows himself to come under the control of his devotees.

---

[36]As the story continues in the BhP (10.9), when Yashoda is not looking, Krishna will drag the mortar to which he is tied out into the courtyard, causing it to become wedged between two trees. Continuing to pull the mortar, he forces these trees to come crashing down, thereby freeing two celestial beings who had been cursed to stand as trees for earlier improprieties. The motif of curse or sinful act, then punishment by lower life form, followed by release by a divinity, is widespread in the Sanskrit epics and Puranas and beyond. Here we may be reminded of the Nriga story of the MBh and BhP. In both cases Krishna's saving grace is the main message, but also, we are reminded of the Indic notion of embodiment—that all living beings, as non-temporal spirit (*atman*), reside temporarily in physical bodies, each body appropriate to previous action (*karma*). This will be further discussed in Chapter 5 in relation to our consideration of Hindu animal ethics in general.

I have saved this final Bhagavata Purana reference to cows (or, more specifically, to dealings with cows' products) for last, as a lead-into the last part of our discussion on the Hindu literary bovine imaginaire. We continue to focus on the bhakti tradition, especially of Krishna-bhakti (often referred to as Vaishnavism—faith in Vishnu as ultimate), moving into its late medieval and early modern manifestations in vernacular languages, particularly Hindi and its Vraja dialect, Vraja-bhasha.[37] Yet for some authors, Sanskrit remains the preferred language. This later Vaishnava tradition invariably draws inspiration from the Bhagavata Purana, often explicitly, and less frequently or explicitly it may also draw from earlier literature. However, at times the later Krishna-*bhaktas* (devotees of Krishna) may explicitly *distance* themselves from Vedic literature such as the Rigveda to highlight the contrast between their own devotional world-transcendence and the perceived mundanity of the latter.

Vraja Bhakti Poetry—The Buttery Sweet Language of Love

We move forward to the sixteenth century to consider a poem attributed to Surdas, an important figure in the late medieval north Indian landscape of Krishna-bhakti. The poet invites his readers/listeners to picture in detail the scene of child Krishna's butter thieving. Gopal (an endearing, popular name of Krishna, meaning "cowherd") is described as being "in the butter," the shimmering color of which contrasts with his own "dusk-toned body." Then ensues a cascade of images mirroring and echoing a sense of divine grace occurring in liquid form, the freshly churned butter "trickling down his face to his chest / As if the far ambrosial moon rained beams on loves below." Then, shifting the metaphor, Surdas suggests a sense of excitement and danger: Gopal has "risen to peer from his lair," perhaps like a lion cub, to look about and confirm that no one is looking, "and then / he cheerfully feeds his friends." Surdas' audience knows (from the Bhagavata Purana

---

[37] In a quite different register of vernacular literature, the Rajasthani oral folk epic of Pabūjī, *Pābūjī ro pavāṛo*, celebrates Pabūjī's heroism often involving the protection of cattle from cattle raiders. He is regarded as a form of the divinity Rama and is worshiped by Rebārī camel herdsmen, see Turek (2006, pp. 300–305).

account) that these "friends" are monkeys, whose impish company points to Krishna's inclination to freely extend his kindness to all beings. The poem's colophon turns our attention to the intense affection of Krishna's beloveds (the "loves below"), the gopi maidens, who have delightedly witnessed Krishna's mischief:

> ... Seeing Sur's Lord in his boyish fun,
>   the maidens start, love-struck and weakened,
> Until their hearts are lost to speech
>   in thought after thought after thought.
> (Hawley and Juergensmeyer 1988, pp. 105–106)

Milk and its derivatives have been prized and praised in Indian literature from the time of the Rigveda. Late medieval vernacular bhakti literature expands this tradition considerably, taking as the seed for further reflection especially the Bhagavata Purana's account of Krishna's yogurt and butter "theft" that we have just seen. Such further reflections may be taken as further "churning" of the milk-as-bhakti motif, whereby the notion of churning to extract something especially desirable, as a creative act, also suggests resonance with a celebrated Puranic churning story— the Churning of the Cosmic Ocean.[38] Yet Krishna's butter theft may also be regarded as an *undoing* of cosmic churning, wherein "the sea of milk products that the butter thief unleashes is the sea of love" (Hawley 1983, p. 305). Whereas the Puranic story is an affirmation of dharma's cosmic order (in which there is a foiled attempt by a demon to steal the ambrosia of immortality from the gods), Krishna's successful butter theft is a playful shattering of dharma's seemingly rigid boundaries, allowing to prevail what the bhakti traditions hold to be essential for dharma to be properly realized, namely divine love.

---

[38]This story has numerous tellings, especially in various Puranas. It is also found in Southeast Asian cultures, famously illustrated for example at Ankor Wat in Cambodia. In the Bhagavata Purana, Book 8, the account features the involvement of several forms of Vishnu, one of which is Mohini, a female form that he manifests to foil the demons' attempt to take for themselves the ambrosia of "immortality" which they, in cooperation with the gods, had churned from the Cosmic Ocean. See Gupta and Valpey (2013, pp. 3–11) for a summary of this episode as representative of broad themes in the BhP.

The poem just quoted, so rich in imagery of savorable fluidity, invites us to partake in a vision of a light-hearted and mildly forbidden sort of divine love. Gopal—Krishna—in his thieving stealth cannot hide his beauty, compared to the moon, which in much Indic literature is associated with ambrosia. That Krishna's moonlike face "rained beams on loves below," implies that Krishna's young cowherdess beloveds (as well as the older mothers, from whose houses Krishna steals butter) are the receivers of his "drop after drop" curd-like flowing love. These maidens are "love-struck" by witnessing Krishna's artless beauty as he freely shares the butter with his monkey friends. The flow of yogurt and butter, as a downpour of mercy, echoes the Rigvedic hope for Indra to bestow blessing in the form of rain. And this flow precipitates a cascading flow of thought ("thought after thought after thought") that arrests speech, possibly alluding to the Rigveda's preoccupation with right and poetic speech by which the divinities may be pleased and bestow their bounty. Here, in the overwhelming power of Krishna's beauty and love, speechless thought prevails, since speech, with all its clumsy limitations and proneness to misunderstanding, fails to do justice to the longing heart.

Ironically, of course, this song of Surdas is constituted of speech. Yet it also alludes to the other essential function of the mouth, namely tasting and eating. The traditions of Krishna-bhakti have a highly developed culture of vegetarian cuisine; and complementary to devotees' alimentary concerns of preparing the most tasty and tasteful food offerings for Krishna is a sophisticated theology of aesthetic taste.[39] Integral to the vocabulary of devotional aesthetic taste, milk and milk products are often referred to as implicit vehicles for the communication of bhakti in the mode of sweetness (*madhurya-bhava*), both because of the literal sweetness of dairy and because they are associated with Krishna's pastoral way of life, in contrast to the mode of lordship (*aishvarya-bhava*) that predominates in the worship of Vishnu.[40]

---

[39] Present-day Vaishnavism, like most other Hindu brahmanical traditions, calls for a strict vegetarian diet. A vegan diet is now becoming increasingly accepted in recognition of current dairy farming malpractices, but Hindu classical traditions do not consider this option, apparently on the assumption that all dairy products will be obtained from well cared for, protected cows. For further discussion of this issue, see Chapters 4 and 5.

[40] A sixteenth-century narrative "commentary" to the Bhagavata Purana, Sanatana Goswami's *Brihad-Bhagavatamrita* (2.6.120–124; Dāsa 2005), celebrates Krishna's festive eating habits with a detailed

We could find any number of later literary works that highlight the aspect of "sweetness" that dominates Krishna-bhakti, but in relation to Krishna's identity as cowherd one or two excerpts may suffice. A Sanskrit work intended as a meditational aid for Krishna-bhakti practitioners is Raghunathadasa's *Vraja-vilasa Stava*, "praise song on the pastimes of Vraja" (sixteenth century), which offers an otherworldly vision of Krishna's cows:

> The hooves of Śrī Krishna's Surabhī cows are decorate with sapphires, their horns are gold-plated, and their white cheeks have broken the snow-capped mountain peaks' pride. I pray these Surabhī cows may protect us. In the company of Balarāma [Krishna's brother] and His other friends, and his own body splendidly covered with the dust raised by their hooves, the prince of Vraja [Krishna] daily enjoys a great festival of protecting and milking the cows. With great happiness he eagerly enjoys pastimes with them in the great forests and on the grand hills and river banks of Vraja. Let me worship these Surabhī cows. Glory to Padmagandha, the favorite bull of the enemy of Baka [Krishna], whose handsome horns are covered with gold and studded with jewels, whose hooves are splendidly decorated with sapphires, and whose fine neck bears a swinging garland of reddish flowers. Sometimes Lord Krishna feeds the calves, attentively placing small bunches of soft fresh grass in their mouths, and sometimes he very carefully massages their legs. I yearn to one day see these calves of Lord Krishna jumping and frolicking in Vrindavan. (Raghunāthadāsa 1922, pp. 108–111, vv. 44–47)

Such eulogistic meditations as this would be used by practitioners of bhakti-yoga—especially by renunciant practitioners—to pursue and enhance their development of constant absorption in remembering Krishna, including his names, forms, attributes, pastimes, and associates, including his cows.

A close associate of Raghunathadasa, Jiva Gosvamin, also includes a meditation on Krishna's interactions with his cows in his lengthy Sanskrit elaboration of the Bhagavata Purana's tenth book, *Gopala-champu*. There he describes how Krishna's foster father Nanda has just decided to permit Krishna to start herding the cows, graduating from herding the calves now

---

description of his rich diet in his atemporal realm, Goloka. His midday meal begins with sweet preparations that include several dairy items, and other dairy items (*go-rasa*) also come later in the meal.

that the boy has turned six years old. The first day performing his new duty is rich with delightful formalities:

> The arrangements for going to the forest were as follows. Putting the priests in front with songs, music, and auspicious verses, bringing the cows near and worshiping them by offering foot-wash and *arghya* [a ritual honorific liquid mixture], feeding them sweet chick peas, respecting them with obeisances and circumambulation, and then offering the same respects to the priests, Kṛṣṇa [Krishna], with his elder brother, remained standing in front of Nanda who had his hands folded. Nanda offered him a jewelled stick and Yaśoda put *tilaka* [ornamental auspicious clay marking] on his forehead. (Swāmi, n.d., p. 207; Gopāla-campū 1.12.34)[41]

Significantly, in this passage the cows take the role of venerable deities and Krishna, despite—or because of—being the supreme *bhagavan*, offers them honor with all the standard ritual forms.[42] That cows come to be regarded as distinctly venerable we have seen from Bhishma's instructions in the Mahabharata, and this notion prompts us to look briefly at a contemporary Sanskrit ritual manual of ritual details for the honoring of cows.

Compilations—Trails Toward Modern Cow Care

The book *Gavārcanaprayogaḥ* ("Procedure for the Worship of Cows") is a compendium of instructions on all formal aspects of cow veneration. It is patterned after other Hindu worship (*puja*) manuals that guide votaries in their service to the various divinities housed in temples throughout India.[43]

---

[41] In Vanamālidās' (2002) edition of Gopāla-campū with Sanskrit and Hindi translation, the same passage is 1.12.26.

[42] See Patton (2009), *passim*, for a germane discussion on the widespread pattern of gods performing religious rites of worship.

[43] Such manuals are typically produced by follows of Hindu Smarta traditions, those whose practices are based on several Puranas, and which enjoin the worship of five deities—Ganesha, Surya, Durga, Shiva, and Vishnu. Also, that the author of this manual is a Smarta is suggested by his title 'Pandita'. This particular manual also includes some elements from Tantric traditions. Both these traditions are

First, there are preparatory procedures such as collecting items for worship, meditation on Vishnu's form, and a short *pranayama* (breathing exercise). The next section provides several mantras—verbal formulas—applicable for remembering, praising, and petitioning cows, including appropriate mantras from the four Vedas, a mantra for protecting cows, and a mantra titled "means for increasing cow milk." This section is followed by procedures for performing ritual fire oblations (*homa*) dedicated to cows. Then come instructions for observing occasional vows (*vrata*) in relation to cows at specific times of the year, followed by detailed instructions on the correct way to give cows (and bulls) in charity, for different purposes (e.g., to counteract sinful acts; to become free from debt; or for attaining liberation). Next is a collection of prayers and hymns, including a *surabhi-kavacham*—a protective mantra that calls upon the various physical features of the cow to protect oneself in all sorts of circumstances. The book concludes with a bovine miscellany that includes instructions such as how to prepare *panchamrita*, "fivefold nectar" consisting of cow's milk, yogurt, clarified butter, cow dung, and cow urine—a mixture commonly used in the worship of temple images, especially of Krishna.

As a Sanskrit ritual manual (with brief Hindi commentary), the *Gavārcanaprayogaḥ* can be seen as a textual record of an effort to establish the full ritualization of cow worship, on par with other Hindu worship practices and objects of worship. The use of Sanskrit further underscores a sense of timeless legitimacy, locating cow veneration as a pan-Indian practice and linking it to the brahmanical, or priestly, milieu.

Our final text to consider in this chapter expands the spirit of the *Gavārcanaprayogaḥ* to promote cow care. This consists of two large hardbound volumes in Hindi, special issues of Gita Press' semi-periodical *Kalyāṇa*. One volume is titled *Go Aṅkh* (Cow Issue) and the second is *Go-seva Aṅkh* (Cow Care Issue). Both are collections of varied texts, mainly short articles by pundits, traditional teachers, gurus, and Indian scholars.[44]

(largely) distinct from that of the Vaishnavas mentioned earlier, for whom the sole object of worship is Vishnu or Krishna. "Sole" object means that nonetheless, on certain occasions, particular divinities or indeed cows might be given veneration by Vaishnavas, albeit as associates of Vishnu/Krishna.

[44] Here are a few samples of subjects treated in these writings, from the *Go Aṅkh* volume (translated article titles): "Prayers to Kāmadhenu by Brahmā, Vishnu, and Shiva"; "Consideration of the Dharma and Non-dharma of Ploughing"; "Mother Cow"; "The Importance of Cow Eulogy and

The aim of these two compilations appears to be to provide Hindi readers with a compendium of Sanskritic cow lore and of later reflection on this lore. Amidst the striking extent and variety of these writings, of particular note for us presently is the occasional article linking cow care with the practice of nonviolence (ahimsa) and with Indian nationalism. How these concerns become linked will be the subject of the next chapter.[45]

In relation to our central concern, namely to discern basic elements for a modern Hindu animal ethics, one might wish to see the focus of this chapter extended beyond the bovine imaginaire. Clearly, the narrow focus maintained here is intentional, but as we proceed, it shall become more apparent both why bovinity is the center of attention and how careful reflection on cow and cow care may serve as a lens through which a comprehensive Hindu animal ethics may be articulated.

Concluding Reflections

In this necessarily brief survey of Hindu textual material related to cows, much has been excluded. Yet from what we have considered, definite themes and motifs emerge. As a preliminary effort to bring these features

---

Cow Protection"; "Cow Killing Is the Same as Human Killing"; "The Glories of Cows in Āryan Literature"; "Worshipable Mother Cow Is Directly Nārāyaṇa (Vishnu)"; "The Story of the Primordial Cow-Mother, Surabhī"; "Cow-Wealth Versus Tractor"; "Cows—The Foundation of the Rajasthan Maru District's Economy"; "Cow Dung, Lakshmi's Residence"; "Cow Care and Cow-Related Vows in the Svāminārāyaṇa Tradition"; "Devotion to Cows in the Sikh Tradition"; "The Position of Cows in Buddhist Literature"; "Testing Milk Cows"; "Cows of Western Countries"; "Advice for Breeding and Protecting Cows"; "Ancient Cow Shelters and Scriptural Rules for Cow Protection"; "Let Cow Killing Be Stopped"; "The Benares Śrī Kāśī Jīvadayā Vistāriṇī Cow Shelter and Animal Shelter"; "A Short History of the Cow Protection Movement"; "The Modern Slaughterhouse 'Al Kabir'"; "Statements of Great Men and Cow Devotees on Stoppage of Cow Killing"; "Greatness of Foreign Cows—Some Memories"; "Cows and Islam"; "Cows and Bulls on Indian Currency"; "Attaining the Lord by Serving Cows."

[45]See Mukul (2017, pp. 289–316) for a summary history of the Cow Protection movement, especially after India's independence (1947) and how Gita Press, especially through its periodical *Kalyan*, took an active role therein. Mukul notes that the special issue *Go Ankh* (663 pages), first published in 1945, and fifty years later the similarly voluminous *Goseva Ankh*, represented the Gita Press' engagement with the cow on three levels: ritualistic, devotional, and economic (pp. 291–296; 422–424). This engagement had started long before 1945 and has continued to the present, especially in the regular issues of *Kalyan*, connecting the importance of the cow to Hindu life and expressly promoting legislation against cow slaughter.

of a Hindu bovine imaginaire together, it may be helpful to conceptualize them in terms of two sorts of polarity. One polarity stretches between the two emic (indigenous) terms dharma and bhakti. These express, on the one hand, the tradition's concern with ethics as an emphasis on maintenance of cosmic order (dharma) and, on the other hand, the tradition's concern to foster devotion (bhakti) toward an ideal being (in our examples, centrally Krishna, who is fondly remembered as a cowherd boy). Put another way, while dharma is concerned with establishment and maintenance of boundaries, bhakti concerns the impulse to extend and go beyond boundaries. How these two valences relate to each other is a central concern of the Bhagavata Purana. This polarity we might designate the "values polarity."

This range of values is served by a second, what we might call "meaning polarity," spanning between literal and figurative meanings of language. The Rigveda's rich referencing of "cow" and "bull" provides a full range of literal to figurative meanings for these terms, unfolding images and ideas that collectively create patterns of human concern that link humanity with nonhuman animals, nature as a whole, and an invisible world of divine beings and powers. Through these meanings, cows—actual cows—are positioned as embodiments of both dharma and bhakti. At the same time, in this range of meanings, cows are symbols, in that they mark boundaries between the finite and the infinite (Neville 1996, p. 69).

By now it may be clear that thus far I have carefully avoided a controversial topic, namely the practice (or alleged practice) of ritual cow sacrifice in the early tradition. Also lacking here is any discussion about the development of ahimsa ideology, which is closely related to early and current cow slaughter controversy. As with the subject of cow care and Indian nationalism, so these will be subjects of our next chapter.

References

Bhāgavata Purāṇa. 1965. *Śrīmad Bhāgavata Mahāpurāṇam*, ed. Kṛṣṇaśaṅkara Śāstrī. Ahmedabad: Śrībhāgavatavidyāpīṭh.
Bhāgavata Purāṇa. 1976. *Śrīmad Bhāgavatam*, trans. A.C. Bhaktivedanta Swami Prabhupāda. Los Angeles: Bhaktivedanta Book Trust.

Biardeau, Madeleine. 1989. *Hinduism: The Anthropology of a Civilization*. New Delhi: Oxford University Press.

Biardeau, Madeleine. 1997. Some Remarks on the Links Between the Epics, the Purāṇas, and Their Vedic Sources. In *Studies in Hinduism: Vedism and Hinduism*, ed. Gerhard Oberhammer. Vienna: Der Östereichischen Akademie der Wissenschaft.

Bowles, Adam (trans.). 2008. *Mahābhārata Book Eight—Karṇa Volume Two*. New York: New York University Press and JJC Foundation.

Brockington, John. 2003. The Sanskrit Epics. In *The Blackwell Companion to Hinduism*, ed. Gavin Flood, 116–128. Oxford: Blackwell.

Calasso, Roberto. 2015. *Ardor*. London: Random House.

Das, Bharat Chandra (Harsha B. Wari). 2013. *Timeless Stories of Gomata from Puranas and Other Classics—In Support of Go-Raksha*. Guwahati, Assam: Center for Traditional Education.

Dāsa, Gopīparāṇadhana (trans.). 2005. *Bṛhad Bhāgavatāmṛta of Śrīla Sanātana Gosvāmī*. Los Angeles: Bhaktivedanta Book Trust.

de Nicolás, Antonio T. 1976. *Four-Dimensional Man: Meditations Through the Ṛg Veda*. Stony Brook: Nicolas Hays.

Feller, Danielle. 2004. *The Sanskrit Epics' Representation of Vedic Myths*. Delhi: Motilal Banarsidass.

Frazier, Jessica. 2017. *Hindu Worldviews: Theories of Self, Ritual and Reality*. London: Bloomsbury.

Ganguli, Kisari Mohan (trans.). 1991 [1970]. *The Mahabharata of Krishna-Dwaipayana Vyasa*. New Delhi: Motilal Banarsidass.

Glucklich, Ariel. 2008. *The Strides of Vishnu: Hindu Culture in Historical Perspective*. New York and Oxford: Oxford University Press.

Go Aṅkh—Kalyāṇa No. 1773. Samvat 2072/2015 [1947]. Gorakhpur, Uttar Pradesh: Gītā Press.

Goldman, Robert P. 2005. *Rāmāyaṇa—Book One—Boyhood, by Vālmīki*. New York: New York University Press.

Gonda, J. 1985. *Pūṣan and Sarasvatī*. Amsterdam: North-Holland.

Gosevā Aṅkh—Kalyāṇa No. 653. Samvat 2072/2015. Gorakhpur, Uttar Pradesh: Gītā Press.

Grimes, John. 1996. *A Concise Dictionary of Indian Philosophy: Sanskrit Terms Defined in English*. Albany: State University of New York.

Gupta, Ravi M. 2007. *The Caitanya Vaiṣṇava Vedānta of Jīva Gosvāmī: When Knowledge Meets Devotion*. London: Routledge.

Gupta, Ravi M., and Kenneth R. Valpey (eds.). 2013. *The Bhāgavata Purāṇa: Sacred Text and Living Tradition*. New York: Columbia University Press.

Hawley, John Stratton. 1983. *Krishna, the Butter Thief.* Princeton: Princeton University Press.

Hawley, John Stratton, and Mark Juergensmeyer (trans.). 1988. *Songs of the Saints of India.* Oxford: Oxford University Press.

Hiltebeitel, Alf. 2011. *Dharma: Its Early History in Law, Religion, and Narrative.* Oxford: Oxford University Press.

Holdrege, Barbara A. 2013. Sacred Geography—Vraja-Dhāman: Krishna Embodied in Geographic Place and Transcendent Space. In *The Bhāgavata Purāṇa: Sacred Text and Living Tradition,* ed. Ravi M. Gupta and Kenneth R. Valpey, 91–116. New York: Columbia University Press.

Holdrege, Barbara A. 2015. *Bhakti and Embodiment: Fashioning Divine Bodies and Devotional Bodies in Kṛṣṇa Bhakti.* London: Routledge.

Jamison, Stephanie W., and Joel P. Brereton (trans.). 2014. *The Rigveda: The Earliest Religious Poetry of India.* New York: Oxford University Press.

Kam, Garrett. 2000. *Ramayana in the Arts of Asia.* Singapore: Select Books.

Knipe, David M. 2015. *Vedic Voices: Intimate Narratives of a Living Andhra Tradition.* Oxford: Oxford University Press.

Macdonell, Arthur Anthony. 1917. *A Vedic Reader for Students.* Madras: Oxford University Press.

'Maithilaḥ' Paṇḍita Gaṅgādharapāṭhakaḥ. Vikram S. 2068/2011. *Gavārcanaprayogaḥ–Saṭīka-ṭippaṇī-vibhūṣita-gosambandhi-vividhānuṣṭhānasamanvitaḥ.* Pathmeḍa, Rajasthan: Śrī Kāmadhenu Prakāśana Samitiḥ.

Maurer, Walter H. 1986. *Pinnacles of India's Past: Selections from the Ṛgveda.* Amsterdam: John Benjamins.

Mukul, Akshaya. 2017. *Gita Press and the Making of Hindu India.* Noida: HarperCollins.

Myers, Michael W. 1995. *Let the Cow Wander: Modeling the Metaphors in Veda and Vedānta.* Honolulu: University of Hawai'i Press.

Neville, Robert Cummings. 1996. *The Truth of Broken Symbols.* Albany, NY: State University of New York Press.

Olivelle, Patrick. 1998. *The Early Upaniṣads: Annotated Text and Translation.* New York and Oxford: Oxford University Press.

Patton, Kimberley Christine. 2009. *Religion of the Gods: Ritual, Paradox, and Reflexivity.* Oxford: Oxford University Press.

Prabhupada, A.C. Bhaktivedanta Swami Prabhupāda, and Hridayananda Das Goswami (trans.). 1993. *Śrīmad Bhāgavatam,* Cantos 1–12 in 18 vols. Sanskrit Text, Translation and Commentary. Los Angeles: Bhaktivedanta Book Trust.

Raghunāthadāsa. 1922 [1329 Bengali Sāl]. Vraja-vilāsa Stava. In *Stāvāvalī*. Murśidābād: Śrī Rāmadeva Miśra.

Rāmsvarūpdās. 2013. *Go Bhaktamāl (Pūrvādh), Gorañjanī Kavittamayī Ṭīkā tathā Bhāvabodhinī Vyākhyā Sahita*. Pathmeḍā, Rajasthan: Śrī Gopāl Govardhan Gośālā.

Ranganathan, Shyam (ed.). 2017. *The Bloomsbury Research Handbook of Indian Ethics*. London: Bloomsbury.

Sathaye, Adheesh. 2011. Magic Cows and Cannibal Kings: The Textual Performance of the Viśvāmitra Legends in the *Mahābhārata*. In *Battles, Bards, Brāhmins: Volume 2, Papers from the 13th World Sanskrit Conference, Edinburgh 2006*, ed. John Brockington, 195–216. Delhi: Motilal Banarsidass.

Smith, Brian K. 1998 [1989]. *Reflections on Resemblance, Ritual and Religion*. Delhi: Motilal Banarsidass.

Srinivasan, Doris. 1979. *Concept of Cow in the Rigveda*. Delhi: Motilal Banarsidass.

Sukthankar, Vishnu S. (ed.). 1966. *The Mahābhārata*, Critical Edition, vol. 17. Anuśāsanaparvan, R. N. Dandekar. Poona: Bhandarkar Oriental Research Institute.

Swāmi, H.H. Bhānu. n.d. *Gopāla-campū [of] Śrīla Jīva Gosvāmī*. Chennai: Vaikuntha Enterprises.

Turek, Aleksandra. 2006. *India in Warsaw. Indie w Warszawie. Tom upamiętniający 50-lecie powojennej historii indologii na Uniwersytecie Warszawskim (2003/2004)*, ed. D. Stasik and A. Trynkowska, 300–305. Warsaw: Dom Wydawniczy Elipsa.

Vanamālidās Śāstrī. 2002. *Śrī Gopāla-campū of Jīva Gosvāmin* (Pūrva-campū). Vrindavan, Mathura, India: Gopinath Gaudiya Math.

Whitney, W.D. 2009. *Atharva-Veda Saṁhitā*, vol. 2. Delhi: Parimal Publications.

Witzel, Michael. 2003. Vedas and Upaniṣads. In *The Blackwell Companion to Hinduism*, ed. Gavin Flood, 68–98. Oxford: Blackwell.

3

Cows in Contested Fields

As with the previous chapter, I begin with an extract from an ancient Sanskrit text. But here, significantly, I draw it from a recent publication, the *Go-seva* (Cow Care) issue of Gita Press' Hindi journal *Kalyāṇa* (January 1995, pp. 15–21). An article therein entitled "Cow's Cosmic Form" (*Gau ka viśvarūpa*) compiles selected Sanskrit scriptural passages, beginning with one from the Atharvaveda (9.7), a hymn consisting of homologies between well-known Vedic divinities, other beings, or natural phenomena, and various features of bovines (initially of the bull, then later of the cow).[1] For example:

> Prajapati and Parameshthin are the two horns [of the bull], Indra is the head, Agni the forehead, Yama the joint of the neck. King Soma is the brain, Sky is the upper jaw, Earth is the lower jaw… (trans. Griffiths 1895, p. 453; see Fig. 3.1)

---

[1]There are other, similar descriptions of divine cosmic forms in the Sanskrit scriptural corpus. Especially well known among these are a cosmic horse description (Brihadaranyaka Upanishad 1.1.1–2) and the revelation of Krishna's cosmic form to Arjuna in the Bhagavad-gita (11.9–49).

© The Author(s) 2020
K. R. Valpey, *Cow Care in Hindu Animal Ethics*,
The Palgrave Macmillan Animal Ethics Series,
https://doi.org/10.1007/978-3-030-28408-4_3

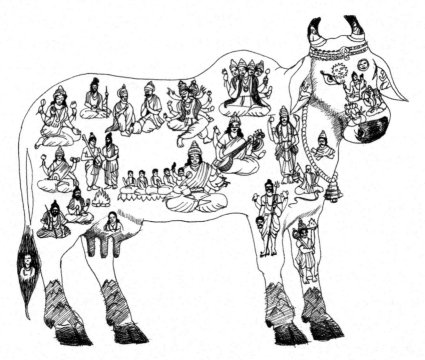

Fig. 3.1 The cow's cosmic form: A typical modern Indian calendar art style of rendering, indicating the presence and specific locations of various divinities in a cow's body (Art rendered by Simo Pejic, used with permission, courtesy of the artist)

After providing a Hindi translation of the hymn, the article's unnamed compiler expresses appreciation for the nineteenth-century British Sanskritist, Prof. Ralph T. H. Griffith, who regarded this hymn as "an example of how the bull and cow are eulogized." The compiler then notes that in this hymn, in addition to several divinities, all different types of human and other beings are mentioned as having their places in this cosmic bovine.[2] Thus, the hymn "shows our oneness with the body of mother cow." "Therefore," suggests the writer, "when a cow encounters harm, we also suffer; hence, with this understanding, cows and bulls should be

---

[2]Identification of various animals and plants with divinities is common in South Asia. For example, different tree types are regarded as embodying different divinities (Haberman 2013, p. 184).

cared for and protected." Further, a person who thus suffers due to a cow's injury "should endeavor to remove the harmed cow's suffering by making a strong retaliation." Implied is that thereby one's own suffering will also be removed.

As this Atharvaveda passage is represented in its modern context, two opposing themes are juxtaposed. On the one hand, there is the image of human diversity finding its locus of unity and presumable harmony in the body of the cow. On the other hand, knowing cows to be vulnerable to abuse, conscientious human beings are called upon to not only care for them but also to protect them, even—presumably—by force that could be violent.[3] This and many similar modern assertions of the importance of cow care and protection partake of the complex history of what began in the late nineteenth and early twentieth centuries as the Cow Protection movement. This movement across northern India expanded rapidly as organizations for this purpose were created. Also, significant momentum for the movement was generated by prominent leaders such as Dayananda Saraswati and, later, Mohandas K. Gandhi.[4] Popular support has led to legislation, and ongoing legal action and discourse have been integral to this history, including the inclusion of Article 48 into the Indian Constitution.[5] Despite, but also because of, legal measures to protect cows and frequent lack of official enforcement, occasions of "communal" violence arise in India to the present day. These are typically acts of violence between persons identifying themselves as Hindus who regard themselves

---

[3]The original intent of the passage might well have been related to ritual: In the consecration of a king, he would have been anointed with liquids—especially milk—thought to be infused with the presence and hence the power of the various divinities. It could be the case that the identification of the cow's body portions with various divinities would mean that the milk of the cow would be the concentrated liquid essence of their presence. See Inden (1998, p. 71).

[4]For a bibliography of the early Cow Protection movement, see Freitag (1980, Chapter 4). For an overview of modern political Hinduism, see Falk (2006, Chapter 11) and, although already slightly dated, see Ram-Prasad (2003). For an historiographical analysis of communalism's rise in India, see Groves (2010). On increasing communal tensions related to cow slaughter in the twentieth century, see Copland (2005).

[5]See Copland (2017) for a detailed account, from a secularist perspective, of the political circumstances under which Article 48 was drafted and included in the Indian Constitution as a Directive Principle of State Policy. The Article reads: "That the State shall endeavor to organise agriculture and animal husbandry on modern scientific lines and shall, in particular, takes steps for preserving and improving the breeds, and prohibiting the slaughter, of cows and calves and other milch and draught cattle." For a Hindu-oriented account, see Lodha (2002).

as duty-bound to protect and defend cows, and (typically) non-Hindus seen or (sometimes falsely) rumored to have slaughtered cows.

We need not delve into the complex and ongoing details of this troubled history. Suffice to consider essential contours, noting that in India the issue persists mainly whether and how Hindus' deference for cows might or might not be respected by non-Hindus or, in a related inflection, whether and how secularity and religion are at cross-purposes regarding the restriction or ban on cow slaughter. At this writing, these issues persist in the Indian public sphere, sustaining the attention of politicians and media, energizing vigilante groups to patrol Indian state border areas to catch and punish cattle smugglers (Safi 2016), and perpetuating smuggling (subjecting bovines to horribly cruel conditions during transport) and illegal slaughter practices (Narayanan 2018, pp. 17–18). On the other hand, public concern for cows also inspires thousands of cow care homes (goshalas) to be financially and organizationally supported throughout India.[6]

The quoted Atharvaveda passage seems to be a vision of unity and cosmic coherence, one that would eventually come to be regarded as expressive of an ideal and practice of nonviolence. Yet in the quoted Hindi article, the author positions this vision as the basis for highlighting divisiveness, the opposite of unity and harmony embodied in the cosmic bovine vision. Going a crucial step further, the author seems to urge action that could involve violence, based on identification of the Atharvaveda's cosmic bovine with actual, living bovines.

Modern divisiveness in relation to cows can be seen as latter-day versions of ancient contentions over cows' ownership. From the previous chapter's picture of Indian literary representations of bovinity, we encountered this trope. As objects of desire and ownership, cows in ancient times held, and cows today hold, special value. The Mahabharata story of Vasishtha's cow of plenty, Nandini (discussed in Chapter 2), is paradigmatic of this notion, even as the story hints at the cow's possessing agency (including giving her a name, suggesting subjectivity rather than mere objectivity). The king's attempt to claim Vasishtha's cow is foiled, as are other attempts to steal cattle (such as the Panis stealing and hiding cows) due to prevailing

---

[6]On the number of goshalas in India, see footnote 10 in Chapter 4.

higher powers (Vasishtha, as a powerful brahmin sage; and Brihaspati, a powerful brahmin priest, respectively).

In this chapter, we consider the contentiousness of bovine ownership in a different register, one that draws us into present-day controversies. Lines of faith tradition and politics have been drawn and group identities (not least caste identities and "Untouchable"/Dalit identities) forged out of the controversies arising from cultural and behavioral differences. This is a long story, going back to Vedic times when cows were prized and, apparently, also ritually sacrificed, as were (apparently) other animals. I say "apparently" because precisely this has been a contentious issue in modern times, whereby in recent years claims are made that ancient textual references to ritual slaughter are either misread or interpolations. And, to complicate matters about what was or was not done in ancient or later times, in early texts we find a distinction made between *killing* and *sacrificing* such that, despite appearances to the contrary, the ritual sacrifice of animals is regarded not only as not killing, but as rewarding them with a better afterlife (Houben 1999). Further, we encounter layers of interpretation—ancient texts interpreted in later texts, and even what may be layered *within* individual texts—all of which are further interpreted by modern writers with varying agendas. What is more, such layering takes place amidst changing economic and cultural influences linked, in turn, to shifting ideologies unfolding in diverse practices.[7]

Dispute over ownership of cows has thus also become dispute over ownership of the dominant narrative of cows. In this arena, cows hold center stage in a polarity of ideologies that interact with each other variously over time and region. At one end of this polarity is the ideology of ritual sacrifice, and the ideology of nonviolence (ahimsa) represents (or is assumed to represent) the opposite end of the polarity. We need to be aware of other polarities as well. There is the opposition between high-caste and low-caste identities and sensibilities, a binary that calls attention to the socially embedded character of ideologies and, importantly in relation to bovines, to dietary practices. And more broadly, there is the opposition between the relative permanence of tradition and the flux of change that characterizes

---

[7]As a comparison of the variety of attitudes regarding animal sacrifice in ancient India, one may note the likely variety of attitudes to animal sacrifice in ancient Israel (over a thousand-year period). See Rogerson (1998, p. 8).

South Asia's present-day rapid transition into modern secular statehood (Larson 1995, pp. 4–6). One important expression of the aspiration for permanence in current Hindu thought is the notion of *sanatana-dharma*, whereby *sanatana* is an adjective denoting eternality, ever-existence, the everlasting. As we will see, in modern times cow veneration and protection are often identified as essential components of the constellation of notions and practices that constitutes *sanatana-dharma*—"eternal law," "ever-existing ethics," or "everlasting cosmic order." By contrast, in the flux of modernity, notions of unchanging dharma are viewed as archaic dreaming, best left to fade with secularization amidst a plurality of religious—particularly Abrahamic—traditions and the triumph of the marketplace. In this shifting landscape, among other loci of Indic veneration, cow sanctity becomes questioned, challenged, and spurned.

So, polarities abound in our field of inquiry. In addition to the value- and meaning-polarities emerging in the previous chapter, and the sacrifice/nonviolence polarity to be discussed in this chapter, we will encounter in this and remaining chapters yet another, what might be called a "perception polarity." On one end of this spectrum is the traditionalist perception that views cow protection as integral to *sanatana-dharma* (generally conceived as having been ever innocent of animal sacrificial practices, while also regarding cow milk use as sanctioned by dharma). On the other end of the spectrum is a modernist view that perceives cows as either objects for commodification and unrestricted consumption or (to be discussed in Chapter 5), alternatively, as rights-bearing subjects with moral status but no religious status.

This chapter has two parts. In the first part, "Hindus' Modern Concern for Cows," I introduce four modern figures of important and differing perspectives in relation to cow care, namely, Dayananda Saraswati (1824–1883), M. K. Gandhi (1869–1948), Bhimrao Ramji Ambedkar (1891–1956), and Bhaktivedanta Swami Prabhupada (1896–1977). Since each of these thinkers and activists make reference to early sacred texts, in the second part, "Ancient Texts, Modern Controversies," I revisit some of the texts discussed in Chapter 2 and also look at or refer to additional early texts. The additional texts are the Manusmriti (Sanskrit: *Manusmṛti*)—the best-known of Hindu "law books," Dharmashastras—and the Bhagavad Gita. Regarding the Bhagavad Gita, we will revisit Gandhi and Swami

Prabhupada in their differing and, in some ways, common interpretations of this text. Finally, we will note Swami Prabhupada's claim, drawing from the Bhagavata Purana, that ahimsa is a "subreligious" principle. In this chapter as a whole, the aim is to show how the sacrificial and nonviolence worldviews collide today, as they seem to have collided in early Indic texts. The difference is that, unlike in ancient and premodern times, today prevails a consumer worldview served by industrial systems of animal "husbandry" (agribusiness) that are utterly removed from both sacrificial and nonviolent worldviews.

Hindus' Modern Concern for Cows

In the previous chapter, we considered how cows were regarded as centrally positioned and valued in three conjoined spheres of concern, namely, the sphere of nature, the sphere of humanity, and the sphere of divinity. This scheme emerged from a survey of mainly Sanskrit literature, stretching in time from the second millennium BCE to the present, with only minimal effort to assign approximate dates for specific texts. Now, as we turn to relatively recent writing on cow care and cow protection, we can keep this conceptual triangle in mind to see how writers elaborate on this cosmic scheme, with cows holding a key role.

Two prominent modern writers and activists of pre-independence India, Dayananda Saraswati and Mohandas K. (Mahatma) Gandhi, are well known as reformers with broad concerns for Indian national mobilization. Both explicitly identified themselves as Hindus, and they both tied this identity closely with their concerns in relation to cows. Seeing systematic development of cow care and protection as integral to their wider aims, both were notably active in promoting this cause, for which they both expressed their ideas in forceful writings. Following a brief look at relevant writings of these two, we turn to consider a similarly forceful—but very differently valenced—counterpoint in the person and writings of Bhimrao Ramji Ambedkar, who raises the disturbing issue of "untouchability" as a product of Hindu casteism, an issue that impinges directly on the subject of cow protection as linked with the dietary taboo against eating beef. Then, as a response—albeit indirect—to Dayananda, Gandhi and Ambedkar, we look briefly at the worldwide missionizing project of Bhaktivedanta Swami Prabhupada, who established farm communities featuring cow care in locations as far-flung as America, Europe and Australia, operated by Westerners, which is to say persons altogether outside the caste system of India and for whom Hindu identity is typically irrelevant.

Dayananda Saraswati: "Cow—Reservoir of Compassion"

Swami Dayananda Saraswati, a *sannyasi* (renunciant) from Gujarat, would become known mainly for the Hindu reform movement he founded in 1875, the Arya Samaj (Noble Society). Five years later, Dayananda published a fifteen-page Hindi tract entitled *Gokaruṇānidhi* (Cow—Reservoir of Compassion).[8] It seems that his writing and organizational efforts were quite effective in awakening considerable sympathy and support for his cow protection cause. Peter van der Veer (1994, p. 92) notes that "Dayananda's ... efforts to ban cow slaughter, found wide support beyond the circle of his followers." This support led to the creation of many cow protection societies throughout India, giving momentum through organization and further use of the printing press to what would become known as the Cow Protection movement from the 1880s.

In the introduction to *Gokaruṇānidhi* (Saraswati 1993, p. 15) Swami Dayananda declares his purpose:

> ... that animals such as the cow be protected as far as possible and, with their protection, agriculture and supply of milk and butter may increase and thereby the comfort and happiness of all may grow more and more. May God grant us success in this goal at the earliest.

---

[8]Quotation and page numbers referred to here are from a 48-page English edition. The translator from the original Hindi, Khazan Singh, renders *Gokaruṇānidhi* as "Ocean of Mercy for the Cow," adding what he considers a better accommodation to English with "In Defense of the Cow: With all Compassion." The writer of this edition's "Introduction," Tulsi Ram, further proposes "Compassion for the cow, (deep and vast) as the ocean." I prefer to render it as "Cow—Reservoir of Compassion," highlighting the sense that it is the cow that is the locus of compassion upon human society, made so by divine arrangement.

In the first of his two-part tract, Dayananda presents reasons why cows in particular are to be protected, beginning with an anthropocentric teleological argument of divine purpose (pp. 18–19): All things created by God have a purpose; if used for their purpose, all is well; nothing should be destroyed instead of being put to its purpose. In particular, cows and other animals have a purpose, by which "the whole world enjoys numerous comforts and pleasures." He then suggests a utilitarian argument against the killing of cows. He calculates that a single cow can provide, in her natural lifetime, some 25,740 persons with one full serving of *khir* (rice pudding made with milk and sugar), and that the grain produced by six oxen (by plowing and threshing) over eight years can feed 256,000 people with a full meal.[9] In contrast, "the flesh of one cow can feed only an estimated eighty beef-eating persons." Then he asks rhetorically, "Why should it not be regarded as a gigantic sin to kill lacs [1 lac/lakh = 100,000] of creatures for a petty gain and thereby deprive countless people?"

In the remainder of the tract, Dayananda makes clear that he regards the unnecessary killing of animals for food—especially cows—as sinful and thoroughly reprehensible. He includes in the first part of his tract an imagined dialogue between a "killer" (*himsaka*) and a "protector" (*rakshaka*), arguing the latter's position by highlighting differences between humans and nonhuman animal carnivores, and by assorted other points (pp. 23–29). In their last exchange, the "killer" agrees that those who kill animals and eat their flesh are sinners, but to purchase meat or to offer meat to Bhairava (a fearful form of Shiva) or Durga (the goddess regarded as Shiva's consort in fearful form), or to accept meat that has been offered in a sacrificial rite as prescribed in sacred texts, is surely not a sin. To this argument, Dayananda replies with an extract from the most prominent of the Dharmashastra texts, the Manusmriti (5.51; Saraswati 1993, p. 29): "One who permits the slaughter, the butcher, the slaughterer, the purchaser of the animal for slaughter, the seller of the animal, the cook who

---

[9]Dayananda bases his calculation on an average daily milk yield of 11 seers (ca. 10 kgs.), an average milking season of 12 months, an average calving number of 13, and an average satisfying meal of *khir* made from two seers of milk. He makes similar calculations for oxen and grain production. Obviously, a more comprehensive calculation would have to include several factors, including time and energy for maintaining the cows, as well as the cow breed and climatic conditions: More discussion on the economics of cow care awaits in Chapter 4.

cooks the meat, the one who serves the meat and the one who eats the meat—these are (all) killers."

Coming to the end of the tract's first part (pp. 32–33), Dayananda insinuates a challenge to Queen Victoria, citing a proclamation of hers to the effect that mute animals should not be subjected to the pain to which they had been at that time subjected. He asks rhetorically, "If the intention (of this provision) is not to give any pain to the animals, then can there be any greater pain than that caused by slaughter?" Further, he chides,

> The ruler receives taxes from his people only to protect them properly and not to exterminate cows and other animals which are a source of happiness both for the ruler and for his subjects...[P]lease keep your eyes open and commit no harmful deeds nor allow such deeds being done by others.

The second part of *Gokaruṇānidhi* is a document setting out the aims, purposes, and rules for membership and decision-making of his newly created organization, the Assembly for the Protection of Cows and Agriculture (Gokṛṣyādirakṣinī Sabhā). Here we see Dayananda's practical thinking for implementing the principles of animal protection he espouses, in particular the protection of cows (indicated by his designating all members of the Assembly as *gorakshakas*—cow protectors).

A striking feature of this pamphlet is Dayananda's employment of ideas from both tradition and modernity to develop his argument. On the side of tradition, the text begins with an invocation from the Yajurveda, followed by two Sanskrit verses (possibly of Dayananda's own composition); similarly, he concludes the work with Sanskrit verses. Within the text, he quotes a stanza from the Sanskrit lawbook, the Manusmriti; he refers to the ancient Aryans as having always regarded violence to animals as a sin; and he longs for a time, some seven centuries prior, before "many flesh-eating foreigners who kill the cow and other animals have come to and settled in this country" (p. 22). The implied resentment in this last comment fixes attention on changing, modern times, in which the current ruler, the foreign Queen Victoria, is challenged in only slightly veiled terms for allowing the killing of cows without restriction in India, while professing compassion for animals.[10] Nor is Dayananda's application of utilitarianism to argue against cattle slaughter without ironic significance, as utilitarianism was James Mill's famous ethical justification for British rule in India.[11] Even so, Dayananda shows readiness to adopt modern ways by setting up a modern-style organization of volunteers (the Gokṛṣyādirakṣa Sabhā), with a markedly western-style documentation of the institution's rules. All of this was set out in Hindi language (for Dayananda, this was a concession to the language's predominance in the north, despite his preference for writing in Sanskrit); and finally, he then had his tract *printed*, thus acknowledging the usefulness of modern Western technology for disseminating his ideas. Significantly, framing his ideas and mission was Dayananda's tradition-laden profile as a Hindu renunciant. This identity served to win him respect while he took the itinerant renunciant's prerogative to travel, enabling him to widely propagate his mission of cow protection along with his broader mission, the Arya Samaj (van der Veer 1994, p. 91).[12]

Mahatma Gandhi: "The Law of Our Religion"

Like Swami Dayananda Saraswati, Mohandas K. Gandhi, later to be honored as Mahatma (great soul), was born and grew up in the northwestern Indian state of Gujarat. Like Dayananda, Gandhi would show great concern for cows, and like him Gandhi would write and speak forcefully on the subject and would make efforts toward implementing his vision of cow care on a national scale.

The name Mahatma Gandhi has become almost synonymous with nonviolence, a key principle on which he based his personal and political life. Less known in the West is that he viewed nonviolence as comprehending human relationships to animals as well as to other human beings. Cows

---

[10]An Indian central government report on cattle cites M. K. Gandhi as contrasting the number of cattle killed during Muslim rule as approximately 20,000 annually, against 30,000 cattle killed *daily* during British rule (Lodha [2002, pp. 10–11], citing Gandhi [CWMG vol. 14, p. 80]).

[11]The irony is compounded further, in that it was Jeremy Bentham's utilitarianism that inspired Mill, the same Bentham who became known for his early championing of animal rights.

[12]See Groves (2010, especially from p. 111) on Dayananda Saraswati's cow protection society and interactions with the British colonial government over cow slaughter.

in particular he regarded as representing all animals, especially deserving to be protected because of the benefits they render human society, and he felt that it was for this reason that ancient sages had singled out cows for special protection. In a letter to Asaf Ali, a fellow activist in the Indian independence movement, Gandhi wrote:

> I have no right to slaughter all animal life because I find it necessary to slaughter some animal life. Therefore if I can live well on goats, fish and fowl (surely enough in all conscience) it is sin for me to destroy cows for my sustenance. And it was some such argument that decided the rishis [sages] of old in regarding the cow as sacred, especially when they found that the cow was the greatest economic asset in national life. And I see nothing wrong, immoral or sinful in offering worship to an animal so serviceable as the cow so long as my worship does not put her on a level with her Creator.[13]

That Gandhi's letter to Ali suggests animal options for human consumption in preference to cows has to do with his interlocutor having been a Muslim. From early on in the independence movement, Muslims were seen by Hindus as cause for concern, partly due to their apparent readiness to slaughter cows which, aside from there perceived inherent sanctity, Hindus were increasingly seeing as a symbol for national unity. In his 1909 tract on Indian independence, Gandhi had written explicitly on this subject, responding to a hypothetical reader's query (in Chapter 10 of *Hind Swaraj*, "The condition of India: The Hindus and the Mahomedans"). First Gandhi notes the cow's practical value, as a "most useful animal in hundreds of ways," and that "Our Mahomedan (sic: Muslim) brethren will admit this." For this reason, Gandhi considers the cow "the protector of India because, being an agricultural country, she is dependent on the cow" (Gandhi 2003, p. 38). He then expounds on how he regards Muslims, namely, as reasonable human beings of whom he holds out the possibility that they may be persuaded to desist from harming cows.

> Am I, then, to fight with or kill a Mahomedan in order to save a cow? In doing so, I would become an enemy of the Mahomedan as well as of the

---

[13]CWMG vol. 19, p. 349 (Letter to Asaf Ali, January 25, 1920).

cow. Therefore, the only method I know of protecting the cow is that I should approach my Mahomedan brother and urge him for the sake of the country to join me in protecting her.

Gandhi was convinced that the importance of cattle as animals to be protected rather than slaughtered was a non-religious, non-sectarian matter. His hope was that his countrymen and countrywomen could become similarly persuaded, whatever their religious convictions and identities. But what if the Muslim would not listen to Gandhi's plea? He continues,

> I should let the cow go for the simple reason that the matter is beyond my ability. If I were overfull of pity for the cow, I should sacrifice my life to save her but not take my brother's. This, I hold, is the law of our religion.[14]

Here the phrase "law of our religion" is a translation of the term *dharmic* ("having to do with dharma"), the early Indic expression we have referred to in the previous chapter as "right behavior," a central concern of the Mahabharata (and of the Manusmriti, mentioned previously in connection with Dayananda Saraswati). As we will see shortly, Gandhi admits his own inability to practice such a perfect level of dharma; yet he does hold it forth as an ideal to be acknowledged, and it is highly suggestive of his conception of nonviolence, a theme that will command our attention later in this chapter.

Gandhi, like Dayananda, was deeply concerned to see cow protection implemented in India. Yet the next point in his *Hind Swaraj* discourse is a striking critique of the cow protection societies existing in India at that time:

> When the Hindus became insistent [by confronting Muslims engaged in cow slaughter], the killing of cows increased. In my opinion, cow protection societies may be considered cow-killing societies. It is a disgrace to us that we

---

[14]Although it is unlikely that Gandhi would have been aware of it, there is a reference, in the Southern Recension of the Mahabharata, to the exaltation to "meritorious worlds" of a kshatriya who sacrifices his life "for the sake of cows and Brahmins or for the sake of the afflicted; even so he obtains meritorious worlds out of regard for non-cruelty (*anṛśaṁsyavyapekṣayā*)" (Hiltebeitel 2016, p. 112).

should need such societies. When we forgot how to protect cows I suppose we needed such societies.

It may be said that Gandhi held Hindus more blameworthy than Muslims for mistreatment of cows. Despite professions of high regard for cows, he found that many Hindus were in fact neglectful of aged cows, over-milking lactating cows, or over-working and harshly treating bulls and oxen. And worse, Hindus were selling unproductive cows for slaughter.[15]

Thus, the level and extent of reform that Gandhi envisioned for realizing his ideal of nonviolent life and livelihood, centered on cow care, was to begin with teaching and learning by example. Gandhi is known for the ashrams (hermitages) he established in Gujarat, places meant to facilitate a self-sustaining way of life based on principles of nonviolence, by maintaining "a strict regimen of vegetarian food, manual labor, social service, celibacy, and sleep" (Thompson 1993, p. 107). Although the economic focus in these ashrams was the production of hand-spun and handwoven cotton products (*khadi*), cows were also maintained. The ashrams were to serve as incubators for training persons who could teach both skills and the ethics of nonviolence in the villages. Further, for developing a nationwide cow care program that would be economically viable, Gandhi gave considerable attention to articulating how cow shelters (*goshalas*) could function by maintaining both dairies and tanneries (leather processing facilities) (Burgat 2004, pp. 224, 227).[16]

Gandhi's concern for cow protection may best be understood in light of his view of an Indian ancient past unsullied by what he regarded as the ravages of "Western civilization." In *Hind Swaraj* (p. 45), Gandhi shows

---

[15]Gandhi could be caustic in his collective self-criticism: "How can we say anything whatever to others so long as we have not rid ourselves of sin? Do we [Hindus] not kill cows with our own hands? How do we treat the progeny of the cow? What crushing burdens do we not lay on bullocks! To say nothing of bullocks, do we give enough feed to the cow? How much milk do we leave for the calf? And who sells the cow [to the butcher]? What can we say of the Hindus who do this for the sake of a few rupees? What do we do about it?" (Gandhi 1999, vol. 24, p. 121, "To the People of Bihar," August 22, 1921). Quoted in Valpey [forthcoming].

[16]We will discuss the economics of goshalas in Chapter 4. Suffice to say here that Gandhi's idea to attach tanneries to goshalas in which only naturally dying cows would provide skins was rather unorthodox, as generally those who maintain cow shelters would consider it highly disrespectful to the dead cow not to leave the animal whole for burial.

a deep aversion for the supposed amenities of modernity, rather giving all credit to Indians' "forefathers" for purposefully rejecting them:

> It was not that we did not know how to invent machinery, but our forefathers knew that, if we set our hearts after such things, we would become slaves and lose our moral fibre. They, therefore, after due deliberation decided that we should only do what we could with our hands and feet. They saw that our real happiness and health consisted in a proper use of our hands and feet.

One may be inclined to read Gandhi's accounts of India's village-centered past as idyllic and his hope to recover such a past as utopian. As Richard King points out (quoting Richard G. Fox), one can discern behind his rhetoric the "Orientalist image of India as inherently spiritual, consensual and corporate." Yet Gandhi also effectively inverted an image of Indian material powerlessness into one of positive mobilization: "The backward and parochial village became the self-sufficient, consensual and harmonious center of decentralized democracy" (King 1999, quoting Fox 1992, pp. 151–152). Moreover, King observes (p. 134),

> Gandhi, quite self-consciously it would seem, inverted colonial presuppositions about Bengali effeminacy, otherworldly spirituality and the passivity of the ascetic ethics of non-violence (*ahimsa*) and reapplied these cultural symbols in terms of organized, non-violent, social protest.

We can add to this picture of politically efficacious nonviolent activity Gandhi's image of the cow, as "a poem of pity" (Gandhi 1999, vol. 24, p. 373). In effect, by virtue of their vulnerability, cows could become powerfully mobilizing symbols for positive change. Thus, we begin to see that for Gandhi cows and their protection formed an integral part of his vision for an enlightened society in which human beings would govern themselves and relate to all creatures on principles of nonviolence— principles, he believed, like Dayananda Saraswati, that were rooted in India's ancient and glorious past.

B. R. Ambedkar: Compassion Denied the "Untouchables"

Both Swami Dayananda Saraswati and Mahatma Gandhi strongly identi-fied reverence for and protection of cows with *Hindu* tradition; Dayananda made this identification implicitly, but Gandhi made the connection quite explicitly, even while he hoped for resolution of differences with non-Hindus regarding cow care. For some, however, the picture of Hindu unity over cow care was not as simple as such champions for cows would have it. In particular, Bhimrao Ramji Ambedkar, Gandhi's contempo-rary and sharply opposed sparring partner in Indian politics surrounding matters regarding Hinduism and the abolition of "untouchability," was outspoken in calling attention to untouchability as being deeply at odds with Hindu ideology.[17]

In his book *The Untouchables: Who Were They and Why They Became Untouchables?* (1948), Ambedkar offers an extended analysis of untouch-ability, especially as he sees it to have emerged and been preserved in India. Important for his argument is to consider ancient India in historical terms, in contrast to the prevailing tendency of Hindus to view ancient India as an undifferentiated past that remains alive and relevant in the present. Thus, a significant element of his argument is that untouchability may be traceable to the ascendency of Buddhism in India after which, according to his analysis, non-Buddhist brahmins during the Gupta Empire (fourth—sixth centuries CE) made cow killing a crime and became themselves (for the first time) vegetarian. This was, he argued, the brahmins' way of regain-ing lost power and prestige, both at the royal court and among the people (Ambedkar 1948, p. 116). He writes,

---

[17]Dr. Ambedkar, who became Chairman of the newly independent Indian constitution drafting committee, identified himself with his caste of origin, the "untouchable" Mahars of Maharashtra. His official conversion to Buddhism shortly before his death was a strong statement of his rejection of Gandhi's plea that untouchables, if they would be properly respected, would be inclined to identify themselves as Hindus. Indeed, he forcefully rejected the notion that there existed a "Hindu Civilization," in light of the existence of what he identified as three classes of "abomination," namely "Criminal Tribes," "Aboriginal Tribes," and "Untouchables." And the culprits for this condition, he felt, have been the self-interested brahmins, who failed to "produce a Voltaire"—a courageous intellectual willing to challenge the brahmins' supposed superiority (Ambedkar 1948, pp. i–iii).

In this connection it must be remembered that there was one aspect in which Brahmanism suffered in public esteem as compared to Buddhism. That was the practice of animal sacrifice which was the essence of Brahmanism and to which Buddhism was deadly opposed. That in an agricultural population there should be respect for Buddhism and revulsion against Brahmanism which involved slaughter of animals including cows and bullocks is only natural.

Ambedkar then sets up his main argument with the question, "What could the Brahmins do to recover the lost ground?" His reply:

To go one better than the Buddhist Bhikshus—not only to give up meat-eating but to become vegetarians—which they did. That this was the object of the Brahmins in becoming vegetarians can be proved in various ways.[18] (Ambedkar 1948, p. 117)

Leading up to this statement, Ambedkar refers extensively to Vedic and post-Vedic texts to conclude that brahmins were, in early times, eating meat, including beef. Aside from brahmins, among others eating meat, those who were involved in any treatment of dead bovines, such as tanners, shoemakers, and so on, were understood to also eat beef, and it is these people, according to Ambedkar, who became demarcated as "untouchables."

But the claim that *brahmins* were eating meat, including beef, has been, to say the least, a controversial claim. We will explore this in greater detail later in this chapter. What is to be noted here is that Ambedkar offers a plausible, if not historically verifiable, explanation for the connection of beef-eating with untouchability.[19] Without assessing the argument's

---

[18]Part of Ambedkar's argument is that early Buddhists were not vegetarians, *stricto senso*, as they merely rejected the animal-sacrificing practice of the Brahmins (see pp. 118–119). Thus, to gain respect, in effect the brahmins decided to go one better than the Buddhists by becoming strict vegetarians. For this, he seems to argue, the first step was to declare cow killing to be a sin on the same level as that of killing a brahmin. Ambedkar quotes at length from one D. R. Bhandarkar, referring to copper-plate inscriptions dated to 412 CE and 465 CE as explicitly referring to the killing of a cow as a *mahapataka*—a mortal sin (Ambedkar 1948, pp. 120–121).

[19]In the beginning of his book (1948, p. vi), Ambedkar recognizes the lack of historical evidence, arguing that in such cases where there are such gaps in the historical record, the historian is called upon to use imagination.

viability, the point here is simply to note that an important voice against a pervasive social violence in India—of upper-caste Hindus against lower or "outcaste" persons—calls attention to a significant problematic condition that persists to the present day in India. On the one hand, the ideal of cow care and cow protection has been strongly voiced from certain Hindu quarters who associate the preservation of bovine sanctity with the practice of nonviolence. But on the other hand, the orthodox brahmanical culture from which this ideal seems largely to spring is also seen as the purveyor of institutional violence in the form of harsh oppression and social exclusion of a substantial portion of India's human population.[20]

Bhaktivedanta Swami Prabhupada: Cow Care for the World

Thus far our sketch of modern Hindu voices concerning the importance of cow care has been confined to pre-independence India. We have also noted an important counter-position in Ambedkar's concern for the untouchables' plight as one that has been perpetuated and exacerbated by the social exclusion resulting directly, in his view, from the high-caste Hindu rejection of cow slaughter and beef-eating. But now we turn attention to one important figure in post-independence Hindu missionizing, in particular because his mission, the International Society for Krishna Consciousness (ISKCON), would take up, with varying degrees of success, his challenge to establish farm projects worldwide in which a central community occupation should be cow care. To this end, the ideological framework invoked by Swami Bhaktivedanta Prabhupada (1896–1977) would be markedly different from that of Dayananda or Gandhi, or indeed of Ambedkar:

---

[20] See Chigateri (2008) for further discussion on this issue of the connection between cow sanctification and violence/oppression against non-Hindus or lower-caste Hindus. Here she discusses the "injustice of the dominant-caste Hindu ethic against cow slaughter and the attendant taboo against the consumption of beef in India by engaging with the associations made between the consumption of beef and the violence of 'untouchability', as well as the arguments that Dalit (downtrodden) communities use to disrupt and subvert such violence" (p. 11). See further, her reference to Nancy Fraser's typology of four strategies for "affirmation" and "transformation" of socioeconomic and cultural/symbolic injustices (p. 14). For a look at a specific present-day relevant situation of Dalits whose profession is skinning dead cattle, see Lahariya (2018).

Cow care should not at all be about so-called Hindu or non-Hindu identity.[21] Rather, it should be rooted in the understanding that cows—whatever their breed[22]—are dear to Krishna, and that they are to be regarded much as one regards one's mother, namely, with care and respect. Further, cow care should be rooted in an understanding of dharma in its deepest, non-sectarian sense—considerate of dharma's outward social dimension, called *varna* and *ashrama* dharma, but not encumbered by any oppressive dynamics of casteism. Such understanding could, according to Prabhupada, be comprehended from the Bhagavad Gita and Bhagavata Purana, in which the term "Hindu" is entirely absent.[23] In these texts, to which Swami Prabhupada would often refer, are important indications that anyone, whatever one's background, may become a practitioner of the highest spiritual caliber while living a life of honest labor, ideally centered in agriculture and cow care.[24]

Swami Prabhupada traveled from Kolkata to the United States in 1965, bringing with him printed copies of his own English translation and commentary to the first of twelve parts or books ("cantos") of the Sanskrit Bhagavata Purana. In the course of his meeting Americans—especially

---

[21] It bears mentioning that Swami Prabhupada, like Ambedkar, subscribed to the narrative of the Buddha having stopped animal sacrifice. However, Prabhupada's understanding of this narrative derived from the Bhagavata Purana account, which briefly refers to Buddha as an *avatara* of Vishnu whose specific and central mission was to curb animal sacrifice.

[22] In Chapter 4, we will consider the distinction made by many champions of cow care in India between "*deshi*" cows—Indian indigenous breeds—and foreign breeds. To be noted here is that, as he made no distinction between Hindu and non-Hindu regarding the potential to practice Krishna-bhakti, similarly Swami Prabhupada made no distinction between different bovine breeds, indigenous Indian and non-Indian.

[23] *Varna* refers to a fourfold scheme of occupational proclivity, including brahmins—priests and teachers, kshatriyas—administrators and rulers, vaishyas—farmers and business people, and shudras—employees and artists. *Ashrama* refers to a fourfold scheme of life stages, including brahmacharin—celibate student, grihastha—householder, vanaprastha—retiree, and sannyasin—renunciant. Although cow care would be specifically the province of vaishyas, Swami Prabhupada emphasized the connection between cow care and what he called "brahminical culture"—a way of life that fosters the cultivation of spiritual (non-temporal) values.

[24] Swami Prabhupada would frequently call attention to a particular verse in the Bhagavata Purana, 7.11.35. In his translation, "If one shows the symptoms of being a brahmana, kṣatriya, vaiśya or śudra, as described [in previous verses], even if he has appeared in a different class, he should be accepted according to those symptoms of classification" (Prabhupada 2017, Vedabase: Śrīmad-Bhagavatam 7.11.35).

young people, initially in New York City—Prabhupada gradually introduced the rudiments of bhakti practices, including strict adherence to a
vegetarian diet. By this and other regulations and practices, he urged his
followers to imbibe the culture and worldview of the particular branch
of the complex of Indic tradition to which he belonged.[25] Essential to
Prabhupada's self-presentation was his connection, through formal initiation, to the Hindu Vaishnava teaching tradition (*sampradaya*) known as
Gaudiya Vaishnavism, traceable through its succession of teachers (*gurus*)
to its sixteenth-century founder, Sri Chaitanya (1486–1534).[26] Prabhupada, prompted by the example of his own guru, Bhaktisiddhanta Sarasvati (1874–1937), eventually began to offer formal initiation (*diksha*) to
young Americans, bestowing on them the mantras and external markers
of the traditional Vedic brahmin. In so doing, he emphasized that this
initiation rite was to be transformative, changing individuals' lives, and
through them gradually building a society that could recover dignity for
human beings as it affirmed dignity for animals, centered in care for cows.
In a letter to one of his students, Prabhupada reaffirmed the strict lifestyle
standards he had set for all his students (in 1972, while visiting India):

> The four sinful activities which one must avoid if there is to be any hope
> for spiritual advancement are the eating of meat, fish and eggs, the use of
> intoxicants, illicit connection with women, and gambling. So these are the
> first four sins which I ask all of my students to strictly avoid committing.
> Practically the entire population of the world is entrapped by these four
> sinful activities. In our Krishna Consciousness Society we are training our
> students up to the standard of brahminical culture. So the great respect
> we are getting here in India and throughout the rest of the world is due
> to these restrictions. Actually our students have surpassed the category of
> brahmana because they are Vaisnavas which means they are transcendental
> to any material position, and brahmana is a material order of life, part of the

---

[25] Swami Prabhupada preferred the term "Vedic" to "Hindu," several times pointing out that the
term Hindu is not found in the sacred texts upon which the tradition is built.

[26] As we will discuss in Chapter 6 in more detail, according to Chaitanya's early seventeenth-century
biographer Krishnadas Kaviraja, in the course of Chaitanya's rich life of proselytizing his message
of Krishna-bhakti, on one occasion he met and spoke with a Muslim government administrator
(Qazi) on the subject of cow slaughter. According to the author, Chaitanya successfully persuaded his
interlocutor to respect the Hindu regard for cows (Prabhupāda 2017, Vedabase: *Caitanya-caritāmṛta*,
Ādi-līlā 17.161–164).

Varna Ashrama system. (Prabhupada 2017, Vedabase: Letter to Niranjana, 5 January 1972)

Swami Prabhupada had counted himself a follower of Gandhi in his college days in the early 1920s. But as Prabhupada took up the devotional path (bhakti) in earnest as a young man, he became disappointed in Gandhi, considering him to be too much absorbed in temporal politics when he should better devote his energy to spread the non-temporal message of the Bhagavad Gita. Prabhupada aimed to show that Krishna's teachings were meant for all people at all times, not just for Hindus, and not just in India. What was most important was the upliftment of souls, whatever political and social conditions might be current. But Prabhupada was convinced that to best facilitate spiritual elevation, the social system outlined in Krishna's teaching to Arjuna—the Bhagavad Gita—should be acknowledged. This was the social system of *varna*, based not on one's birth in a particular family as had come to be generally (mis)understood, but rather on individuals' qualifications and propensities. And since, according to the Gita, one of the naturally appropriate activities of those who show the propensities of the vaishya *varna* is to take care of and protect cows (*go-rakshya*—Bg 18.44), it followed—Prabhupada would emphasize—that cow care should be included as a component of implementing the Gita's teachings—not just in India, but throughout the world.

But for the *varna* system to be successful, there would need to be persons qualified as brahmins to lead the society. And to be a qualified brahmin meant, first of all, to be self-controlled. Self-control, in turn, meant to strictly renounce the four types of indulgence already mentioned—meat-eating, gambling, intoxication, and illicit sexuality—activities that are associated in the Bhagavata Purana (as we noted in the previous chapter) with degrading influences of Kali, namely, loss of mercifulness, loss of truthfulness, loss of austerity, and loss of purity.

To develop such a society where all these ideals and practices could be fostered, the best would be to have places in the country where cows could be maintained, and agriculture could be practiced with the help of trained oxen. Such an opportunity came for Prabhupada and his followers initially in 1968. Writing from America to an Indian acquaintance about a recently acquired farm near Moundsville in West Virginia, Prabhupada explained:

> This site situated in the midst of the beautiful West Virginia mountains provides an ideal setting for demonstrating the simplicity of naturalistic living based on brahminical culture and cow protection in Kṛṣṇa consciousness. Cow protection practically solves the problems of sustenance and the greater portion of time of the devotees, being not engaged in the frantic scramble of materialistic competition for food and shelter, is kept engaged in the pursuit of spiritual perfection. (Prabhupada 2017, Vedabase: Letter to Nevatiaji, 16 July 1970)

Prabhupada's idyllic picture of "naturalistic living" that should free people from the kinds of struggle characteristic of modern city life drew considerably on pastoral imagery of the Veda that we considered in the previous chapter. The more immediate sources of this vision—the Bhagavad Gita and the Bhagavata Purana—were taken as blueprints for a way of life that would focus entirely on devotion to Krishna, the divine cowherd. Such devotion was to unfold naturally, through practical activities, including the herding of cows (to be regarded as Krishna's cows) and preparing vegetarian food, including milk products, from the cows thus cared for—food preparations to be ritually offered to Krishna in a regular manner as part of one's daily routine.[27]

Following Prabhupada's Gaudiya Vaishnava teaching tradition, such daily routine consisting in service to Krishna was to be understood as service directly to *bhagavan*, the supreme person. And taking this to be the case, the problem of determining what is dharma (as we saw in Chapter 2 in relation to the Mahabharata) becomes largely solved: From the Bhagavata Purana's bhakti perspective, dharma is fully comprehended in the practice of "unmotivated and uninterrupted" devotion to this supreme person, Krishna (Bhagavata Purana 1.2.6). Thus, with devotion to Krishna as the center of meaningful human pursuit, the prescriptive aspect of dharma

---

[27] Considering his early admiration for Mahatma Gandhi, a more immediate influence on Prabhupada for establishing farm communities may well have been Gandhi's ashram experiments. On the theology and practice of daily ritual service to Krishna in the Gaudiya Vaishnava tradition and the challenges of translating this tradition in the West, see Valpey (2004, 2006).

would become clear and practically applicable in light of its descriptive aspect. As description, Prabhupada emphasized, dharma should be understood as the essential and perpetually existent, inalienable feature of all living beings, namely, that of service.[28] All prescriptions for action—all ethical guidelines—were then to be understood and adjusted to facilitate the full comprehension of one's identity as servant of God, *bhagavan*, beyond all temporal identities such as gender, race, caste, ethnicity, or nationality. The upshot of this bhakti-centered questioning of temporal designations was that, ironically, anyone could become qualified as a true brahmin (as one who comprehends, or lives in, *brahman*, or atemporal reality). Thus, anyone could become a custodian of dharma (in both descriptive and prescriptive senses) and, as such, anyone could become favored by Krishna, for whom (following the Bhagavata Purana) brahmins and cows were particularly objects of affection and protection.

In Chapter 6, we will look at two of ISKCON's existing cow care projects in some detail. Here we can conclude the present sketch of Hindu cow care and cow protection ideology in its modern contexts by reviewing commonalities and differences in perspective. Dayananda, Gandhi, and Prabhupada seem to have held in common a marked valuing of hoary Indian tradition as the basis for belief in the importance of cow care as sacred duty. Gandhi's references to tradition are highly generalized, whereas Dayananda and Prabhupada base their ideas on specific sacred texts, or selected extracts from these texts. Yet all three have, ironically, a similar investment in modernity, either by use of modern (utilitarian) reasoning, or of technology (grudgingly used by Gandhi, especially for transportation; welcomed by Prabhupada, who applied a principle found in his tradition that accommodates such use in a positive way). And, of course, all three embraced print technology to propagate their ideas.

---

[28] A key prooftext for this notion of identity in eternal service is found in Chaitanya Charitamrita (CC), a definitive sacred text for the Gaudiya Vaishnava tradition: "It is the living entity's constitutional position to be an eternal servant of Kṛṣṇa because he is the marginal energy of Kṛṣṇa and a manifestation simultaneously one with and different from the Lord, like a molecular part of sunshine or fire" (Prabhupada 2017, Vedabase: CC Madhya 20.108–109, Sri Chaitanya speaking to Sanatana Gosvami, Prabhupada's translation).

Ambedkar's writing may be seen as challenging all three of these activists with his concern for the plight of untouchables. Perhaps the most challenging question has to do with the place and proper understanding of ahimsa, nonviolence. According to Ambedkar's reading of ancient sacred texts, not only was cow sacrifice practiced routinely by ancient brahmins, but also meat-eating—including beef—constituted some of their standard diet. Beyond these claims is his charge that the entire Hindu system of social stratification, which is thought to be based on ideas of purity and pollution, amounts to a system of exclusion and violence against the disenfranchised classes. And this state of affairs would seem to directly implicate the ethos of cow care and cow protection as widely understood and practiced today.

Ancient Texts, Modern Controversies

"Sacrifice and murder, offering and killing: a conundrum from the very beginning, which history cannot unravel. Indeed, history will be marked by failures to unravel it" (Calasso 2015, p. 258). Robert Calasso pauses to make this trenchant observation in his study of the ancient Sanskrit text on sacrificial ritual, the Shatapatha Brahmana. The question that drives his study is simple: Why is killing considered necessary in the Vedic sacrifice?[29] His answer is that it is a conundrum, one that forces us to consider the paradoxical nature of the human condition, and to reflect on a similar, pressing question for today: Why it is that our species routinely kills millions of animals daily. The Shatapatha Brahmana is a long work that has confounded and largely repelled scholars for its exasperating sacrificial ritual detail and seemingly far-fetched stories that explain the rituals. For us to note is, as Calasso shows, the deep discomfort the text maintains about killing, even as it insists on its necessity.

Here we want to attend to the matter of ritual killing (in sacrifice) and its apparent opposite practice, that of ahimsa or non-harming, especially

[29]Calasso's question is actually about killing and ritual sacrifice in general, and he finds the Vedic sacrifice and its treatment in the Shatapatha Brahmana to be the most elaborate and detailed, hence most conducive for applying his reflections (2015, pp. 279–294).

as the subject has been treated from the late nineteenth century in relation to cows and special regard for cows.[30] Since modern concern for cows has been predicated largely on passages in the ancient Vedic and post-Vedic texts that are regarded as more or less revelatory, it becomes imperative to clarify the meaning of these texts as thoroughly as possible, preferably such that all ambiguities are removed. To complicate matters is the question of qualification and authority to interpret. We find ourselves treading in areas that have surely been well charted, but in radically different ways by different map-makers.[31] And although "map is not territory," one naturally seeks competent guidance to traverse this rugged terrain.

In 1881, the year after Swami Dayananda Saraswati published his cow protection tract *Gokaruṇānidhi*, the librarian of the Asiatic Society, Rajendralala Mitra (1824–1891) published a collection of his own previously published articles (all in English) in a two-volume work *Indo-Aryans: Contributions towards the Elucidation of their Ancient and Medieval History.* Therein, amidst articles on relatively innocuous subjects such as "Principles of Indian Temple Architecture" or "Dress and Ornaments in Ancient India" Mitra included in volume I, as the sixth chapter, an essay entitled "Beef in Ancient India," an article he had published nine years earlier in the *Journal of the Asiatic Society of Bengal.* Mitra opened his essay with this observation (Mitra 1881, p. 354):

> The title of this essay will, doubtless, prove highly offensive to most of my countrymen ... The idea of beef—the flesh of the earthly representative of the divine Bhagavatī—as an article of food is so shocking to the Hindus, that thousands over thousands of the more orthodox among them never repeat the counterpart of the word in their vernaculars, and many and dire have been the sanguinary conflicts which the shedding of the blood of cows has caused in this country.

---

[30] See Bryant (2006) for an excellent discussion of textual evidence of animal sacrifice in India and the development of an ethos of avoiding the same, with detailed references and clear account of a historical trajectory toward nonviolence.

[31] See Leslie (2003, pp. 17–23), for a discussion titled "Fact, Text and Religious Meaning," relevant to the present issue, as she deals with conflicting views of Hindu practitioners and Indologist textual scholars over a controversy having to do with the identity of a contemporary Hindu tradition and differing views of their founder, the sage Valmiki.

And yet, he writes, the texts he will refer to "are so authentic and incontrovertible that they cannot, for a moment, be gainsaid" (p. 355). He then proceeds to provide several references from ancient and medieval texts that indicate the practice both of sacrificial cow slaughter and the eating of the slaughtered meat. Especially extensive are references from the Taittiriya Brahmana (TB, associated with the Black Yajurveda): Oxen or bulls of particular color or markings, or with drooping horns; cows of one or two colors, barren or able to conceive, or having suffered miscarriage—each are to be immolated and offered to particular divinities, including Vishnu, Vayu, Indra, Agni, Pushan, Rudra, and Surya, at appropriate times in appropriate sacrifices. Most such sacrifices would have involved the immolation of single animals; according to the texts, however, some required the immolation of dozens of animals. In the case of the grand *ashvamedha* sacrifice, writes Mitra (citing TB 2.651), 180 animals should be sacrificed, including horses, bulls, cows, and goats. That the sacrificed bovine's meat would have then been eaten is indicated, Mitra argues, by the detailed injunctions on how the carcass should be cut up. Further, the Gopatha Brahmana text specifies to which of the sacrificial priests and assistants which of the cut pieces should then be distributed for eating (Mitra 1881, pp. 373–375).[32]

One Vedic ritual Mitra reports on concerns hospitable reception of an honored guest, which includes an offering called the "honey mixture" (*madhuparka*), regarded as a simplified version of more elaborate sacrificial rites. According to the author's summary of the Ashvalayana Sutra, an early ritual text, after some preliminary gestures of welcoming (including providing a drink of yogurt mixed with honey), Mitra writes (p. 381),

> A cow was next brought forward and offered to the guest; whereupon he [the guest] said, "My sin is destroyed, destroyed is my sin," and then ordered the immolation of the animal with the words *Om kuru*, "accomplish, Amen."

---

[32] See also Denny (2013) for a brief examination of similar Vedic/post-Vedic textual prescriptions in the context of Christian reflections on sacrifice. See also Knipe (2015, pp. 209–218) for descriptions of current Vedic sacrifices, including a goat sacrifice, by an orthodox brahmin community in Andhra Pradesh.

In other words, according to Mitra, the guest was to consent to having the animal slaughtered for his, the guest's, meal. But the guest could, alternatively, order the cow to be released, a gesture for which he should intone the appropriate Rigvedic mantra: "This cow is the mother of the Rudras and the daughter of the Vasus, the sister of the Adityas, and the pivot of our happiness; therefore I solemnly say unto all wise men, kill not this harmless sacred cow. Let her drink water and eat grass" (pp. 381–382).[33] But then Mitra tells his readers that the ritual text in question, with further emphasis by its traditional commentator Ganganarayana, insists that even if the guest orders the cow released, the ensuing feast *must* nonetheless include meat acquired by some other means.

As it happens, though, the commentarial tradition continues after Ganganarayana, with different ideas. One later ritual text, Mitra informs us, quotes the Ashvalayana Sutra on the method of offering the honey mixture to an honored guest, but then quotes from Upapuranas—regarded as less authoritative, much later texts—to the effect that in the present age, the *kali-yuga*, the rite should be done without slaughtering a cow.[34] Finally, coming to the end of his essay, Mitra notes further steps taken in later times by the brahmanical orthodoxy to enjoin avoidance of ritual animal slaughter, recognizing that times had changed, such that animal slaughter was strongly disapproved by the public. Mitra suggests (somewhat similar to Ambedkar), that the public referred to must have been such that Buddhist presence, with its strong rejection of brahmanical sacrificial practices, had prevailed. In Mitra's estimation, by the influence of the Buddhists, "… [the Brahmins] found the doctrine of respect for animal life too strong

---

[33]The Ashvalayana Sutra (1.24.32) here refers to a Rigveda verse, 8.101.15. Jamison and Brereton's translation (2014, p. 1213): "Mother of the Rudras, daughter of the Vasus, sister of the Adityas, navel of immortality—/I now proclaim to observant people: do not smite the blameless cow—Aditi."

[34]Mitra (pp. 384–385) gives the relevant reference from the Aditya Purana and the Brihannaradiya Purana (without verse numbers), both of which would be counted as Upapuranas, or supplementary Puranas. The Aditya Purana citation is part of a longer list of several activities prohibited in consideration of the present age. Notably, the list concludes (Mitra's translation), "[these practices] have been abstained from by noble [*mahatmas*] and learned men at the beginning of the Kali Yuga for the well-being of mankind. The practice of revered persons is proof [*sādhūnāṁ pramāṇam*] as potent as that of the Vedas." The Brihannaradiya reference, Mitra notes, includes some additional items to be rejected in the present age, including horse sacrifices and cow sacrifices (*ashvamedha* and *gomedha*).

and too popular to be overcome, and therefore gradually and impercep-
tibly adopted it in such a manner as to make it appear a part of Śastra
[scripture]" (p. 387).[35]

Although we don't know to what extent there may have occurred the
sort of reaction Mitra anticipated to his article, the book *A Review of
'Beef in Ancient India'*, written by an unidentified author, was published
by Gita Press ninety years later, in 1971, as an explicit critical response
to it.[36] For its refutational purposes, the book makes considerable use of
extracts from ancient and medieval ritual and other sacred Sanskrit texts,
though the author also ranges over other types of argumentation.[37] And
while the book addresses some specifics of Mitra's article, it also raises and
challenges related issues and claims for ancient practices of cow sacrifice
and beef-eating from other sources.

The Gita Press book devotes seventy pages—almost one-third of the
work—to one topic that Rajendralala Mitra discusses in his article, namely,
the "honey mixture" (*madhuparka*) rite of hospitality. Martialing numerous references from a wide variety of post-Vedic texts, the author first shows
that the ingredients of the *madhuparka* drink surely include no meat, what
to speak of beef (although Mitra never argued that the drink was expected

---

[35]See Stewart (2014) for a discussion of Buddhist anti-sacrificial attitude in relation to Hindu
practices.

[36]Like the article it reviews, this book is in English. The title page includes reference to two editions, of
5000 and 1100 copies respectively, and invites its readers to freely share its content: "(No permission
is required to publish, reproduce or translate the whole or any part of this book by anyone in any
language)." The first edition was published by Gita Press and the second, with additional material
included by "the compiler" (p. 2), was published as noted in our "References"; page references here
are to the latter edition. Further investigation has indicated to me that the author was the late
Haridas Shastri (1918–2013), a Gaudiya Vaishnava scholar of Vrindavan, respected for his extensive
knowledge of Hindu sacred texts and his prolific writing and translations. I refer to his cow care
practices in Chapter 4.

[37]One notices a possibly well-justified post-colonial resentment to foreign influence: The
author/compiler clearly aims to cast suspicion on Western Indologists with an early chapter, "Western Indologists: A Study in Motives," for which an author attribution is provided, "Pt. Bhagawad
Datt (with minor additions)." Whatever Western Indologists' motivations, we may also note the
meticulous research done in the mid- to late nineteenth century by German Indologists, some of
whom focused specifically on the details of Vedic textual accounts of ritual procedures for animal
sacrifice. It is unlikely that Indian critics of Western Indology would have had access to these German
writings (one of which has just been made available as a facsimile in 2018. See Schwab [1886] n.d.).
For an overview of scholarship on the issue of beef-eating in ancient India, followed by his own,
expanded scholarship on the same, see Jha (2009).

to contain meat). Next are several references from the later Ramayana and Mahabharata epics, indicating that a cow has been merely gifted to the honored guest immediately after the guest has received and drunk the *madhuparka* (*Review* 1983, pp. 94–110). The author then reviews the relevant Sanskrit passages of the particular text to which Mitra refers, the Ashvalayana Sutra, examining quite technical issues of translation, multiple meanings of words, and also comparison of similar passages in another, similar text. Essentially, the claim is that it is either a mistaken reading or an interpolation that a cow might be offered for slaughter to a guest. An analogy is suggested: As a host will show hospitality to a guest by saying "My house is yours, do feel at home," it is never expected that the guest will then actually behave as if it is indeed his or her own home. Similarly, a cultured host will offer a cow as a gift to an honored guest, but it would not be expected that the guest would actually accept the cow, much less order it to be killed (p. 138).

Or would he? At a certain point we run up against the limiting wall that unavoidably looms when dealing with ancient texts—the difficulty or impossibility of seeing through the texts to the practices of actual persons of ancient times: To what extent are the ancient injunctive texts of India practice-descriptive, or to what extent are they ideal-prescriptive?[38] The Gita Press's *Review* does not consider the prescriptive Taittiriya Brahmana passage referred to by Mitra (which, we recall, quite explicitly enjoins various types of cows to be selected for immolation in specific sacrifices). Assuming that these injunctions were to be taken literally (and the *Review* author would likely question this, considering his arguments on other texts), one wonders where and when and for whom these injunctions were intended. As far as the Gita Press's *Review* is concerned, the primary, broader point to be understood is the intent or spirit of the Vedic corpus as a whole. The *Review* declares, "The primary principle of the Veda is to view all beings in friendly compassion" (p. 163), providing a few short passages

---

[38]An intriguing reference that could indeed have historical significance comes from the Chinese Buddhist visitor to India, Hsuang Tsang (Xuanzang, fl. c. 602–664): Indians "are forbidden to eat the flesh of the ox, the ass, the elephant, the horse, the pig, the dog, the fox, the wolf, the lion, the monkey, and all the hairy kind. Those who eat them are despised and scorned, and are universally reprobated." The word for "ox" (niu) can also mean "cow" (Beal [1884] 1983, p. 89; quoted in Wedemeyer 2007, p. 400 and note).

from diverse texts as support for this claim. It is through this hermeneutic lens, the *Review* urges, that it becomes easy to accurately interpret all questionable passages (those seeming to indicate animal immolation or cow immolation) as something other than violence to animals, especially given the multiple meanings of many critical terms.

And yet even if one accepts a reading of the Vedas' primary principle as being "friendly compassion" for all beings, one cannot ignore the pervasive presence of sacrificial language in the ancient texts, nor the mention of sacrificial animals. Clearly a sacrificial cult existed, rooted in the Veda, and it is not unreasonable to suppose that animals—including bovines, precisely because they were highly regarded—were immolated in certain sacrificial rites at some early period. But there also appears to have been a current of discomfort with the sacrificial cult that nonetheless would not, unlike such movements as those of the Jains and Buddhists, dare to reject the Veda outright. This current can be seen in later, post-Vedic literature, beginning with the Hindu "law books," the Dharmashastras.

Nonviolence Preferred in Dharmashastra

As we have seen in Chapter 2, it bears repeating that the ancient Vedic and later post-Vedic religious culture—which regarded various divinities as integral actors in the cosmos—revolved around the practice of *yajna* or sacrifice (with or without the immolation of animals). The three spheres of existence—nature, humanity, and divinity—found their connecting point in sacrificial rites performed by humans, as the core practice for realizing dharma—the principle of cosmic sustenance and order. Providing what may be called "legal affirmation and support" of the dharma of sacrifice are the genre of texts called Dharmashastras, several—but predominantly four—prescriptive works that cover a wide range of topics, with emphasis on observances in terms of *varna* and *ashrama*—occupation and life stages. Among these texts, the Manusmriti (Ordinances of Manu) came to be regarded as most important and the most representative of brahmanical orthodoxy.[39]

We are concerned with the first part of Manu's fifth chapter, which delineates proper and improper food, in particular for "twice-born" (*dvija*) persons—those of the brahmin, kshatriya, and vaishya *varnas* who have undergone a "second birth" initiation into Vedic study in their youth. Famously, this section shows apparent ambiguity, with some statements sanctioning the eating of meat, and other statements forbidding or condemning it. Commentators, beginning already with Medhatithi in the tenth century, have puzzled over it. We will view Medhatithi's comments in Chapter 5, but here we can see how Manu shows a preference for nonviolence and abstention from meat, while still honoring the Vedic sacrificial principle and practice.

Manu's fifth chapter begins with a list of foods, identifying them as either pure or impure (5.5–21).[40] Then, at the end of this list (v. 22–23), is a reference to practices of earlier times—obviously prior to this particular text—as sanctioning animal sacrifice:

> To perform sacrifices Brahmins may kill sanctioned animals and birds, as also to feed their dependents; Agastya did that long ago. For, at the ancient sacrifices of seers and at the Soma offerings of Brahmins and Kṣatriyas, the sacrificial cakes were prepared with the meat of permitted animals and birds. (transl. Olivelle 2005, p. 139)

---

[39]The Manusmriti, also known as the Manavadharmashastra, is generally dated from 200 BCE to 200 CE (Rocher 2003, p. 110). For a broad theoretical discussion of animals in Dharmashastra, see Gutiérrez (2018).

[40]Noteworthy here is the *non*-inclusion of bovine animals as forbidden food, while the specification of certain forbidden animals (such as single-hoofed animals, and several types of birds) suggests that other animal flesh—of animals *not* listed—was permitted for such persons' consumption. Countering the idea that the absence bovines in the list of forbidden food indicate its allowance, I have heard the argument that there is no mention of cows because no one would have dared even think of slaughtering a cow. However, verse 26 concludes the passage with the statement, "I have described above completely (*aśeṣataḥ*) what foods are forbidden and what permitted to the twice-born." Further, Heesterman points out that the list is based on purity/impurity identifications of animals, and therefore cows, which are considered pure animals, could hardly be expected to be included in a list of animals forbidden to be eaten (because they are impure) (Heesterman, in Alsdorf 2010, p. 91).

The next section introduces nonviolence with exceptions for sacrifice, conditions under which the eating of permitted meat is sanctioned. These conditions have mainly to do with requirements to perform prescribed sacrificial rites in which the animal(s) to be eaten would be ritually immolated. Although Manu seems to waver here by including statements suggesting divine sanction for unrestricted flesh consumption (vv. 5.28–30), he clearly wants to set boundaries (v. 5.31):

> "The sacrifice is the reason for eating meat"—this, the tradition says, is the rule of gods. Doing it for any other purpose is called the rule of fiends [*rakshasas*—man-eating ogres]. (Olivelle, p. 139)

Conforming to the law regarding meat-eating assures that one remains sinless, whether one has bought the meat or directly killed the animal. However, Manu warns (v. 5.33), "Except in a time of adversity, a twice-born man who knows the rules must never eat meat in contravention of the rules; if he eats meat in contravention of the rules, after death he will be eaten forcibly by those very animals." And again, we see affirmation of Vedic sacrificial authority when Manu enjoins, quite surprisingly (v. 5.35),

> If a man refuses to eat meat after he has been ritually commissioned according to rule, after death he will become an animal for twenty-one lifetimes.[41] (Olivelle, p. 140)

And then, just two stanzas later, appears an intriguing shift toward ahimsa with a suggestion to make a substitution (Manu 5.37–38):

---

[41] Jan Heesterman's (in Alsdorf 2010, p. 92) explanatory surmise may be helpful: The Vedic ritual system is comparable to the social system (particularly in early Buddhism) wherein the monk, who does not kill, can remain sinless thanks to the sin of the layman, who kills and offers to the monk. Within the Vedic ritual system, the one who is "ritually commissioned" (in Manu 5.35) refers to a priest, who is commissioned by a sponsor, a sacrificer (a householder, usually a kshatriya), who must abstain from the meat of the sacrifice. Thus, there is a sort of sacrificial "division of labor" that, by its own logic of cosmic order and affirmation of life, must include affirmation and enactment of death, but in such a way that both victims and priests (who are simultaneously regarded as guests at the "banquet" of the sacrifice along with the gods) are guaranteed elevation after death (provided—and this is crucial—that the priests perform the rituals and pronounce the mantras correctly).

If he gets the urge [for meat], let him make an animal [replica] out of butter or flour; but he must never entertain the desire to kill an animal for a futile reason [*vṛthā*].[42] When a man kills an animal for a futile reason, after death he will be subject in birth after birth to being slain as many times as the number of hairs on that animal.[43] (Olivelle, p. 140)

One might well ask what Manu would consider to be the crucial difference between lawfully sacrificed animal flesh eating and unlawful, not ritually sacrificed animal flesh. This is hinted in verse 44, which assures that the mantras of the Vedic texts have the power to consecrate an animal for sacrifice, thus inoculating it from actual harm: "When a killing (*hiṁsa*) is sanctioned by the Veda and well-established in this mobile and immobile creation, it should be regarded definitely as a non-killing (*ahiṁsām eva*); for it is from the Veda that the Law (*dharma*) has shined forth." Further, verses just prior to this explain what makes prescribed sacrifices so much different from non-sanctioned animal killing (vv. 5.39–40, 42):

The Self-existent One himself created domestic animals for sacrifice, and the sacrifice is for the prosperity of this whole world. Within the sacrifice, therefore, killing is not killing. When plants, domestic animals, trees, beasts, and birds die for the sake of a sacrifice, they will in turn earn superior births … When a twice-born man who knows the true meaning of the Veda (*veda-tattvārtha-vit*) kills animals for these purposes, he leads himself and those animals to the highest state (*uttamaṁ gatim*). (Olivelle 2005, p. 140)[44]

---

[42] *Vṛthā* means "at will, at pleasure, at random, easily, lightly, wantonly, frivolously" (Monier-Williams 1995).

[43] To "make an animal out of butter or flour" would be an example of "double substitution" according to Brian K. Smith, who extensively discusses substitution as a central concept in modern theories of sacrifice (Smith [1989] 1998, pp. 172–193). The substitution of butter or flour for an animal, when properly done (presumably by making a form *resembling* the animal in some way—*samanya*—pp. 183–184) would be entirely within the fold of the Vedic procedure, whereby the exact same mantras and actions would be performed "as if" the actual animal were offered. And yet, Calasso (2015, pp. 285–286) warns, one should not think that an offering of rice and barley as substitute for animals is not killing. The Shatapatha Brahmana (11.1.2.1) states: "Now when they lay out the sacrifice, celebrating it, they kill it; and when they press King Soma, they kill him; and when they obtain the victim's consent and cut it up, they kill it. It is by means of a pestle and mortar and with two millstones that they kill the offering of grain."

[44] This and similar statements of Hindu sacred texts may be the inspiration for some later Hindu traditions maintaining the idea that ancient Vedic sacrificial priests had the power, through correct recitation of mantra, to in effect bring sacrificial animals back to life immediately after immolation.

Thus, in this section of Manusmriti, the propriety of Vedic ritual animal slaughter would seem to be strongly affirmed at the same time that an alternative to it (involving self-restraint and substitution of butter or flour for animals) is suggested. And the clear distinction between ritually sanctified meat and non-sanctified meat points strongly to the value of restraint from meat-eating. And yet, here there seems to be suggested a coexistence of two moralities—a ritual morality (in which "time and again life has to be rewon out of death") and an ascetic morality (in which "death is no longer periodically conquered, but permanently eliminated") (Heesterman, in Alsdorf 2010, p. 92).[45]

A third section of this Manusmriti passage most strongly affirms ahimsa *and* vegetarianism, showing an almost—but not entirely—unambiguous endorsement of complete abstention from animal flesh. Stanzas in this last phase appeal to a consideration of negative consequences and a sense of disgust at the slaughtering process (vv. 5.48–49). It also includes the grave declaration quoted by Swami Dayananda that we previously encountered (5.51). In Olivelle's translation (p. 140):

> The man who authorizes, the man who butchers, the man who slaughters, the man who buys or sells, the man who cooks, the man who serves, and the man who eats—these are all killers.

And then, to highlight the contrast between the sacrificial culture and the culture of abstention (without rejecting the former), the text equates the benefit of entirely abstaining from meat to the benefit of performing an annual horse sacrifice for one hundred years (a sacrifice in which, according to prescriptions found in other texts, many animals are immolated). I have said *almost* completely unambiguous because stanza 56, the last in this

---

This notion is underscored in the central Gaudiya Vaishnava text, Chaitanya Charitamrita (Adi 17.160–165). Here Sri Chaitanya quotes and explains a stanza from the Brahma-vaivarta Purana which lists five acts forbidden in the present (Kali) age. Two of these—the performance of horse sacrifice and of cow sacrifice—are prohibited because no priests are qualified enough to bring immolated animals back to life (Rosen 2004, pp. 24–25; Prabhupāda 2017, Vedabase: *Caitanya-caritāmṛta*, Ādi-līlā 17.161–164).

[45] "Ritual morality": Nicholas Sutton uses this phrase in reference to the Mahabharata, noted by Hiltebeitel (2016, pp. 27–28). "Coexistence" may be too mild. Sutton (2000, pp. 317–325) notes the sharp critique of ritual morality in the Mahabharata, Moksha-dharma Parva, to be discussed in the next section.

passage, holds out that "There is no fault in eating meat, in drinking liquor, or in having sex; that is the natural activity of creatures. Abstaining from such activity, however, brings great rewards" (Olivelle, p. 141).

There is a sense in which, because these three sections of Manusmriti are back to back, the text as a whole is offering a spectrum of positions from which persons or groups from varied dispositions might find acknowledgment of their propensities and direction for human fulfillment. Seen in this way, it reflects the inclusivism of the tradition—retaining all layers of culture in a multidimensional present.[46] At the same time, the Manusmriti seems to appeal to one's reason to choose the way of abstention as the best, even if only for selfish reasons. Further, that we find such an appeal to reason within an ancient Hindu lawbook is important, showing—in our context of Hindu dietary regulation—that its rules, regulations, and laws admitted of the human capacity and demand for reasoning, in turn rooted in the necessity to find and uphold value and meaning beyond immediate, selfish desire.

Thinking Aloud in the Sacrifice of War

The Manusmriti is one of several law texts concerned largely with prescriptive dharma. In contrast to these Dharmashastras in terms of genre are the great Sanskrit epics, the monumental narratives, the Ramayana and the Mahabharata, the latter of which we have examined briefly in the previous chapter. As already noted there, the Mahabharata shows "a sense of increasingly pressing need to establish clearly the principles and practices

[46]Ludwig Alsdorf expounded his theory that these three sections betray three layers of diachronic development (Alsdorf 2010, pp. 17–22). In his review of Alsdorf's text (Alsdorf 2010, pp. 90–93), Heesterman voices reservations about the theory to the reality of India where, much as today, one can expect to see simultaneous differing attitudes and practices in ancient times. In any case, while there may be some truth to chronological progression of the text's development, the final redaction's inclusion of all three perspectives suggests a concern to be inclusive and to show the existence of options within the law. Olivelle (2005, p. 279) see the passage as having two positions—a traditional one that regards meat-eating as the natural order of creation—and an ethic of vegetarianism and noninjury that nonetheless acknowledges restrictive parameters of the Vedic sacrifice. The latter view, he suggests, may be taken as Manu's, considering that it follows the first (unfavored or rejected—*pūrvapakṣa*—view), and does so in much more elaboration. In Chapter 5, we will see how the traditional commentator Medatithi deals with the passage, coming to much the same conclusion.

for human well-being, due to a felt acceleration of time's degrading influence." This story of fratricidal war is no less concerned with dharma than the Manusmriti. Indeed, as Vishwa Adluri writes (2017, p. 386), "Next to the *Manusmṛti* (which it frequently invokes), there is no other work as central for the formulation of *dharma* in the Indian tradition."[47] The epic's context in cosmic time—of a fast-approaching Kali age—conjoins with its occasional rendering of the story's tragic fight between the two sides of a family as a cosmic battle, one that is occasionally represented in the text as a grand "sacrifice of war" (*rana-yajna*).[48] It thus tells of one episode in the perpetual battle between the gods and anti-gods, of dharma and *adharma* (acts in opposition to or negligent of dharma) as they collide on the plane of the temporal world. And as they collide, questions arise as to what constitutes dharma, the questioning frequently unfolding in the form of stories, typically presenting a dharma conundrum, as we saw with the story of King Nriga, whose generosity in gifting cows got him into trouble by no fault of his own. There is another story in the Mahabharata involving correct performance of ritual sacrifice that concerns our present issue, the development or unfolding of the ahimsa concept and ethos in Hindu literature. This story is about the elevation, degradation, and again elevation to heaven of an important figure in the Mahabharata, King Vasu. As summarized by Simon Brodbeck (2009, p. 387, from MBh 12.324),

> The *ṛṣis* [rishis—sages] and *devas* [gods] argued about whether sacrificial offerings should be vegetarian (thus the *ṛṣis*) or not (thus the *devas*). Vasu, asked to arbitrate, decided in favour of the *devas*, and the *ṛṣis* expelled him. The *devas* arranged for him to be fed while in his hole (12.324:23-5), and eventually Nārāyaṇa [identified as Vishnu] sent Garuḍa [his eagle carrier] to fetch him to Brahmaloka [the divine abode].

The point of contention between the sages and the gods is the interpretation of one word in a Vedic ritual text, namely, the word *aja*. Does it mean "he-goat," as the gods contend, or does it mean "a kind of rice,"

---

[47]One might even argue that the Mahabharata comes *prior* to the Manusmriti in centrality for matters of dharma, in terms of popularity and familiarity for contemporary Hindus.
[48]One instance of calling the battle a *rana-yajna* is MBh 5.57.10–18, noted by Feller-Jatavallabhula (1999).

as the sages insist?[49] The fact that Vasu is otherwise known in the text for his nonviolent behavior complicates the story. And it is this narrative complexity that serves as one expression of the tradition "thinking aloud" about sacrificial ethics and the problematic of killing supposedly for the sake of maintaining dharma.[50]

Mahabharata's strongest pronouncements on the virtue of ahimsa are undoubtedly those in the so-called *Ahimsa-Phalam,* "Fruit of Nonviolence" section of the Anushasana Parva (13.115–17). In this section, the dying grandsire Bhishma instructs Yudhishthira that nonviolence should be practiced in speech, thought, act, and eating; then he speaks extensively on the evils of meat-eating, citing the Seven Rishis and others. Yet even after elaborating on the evils of meat-eating, he still allows for it at Vedic sacrifices and in hunting. Despite this concession, he concludes unambiguously (13.117.37–38; Hiltebeitel 2016, p. 136),

> *Ahiṁsā* is the highest *dharma, ahiṁsā* is the supreme restraint, *ahiṁsā* is the highest gift, *ahiṁsā* is the highest penance, *ahiṁsā* is the highest sacrifice, *ahiṁsā* is the supreme force, *ahiṁsā* is the highest friendship, *ahiṁsā* is the highest happiness, *ahiṁsā* is the highest truth, *ahiṁsā* is the highest revelation.

It will be helpful to appreciate the richness of the Mahabharata's approach to nonviolence and to dharma in general by recognizing its clear emphasis on a twofold typology of dharma, namely, that of worldly engagement (*pravritti dharma*) and that of disengagement from the world (*nivritti dharma*). As Adluri notes (2017, p. 387), the Mahabharata never claims that *pravritti dharma* can lead to freedom from suffering. Rather, the human world of activity for which ritual sacrifice is considered integral will always be such that the best one can hope to achieve is a modicum of propriety that will, ideally, lead one to question and finally reject this

---

[49] *A Review of 'Beef in Ancient India'* (N/A 1983, p. 178) quotes this Mahabharata verse (compiler's translation, 12.337.4–5; 12.324.4–5): "*Yajñas* should be performed with seeds—this is the Vedic tradition. *Aja* are a variety of seeds, therefore it is not proper to slaughter he-goats. Wherever there is animal-slaughter in *yajñas,* that is not the way of good men."

[50] See Adluri (2018) for a detailed discussion of this episode.

orientation in favor of renunciation.[51] And the Mahabharata gives ample representation of *nivritti dharma* followers who overtly challenge those engaged in acts of *pravritti dharma*, specifically in relation to the latters' engagement in ritual acts of animal sacrifice. One example is in the Ashvamedha Parvan (14.28, summarized by Sutton [2000, p. 323]):

> Kṛṣṇa recounts a conversation between a priest and a renunciant (*adhvaryu* and *yati*). Seeing a goat about to be slaughtered in a *yajña*, the *yati* condemns the priest by saying, 'This is an act of violence' (v. 7). To this the priest replies that the goat will not cease to exist and will benefit from being offered; this is the version of the Vedas which approve of the ritual he is about to perform. The ascetic responds by sarcastically asking whether, as the whole performance is for the goat's benefit, he has the support of the animal's parents and relatives (vv. 12-15). He then asserts that not harming is the highest of all types of dharma, before moving on to an exposition of Sāṃkhya philosophy.[52]

In concluding for the present our discussion of the Mahabharata, there remains for our attention its most quoted portion, the Bhagavad Gita. This seven-hundred verse interlude in the Mahabharata's dramatic story consists of Krishna's famous dialogue with his friend and devotee, the warrior Arjuna. The Bhagavad Gita is of particular concern with respect to the issue of violence versus nonviolence that bears directly on our present subject of modern Indian controversy related to cows and cow care.

---

[51] Adluri (2018, p. 59n3) offers an apt definition of *ahimsa* to highlight its function in the Mahabharata: "*Ahiṃsā* is the vantage point from which *pravṛtti* [worldly engagement] is critiqued." Thus, *ahimsa* is more than "non-harming" or "noninjury." Rather, it is the key term for "a hermeneutic that hints at and enables the transition to a peaceful *nivṛtti* [disengagement from the world] register…"

[52] The celebrated Bengali author Rabindranath Tagore (1861–1941) portrayed a similar debate over the right versus wrong of ritual animal sacrifice in his 1917 English play, *Sacrifice*. See Burley (2019) for a summary and analysis of the play. Burley calls attention to its complexity and its occasional echoing of the Bhagavad-gita's Vedantic expressions of time and the indestructible self.

Violence, Nonviolence—And Cows in the Bhagavad Gita and Bhagavata Purana

Aside from its long commentarial tradition (running back to the eighth century CE), in the last 150 years the Bhagavad Gita has enjoyed prominence in Indian public discourse. Both Mahatma Gandhi and Swami Prabhupada had high regard for the "Gita" and both considered Krishna's teachings therein to be important or foundational to their views on proper regard for bovines. And yet, Gandhi and Prabhupada appear to have had entirely contradictory interpretations of the work in important respects, specifically regarding its teachings about nonviolence. Before examining this divergence, let us note briefly that "cow" appears thrice in Krishna's Gita discourse, in each case included in lists of different contents. The first instance concerns the way a pundit—a learned person—perceives other beings: Whether a learned brahmin, a cow, an elephant, a dog, or a "dog eater," the true pundit sees them all with "equal vision" (Bg. 5.18). The second instance is a passing reference to the celestial Kama-dhuk ("Wish-yielder," 10.28) cow with which Krishna identifies himself, in relation to all cows. The third instance is within a list of qualities and duties for members of the four *varnas* (social-occupational orders—see footnote 23 in this chapter), simply stating that a *vaishya* may engage in farming, cow protection (*go-raksha*), or business (Bg 18.44). These references all relate to different aspects of dharma. No less so, they are related to the Gita's major theme of bhakti—devotion—with important ramifications that we will consider here and in Chapter 5.

Gandhi's first encounter with the Gita, in 1889, was in Sir Edwin Arnold's English verse translation *The Song Celestial* (1885). The Gita would come to occupy a central place in his reading life, and he would come to consider himself as a dedicated practitioner of its tenets. Indeed, he would consider himself qualified to expound on the Gita's meaning because of his experience in its practice, which led him to find within its pages, despite appearances to the contrary, a central place for the principle of ahimsa (Clough 2002, p. 68). One way he arrives at this understanding is by an allegorical reading:

I regard Duryodhana [the arch-enemy of Arjuna, the main antagonist in the Mahabharata] and his party as the baser impulses in man, and Arjuna and his party as the higher impulses. The field of battle is our own body. An eternal battle is going on between the two camps and the poet seer has vividly described it. Krishna is the Dweller within, ever whispering in a pure heart. (*Discourses on the Gita*, pp. 12–13; quoted in Clough 2002, p. 73)

Gandhi's allegorical reading allows him to, in effect, shift the violence of battle from the external world in which Krishna urges Arjuna to fight, instead making of the conflict a battle within, of opposed "baser" and "higher" inner impulses. By this hermeneutical move, he can argue that the practice of self-control—which Krishna surely also advocates in the Gita—is the pivotal teaching. For Gandhi, from this perspective, the assiduous *yogi* (yoga practitioner) becomes naturally nonviolent in the outer world. Such a person, guided by the "whispering" of the "Dweller within," will always act beneficently in all circumstances.

In contrast to Gandhi, whom he explicitly criticized for his allegorical interpretation of the Gita, Swami Prabhupada was, in many respects, a literalist. Indeed, as suggested in the title of his English Gita translation and commentary—*Bhagavad Gita As It Is*—he urged readers to take the dialogue of Krishna and Arjuna as historical—though surely very ancient—reality, that had occurred on an actual battlefield in present-day northern India. And whereas Gandhi claimed qualification for interpreting the Gita on the basis of his own lifelong experience practicing the Gita's tenets, Prabhupada insisted that full qualification comes only if one submissively receives the teaching through Krishna's recognized representative. And such a representative would need to be connected to Krishna by an unbroken succession of teachers (*guru-parampara*) extending back in time to Vyasa, the original writer of the text (who, it is understood, had directly audited Krishna's dialogue with Arjuna) (Prabhupada 1983, pp. 3–4).

Thus, for Swami Prabhupada, the salient message of the Gita can hardly be considered nonviolence, since throughout the dialogue Krishna martials reasons for Arjuna to take up weapons and fight in the ensuing battle. Rather, the core message is to be realized by recognizing the special, devotional (bhakti) relationship between Krishna and Arjuna—between the supreme, divine person, and the human devotee. To be sure, the virtue of ahimsa is extolled in the Gita, as one of several virtues of the self-controlled yogi (which Arjuna is advised to become); and surely it is a virtue of great importance, both for self- and world-maintenance.[53] However, Prabhupada would insist, one cannot ignore the fact that Krishna commands Arjuna to fight. Rather, one does well to take all of Krishna's instructions in the Gita into account, one of which is the simple method Krishna prescribes for pleasing him. In Prabhupada's translation,

> If one offers Me with love and devotion a leaf, a flower, a fruit or water, I will accept it. (Bg. 9.26)

For Prabhupada, aside from the simplicity and inclusivity that this verse suggests, it also suggests dietary restriction, which is to say that Krishna is vegetarian, and *therefore* a Krishna-*bhakta*—one who is dedicated to the life of service to Krishna—will necessarily be likewise vegetarian. Prabhupada wrote in his commentary to this verse,

> One who loves Kṛṣṇa [Krishna] will give Him whatever He wants, and he avoids offering anything which is undesirable or unasked. Thus meat, fish and eggs should not be offered to Kṛṣṇa. If He desired such things as offerings, He would have said so. Instead He clearly requests that a leaf, fruit, flowers and water be given to Him, and He says of this offering, "I will accept it." (Prabhupada 1983, p. 488, Bg. 9.26 Purport)

Such vegetarian offerings to Krishna are to be understood as sacrificial practices, as an aspect of the ritual component to the devotional form of sacrifice outlined by Krishna in the Gita, especial in its third chapter. Based on this devotional context of Krishna-bhakti, the pundit previously mentioned is understood to have such vision by which one views all

---

[53] In emphasizing the necessity to act, Krishna distinguishes "ignorant" from "learned" persons in terms of attachment to and detachment from results, respectively. Those who are detached are enjoined to act for the benefit of the world, by showing example of detached action (Bg. 3.25). This is a different concept from the dichotomous engagement/disengagement typology mentioned previously (*pravritti/nivritti*), as Krishna insists that it is not possible for anyone to desist from action (*nivritti*) for even a moment (Bg. 3.5); rather, a self-controlled person must act out of duty, without attachment (Bg. 3.19). Such duty could, as in the case of Arjuna, call for violent action, but certainly never against innocent creatures.

humans—cultured or otherwise—and animals of all varieties as "equal" (*sama*): Because Krishna "stands in the heart of all beings" (Bg. 18.61), Krishna's devotee is pleased to remember this by treating all beings appropriately. Similarly, Prabhupada would explain, in a spirit of service and sacrifice to Krishna and adherence to his directions in the Gita, Krishna's devotees (especially those with the propensities of the *vaishya*) care for cows: Taking cues from descriptions in the Bhagavata Purana that we have seen in the previous chapter, devotees who follow this Vaishnava Hindu tradition regard the cows they care for and protect as Krishna's cows.

Further, such understanding of equality would mean that anyone, anywhere in the world, could be a Krishna devotee and that all the cows they would care for—not just Indian indigenous cows—would be regarded as Krishna's cows. Both Mahatma Gandhi's and Swami Prabhupada's Gita interpretations show a strong faith in the text's universal applicability. Thus, both found in the Gita essential ideological foundations for their respective lives and for the ethical visions they sought to share for making worldwide well-being possible. For both Gita spokesmen, this would call for positive action in the world rather than withdrawal from the world. For Gandhi, his own political engagement would be his positive action. For Prabhupada (who, in letters, twice urged Gandhi to withdraw from politics to focus on spreading the teachings of the Gita), action in the world would mean developing a worldwide mission as a network of devotional communities that would include cow care among their activities. Finally, both saw themselves as grounded in tradition, one that Gandhi identified with as Hindu and that Prabhupada identified with as Vaishnava, although both would also regard their traditions as *sanatana-dharma*, as an ever-present ethical principle that urgently called for its recovery, preservation, and renewal in current times.

As an addendum to this discussion of the Bhagavad Gita with respect to violence, nonviolence, and cow protection, a few words remain to be said about these issues in relation to the Bhagavata Purana. As mentioned in Chapter 2, the Bhagavata Purana enjoys high regard throughout India, and especially Vaishnava Hindus take it as the final word of sacred literature. Therefore, the Bhagavata's clear affirmation of nonviolence with respect to sacrificial practice conjoined with its message of bhakti becomes decisive. By describing various tortures an animal slaying ritualist should expect to experience after the present life, as Edwin Bryant puts it, the Bhagavata "supplies the fine print of the Vedic contract—violence performed in the pretext of sacrifice produces temporary benefits, but at a horrible price" (Bryant 2006, p. 201). Further though, in relation to Ambedkar's comments on Buddhism and Brahmanism, the Bhagavata Purana refers twice to a Buddha as an avatar of Vishnu. In the second reference (2.7.37), Buddha is referred to as one who propagated *upadharma*—supportive religious principles. Relevant for us to note here, in connection with his differences with Mahatma Gandhi on Gita interpretation, is Swami Prabhupada's comment to this Bhagavata verse:

> Lord Buddha incarnates at a time when the people are most materialistic and preaches common-sense religious principles. Such *ahiṁsā* is not a religious principle itself, but it is an important quality for persons who are actually religious. It is a common-sense religion because one is advised to do no harm to any other animal or living being because such harmful actions are equally harmful to him who does the harm.

Prabhupada's calling ahimsa "common-sense" religion suggests that it should be taken for granted by people claiming to be religious that they must be grounded in nonviolence. Whereas Gandhi, following Bhishma in the Mahabharata, considered nonviolence the highest principle of dharma, Prabhupada, following the Bhagavata Purana, considered it an essential but secondary, "common sense" principle, supportive of the all-encompassing principle of bhakti, devotion to the supreme person who, as we have noted, the Bhagavata insists, is the primordial cowherd, Krishna.

Before closing this chapter with concluding reflections, let us summarize: Cows in modern India are situated in "contested fields" of differing convictions about their proper place in ethical discourse and practice. Champions of the Cow Protection movement in early and later forms insist on bovines' integral position with respect to traditional Hindu ethics, dharma. Counter-voices are heard, saying that (1—Ambedkar) Hindu dharma's protection of cows comes at the cost of oppression for lower-ranked people, and (2—Mitra) Hindu dharma in the past has not been the nonviolent, non-meat-eating tradition it is claimed to be. A learned attempt to refute the latter claim has taken us back into ancient texts, there to see how the Manusmriti and the Mahabharata indicate preference for ahimsa on the basis of a distinction between the way of worldly engagement (*pravritti*), which may call for violent sacrificial rites, and the way of disengagement from the world (*nivritti*), which calls for renunciation of such rites. Then we noted how the Bhagavad Gita seeks to bring these two ways, or worldviews, together in detached action, as the basis for a society of care, in which cows are protected as a matter of course. Finally, revisiting the Bhagavata Purana, we are reminded of its bhakti message as the encompassing principle, in which cow protection as a negative practice of avoiding harm becomes a positive practice of cow care.

Concluding Reflections

In revisiting early texts (and in considering additional texts that we bypassed in Chapter 2), we must recognize the extreme limitations of our ability to comprehend the tradition as a whole, due to the vast expanse of time and breadth of geographical space.[54] We should also see that what we are calling Hindu tradition is multidimensional and multi-vocal—in the past as it is very much so in the present. But given these considerations, we can also see a strong voice persisting from earliest times, that cows in particular, and animals more generally, call for special consideration by humans. The "special consideration" is typically articulated negatively in terms of "nonviolence," but nonviolence is closely linked to regard for

---

[54] It is surely useful to consider present-day theories of sacrifice—many of which have given special attention to the Vedic model—to gain a sense of the bigger picture in which these texts and practices are situated. But whichever of the several contemporary theories of sacrifice one might favor, the point for us to keep in mind is the Vedic and post-Vedic culture's sense of the necessity and centrality of ritual sacrifice *and* the presence of a strong, eventually predominating, moral impulse to remove violence from the sacrifice. See McClymond (2008, pp. 3–17) for an overview of six major approaches to sacrifice in contemporary scholarship. See Calasso (2015, pp. 251–252) for a discussion of two major divisions in theories: Either sacrifice is "a device used by society to ease certain tensions or to satisfy certain needs … or it is an attempt by society to blend with nature, taking on certain irreducible characteristics, in which case it must be seen as a form of metaphysics put into action, celebrated and displayed in a formalized sequence of gestures." I am inclined toward the latter view, though "to blend with nature" may not adequately describe the impulse of Vedic sacrifice, which certainly comprehends a vital divine dimension. See also Calasso (2015, p. 245) on the sacrificial vision originating in "the recognition of a debt contracted with the unknown and a gift that is bestowed upon the unknown."

humans as possessing the rare opportunity to elevate themselves spiritually, especially by conscientious practice of self-restraint and thus minimizing of violence. The opposite applies as well: The slaughter of cows for human consumption is regarded by many present-day Hindus as an abomination in defiance of a cosmic order that requires human vigilance, particularly in the form of cow protection. This is hinted in the Bhagavad Gita, with its reference to the same (*go-raksha*) as the duty of vaishyas. But even if it is granted that animal sacrifice, including cow sacrifice, has been practiced in earlier times, the texts suggest by virtue of their attention to detail and by occasional allusion to the animal victims' subjectivity, that these sacrifices were done—or were supposed to be done—with "special consideration" for the animal victims. More broadly, sacrificial animals were considered to be "special" as fulfilling a role in the cosmic order of dharma, such that by their sacrifice, if properly performed, that order would be sustained.

Economic and political forces impacting cow care in modern India have been deeply affected by the shifting landscape of circumstances that we identify as globalization. This has been the case throughout the time of European presence and domination in South Asia. To better grasp the complexity of our subject, it may be helpful to draw on Gerald Larson's notion of historical "layers," whereby the Indian landscape we have considered in the first part of this chapter is that of the "Indo-Anglian layer," dated from c. 1757 to the present.[55] In the second part ("Weighing Texts, Debating Cows"), we revisited (from Chapter 2) what Larson would call the "Indo-Brāhmaṇical layer" (c. 1500–600 BCE), the "Indo-Śramaṇical layer" (c. 600 BCE–300 CE), and the "Indic (Hindu-Buddhist-Jain) layer" (c. 300–1200 CE). Looking back on these earlier layers, we are attempting to do what concerned Hindus have been doing over the last two centuries—to discern the voice of a continuous tradition from ancient times, even as globalization has brought in so many other voices.

---

[55]Larson (1995, pp. 52–53) notes the geological character of this imagery, such that one can speak of major changes as the shifting of tectonic plates. He identifies six "layers," all of which color the present to varying degrees. These are, from earliest to latest, the Indus Valley layer (c. 3000–1500 BCE), the Indo-Brāhmaṇical layer (c. 1500–600 BCE), the Indo-Śramaṇical layer (c. 600 BCE–300 CE), the Indic (Hindu-Buddhist-Jain) layer (c. 300–1200), the Indo-Islamic layer (c. 1200–1757), and finally the Indo-Anglian layer (c. 1757–present).

Indians experienced British rule as increasingly oppressive in the late nineteenth and early twentieth centuries, responding with intensified agitation for independence. The accompanying growth of national identity was thereby increasingly associated, for many, with being Hindu, and this identification was to play a major role in the story of how India's eventual political independence (officially assumed in August 1947) would unfold. This complex story, as well as that of post-independence India (with the concomitant creation of the Islamic State of Pakistan), is marked by pronounced efforts to articulate a generic Hindu identity that might subsume and include the widely diverse ethnic, caste, and other groups more or less considered as Hindu—groups that nonetheless would invariably privilege more immediate markers of identity among themselves (Larson 1995, pp. 176–177). Such a generic identity would necessarily look back to and emphasize the importance of earlier "layers" of India's past, back to the Indo-Brahmanical layer and even, occasionally, to the prior Indus Valley layer. And this renewal of tradition involved a considerable blending of these layers, such that what was described in ancient texts (but only those considered authentic) were by no means outmoded; rather they were seen to express eternal truths of right living, cosmic order, and divine law—*sanatana-dharma*. But, much as reinterpretation of earlier texts is evident within later texts, so present-day efforts to reinterpret the early texts have at times yielded creative strategies that have partaken, perhaps unwittingly, of Western historical-critical methods of analysis.

Cows served as a vital, unifying symbol to fuse Hindu identity with Indian nationhood. With the deep and enduring associations of cows with sanctity, piety, and selfless motherly giving, their lifelong protection from harm would come to be seen as essential. In particular, the cow was thought to embody the unchanging truth of *sanatana-dharma*. And quite the opposite of cows as embodiments of dharma were the overbearing, beef-eating, British Raj administrators, seen as veritable embodiments of *adharma*. Implicated as well in notions of adharma were non-Hindu Indians—especially Muslims, for whom the slaughter of cows for meat and leather seemed to hold no taboos.

Again, of great importance in modern Indian cow semiotics has been the symbol of cow-as-mother, woven closely together with the image of the

Indian nation-as-mother.[56] We have noted (in the previous chapter) the association of the female cow with the earth in the Bhagavata Purana's allegory of Kali's torturing the earth-cow. Increasingly in the modern period, "earth" would become reconceived as a geographically defined area of earth, Bharata Bhumi—the land of Bharata (India), the Indian nation. And as the Indian independence movement gained momentum, continuing after independence to the present day, it would not be difficult to sustain in the public mind a connection between "mother cow" and "Bharat Mata" (Mother India).[57]

Yet also to be noted, in the logic of Indian feminine symbolism and Hindu nationalist iconography, popular counterparts to mother cow imagery have been those of the dark goddess Kali and the fierce tiger-riding Durga.[58] As mother cow has embodied India's sheltering and nurturing nature, the centuries-long tradition of Shaktism—reverence for a feminine divinity as ultimate—became an important resource for articulating a wrathful and destructive feminine counterpart to the submissive and easily victimized cow. Indeed, Durga, in her divine wrath, would fuel the impulse of some Hindus to show "strong retaliation" for the killing of cows, even showing readiness to kill human beings for the sake of protecting cows (van der Veer 1994, p. 89).[59]

---

[56]As Mukul notes (2017, p. 290) and Peter van der Veer (1994, pp. 86–88) identifies four levels of cow symbolism: (1) related to brahmanical ritual, wherein the cow symbolizes earth, nourishment, wealth and good fortune (*lakshmi*), as well as the vehicle for crossing beyond death and yielder of substances essential for devotional worship; related to this last; (2) the cow's substances—milk, dung, and urine—carry sacredness for their benefits to humans (more on this in Chapter 4); (3) the association of cow with Krishna links her to the tradition of devotional (bhakti) culture; and (4) cow as mother associates her with family and community.

[57]Even well after independence was gained, the 1957 Hindi film *Bharat Mata* (Mother India) became one of the highest-grossing films of Indian cinema history (D. Smith 2003, p. 108). Although no explicit connection is made in this film between its heroine Radha (implicitly the instantiation of "mother" connected to India) and the cow, when she shoulders the plow of the family farm following the death of the family's buffalo, one can easily make this identification.

[58]Ironically, most Durga iconography shows her killing the buffalo demon Mahisha with her spear. Domestic water buffalo, widely found throughout South Asia, though providing richer milk than cows and providing traction for plowing and transport, by no means enjoy the same degree of regard as the cow in religious terms.

[59]Peter van der Veer refers to the first agitation against cow slaughter during British rule in India as having taken place in Punjab in 1871, following British victory over the Sikhs. A Sikh reform group, the Namdharis, killed Muslim butchers in Amritsar and Ludhiana. Although the immediate victims were Muslims, van der Veer notes (p. 91), "It is important to note that from the start cow

In modern times, all these cow-related considerations have been within a context of consuming public attention in which a pivotal factor has been the Indian state. From the late nineteenth century through independence and into the present day, appeals have been continuously made for legislation on various levels of government to ban bovine slaughter, to tighten ban enforcement, or to impose greater punishment on offenders. Since the Indian Constitution was ratified in 1949, all Indian provincial governments except Kerala, West Bengal, and the northeastern provinces have enacted laws restricting or prohibiting bovine slaughter in varying ways and degrees. More recently, attempts to institute a national ban have been made and then defeated by appeal to minority rights and secularism. Yet all such measures and appeals are grounded in a certain mindset that is, as Donald Davis observes, a "hopelessly exceptional" notion of law as legislation in the form of codes (Davis 2007, p. 243). As Kelsy Nagy aptly observes (Nagy 2019, p. 254),

> To someone outside the dairy, leather, or meat industries, the perception of the cow as a sacred symbol combined with the existence of anti-slaughter laws may contribute to the illusion that cattle are cared for and protected, which may contribute to the prevalence of cattle welfare problems remaining hidden in plain sight.

I have several times mentioned the Hindu notion of dharma, and we have seen that it is often with an appeal to dharma that Hindus argue for cow care and protection. Since one important meaning of dharma is "law," what may be called for is a careful examination and cautious, nuanced application of the traditional, arguably non-sectarian, notion—or notions—of dharma to present conditions.

But let us recall that, in considering the Hindu imaginaire of bovinity as a whole (in Chapter 2), a major impulse for its composition and endurance is to be found in the bhakti dimension, or bhakti paradigm, of Hindu religious thought and practice. Further, we noticed a polarity of values constituted of dharma at one end and bhakti on the other—what we termed a "values polarity." Thinking of dharma as law in a broader sense

---

protection challenged the legitimacy of British rule, although the immediate violence was directed at Muslims who killed cows. Cow protection was clearly a sign of the moral quality of the state."

than in modern usage as "legislation," it may be useful to consider insights from the bhakti tradition, as the complementary *counterpart* to dharma in the Hindu calculus of cultural meaning. Thus, the important bhakti texts show deep concern with dharma; at the same time, the sense of rigidity often associated with dharmic injunctions is mitigated by the fluidity of emotion and the sense of humble care that bhakti celebrates. In bhakti texts, "*dharma* as law serves this baseline function" of "giving meaning and connection to broader religious and theological patterns" (Davis 2007, pp. 248–251). Bhakti is seen as the full blossoming of dharma's purpose and meaning.

With this connection in mind, we may again recall the episode in the seminal bhakti text, the Bhagavata Purana, discussed in Chapter 2: While inspecting his kingdom, King Parikshit confronts the personified current age, appearing as a *shudra* disguised as a king (BhP 1.16–17). Despite Kali's deplorable crime against the earth embodied as a cow, Parikshit restrains himself from slaying the offender. Instead, he assigns for him restricted places of residence, namely, where specific types of degraded and degrading activities are practiced. The message would seem to be that ignorance and degradation have their rightful place in this world, even—or especially— in the present degraded age. They have a place, but it should be a limited, circumscribed place, one that is set by a widely understood grasp of law as dharma which is, in turn, tempered with bhakti. How such a place should be circumscribed is by the firm but wise actions of truly qualified rulers, whose grasp of dharma is such that they exhibit the highest caliber of virtue that rulership demands—virtues understood to show forth as a result of rulers' humble spirit of dedicated devotion (bhakti) for a supreme divinity. Krishna summarizes this point in the Bhagavad Gita: "Whatever the greatest one does, common people do just the same, following the standard he sets" (Bg 3.21).

Aside from political mobilization for cow protection in India, there is, like nowhere else in the world, a widespread practice of cow care and protection, or sheltering, in a wide variety of settings, including but not limited to institutional *goshalas* and similar establishments. Not only Hindus, but also Sikhs and Jains are involved in these projects, as are various non-religious animal activist organizations (Nagy 2019, pp. 254–257). One often hears the expression *go-seva* (Sanskrit/Hindi: *go-sevā*)—care or service for cows—and one may be reminded of the bhakti principle of *seva* to a divinity. The many persons in India who dedicate themselves to *go-seva* may be regarded by Hindus as such exalted persons as Krishna mentions in the Gita, and by their practices one can get a sense of just how bhakti, rooted in dharma, is understood as a way of practically caring, day by day, for cows. In the next chapter, we will meet some of these people and their cows, to understand something about the ethos and the practicalities—and the practical challenges—of cow care. Yet we must also face the harsh reality of wretched conditions for the vast mass of bovines in India today. We must wonder and bemoan the gaping disconnect between the culture of cow reverence on one side and the reality on the ground: India is the world's top dairy producer, and since modern dairy production is an extension of the bovine meat industry, India is also one of the top producers of meat and leather in the world. How these two realities collide yet persist in India will concern us in the next chapter.

References

Adluri, Vishwa. 2017. Ethics and Hermenuetics in the *Mahābhārata*. *International Journal of Hindu Studies* 20: 385–392. https://doi.org/10.1007/s11407-016-9200-y.

Adluri, Vishwa. 2018. *Ahiṁsā* in the Mahābhārata: Sacrifice, Violence, and Salvation. *Journal of Vaishnava Studies* 26 (2, Spring): 45–75.

Alsdorf, Ludwig. [1962] 2010. *The History of Vegetarianism and Cow-Veneration in India.* Translated from the German by Bal Patil, edited with additional notes, a bibliography and four appendices by Willem Bollée. London: Routledge.

Ambedkar, B.R., Dr. 1948. *The Untouchables: Who Were They and Why They Became Untouchables?* New Delhi: Amrit Book Company.

Beal, Samuel. [1884] 1983. *Buddhist Records of the Western World.* New Delhi: Motilal Banarsidass.

Brodbeck, Simon Pearce. 2009. *The Mahabharata Patriline: Gender, and the Royal Hereditary.* London: Routledge.

Bryant, Edwin. 2006. Strategies of Vedic Subversion: The Emergence of Vegetarianism in Post-Vedic India. In *A Communion of Subjects: Animals in Religion,*

Science, and Ethics, ed. Paul Waldau and Kimberley Patton, 194–203. New York: Columbia University Press.

Burgat, Florence. 2004. Non-Violence Toward Animals in the Thinking of Gandhi: The Problem of Animal Husbandry. *Journal of Agricultural and Environmental Ethics* 14.

Burley, Mikel. 2019. 'Mountains of Flesh and Seas of Blood': Reflecting Philosophically on Animal Sacrifice Through Dramatic Fiction. *Journal of the American Academy of Religion* 85 (3, September): 806–832.

Calasso, Roberto. 2015. *Ardor*. London: Penguin Random House.

Chigateri, Shraddha. 2008. 'Glory to the Cow': Cultural Difference and Social Justice in the Food Hierarchy in India. *South Asia: Journal of South Asian Studies* 31 (1): 10–35. https://doi.org/10.1080/00856400701874692.

Clough, Bradley S. 2002. Gandhi, Nonviolence and the *Bhagavad-gītā*. In *Holy War: Violence and the Bhagavad Gita*, ed. Steven Rosen. Hampton, VA: A. Deepak Publishing.

Copland, Ian. 2005. *State, Community and Neighbourhood in Princely North India c. 1900–1950*. New York: Palgrave Macmillan.

Copland, Ian. 2017. Cows, Congress and the Constitution: Jawaharlal Nehru and the Making of Article 48. *South Asia: Journal of South Asian Studies*. https://doi.org/10.1080/00856401.2017.1352646.

Davis, Donald R., Jr. 2007. Hinduism as a Legal Tradition. *Journal of the American Academy of Religion* 75 (2, June): 242–267.

Denny, Christopher. 2013. Christians and Vedic Sacrifice: Comparing Communitarian Sacrificial Soteriologies. *Journal of Hindu-Christian Studies* 26 (Article 8). https://doi.org/10.7825/2164-6279.1547.

Falk, Nancy Auer. 2006. *Living Hinduisms: An Explorer's Guide*. Belmont, CA: Thomson Wadsworth.

Feller-Jatavallabhula, Danielle. 1999. Raṇayajña: The Mahābhārata War as a Sacrifice. In *Violence Denied: Violence, Non-Violence and the Rationalization of Violence in South Asian Cultural History*, ed. Jan E.M. Houben and Karel R. van Kooij, 69–103. Leiden–Boston–Köln: Brill (Brill's Indological Library 16).

Fox, Richard G. 1992. East of Said. In *Edward Said: A Critical Reader*, ed. Michael Sprinker, 144–156. Oxford: Basil Blackwell.

Freitag, Sandria B. 1980. Religious Rites and Riots: From Community Identity to Communalism in North India. Ph.D. dissertation, University of California, Berkeley. ProQuest Dissertations and Theses Global.

Gandhi, Mohandas K. [1909, 1938] 2003. *Hind Swaraj or Indian Home Rule*. Translation of "Hind Swaraj," Published in the Gujarat columns of Indian

Opinion, 11 and 18 December 1909. Ahmedabad: Navajivan Publishing House.

Gandhi, Mohandas K. 1999. *The Collected Works of Mahatma Gandhi* (CWMG) (Electronic Book). New Delhi: Publications Division Government of India.

Griffiths, Ralph T.H. 1895. *The Hymns of the Atharva Veda*, vol. 1. London: Lazarus.

Groves, Matthew. 2010. Law, Religion and Public Order in Colonial India: Contextualizing the 1887 Allahabad High Court Case on 'Sacred' Cows. *South Asia: Journal of South Asian Studies* 33 (1): 78–121. https://doi.org/10.1080/00856401003592495.

Gutiérrez, Andrea. 2018. Embodiment of *Dharma* in Animals. In *Hindu Law: A New History of Dharmaśāstra*, ed. Patrick Olivelle and Donald R. Davis, Jr., 466–479. Oxford: Oxford University Press.

Haberman, David L. 2013. *People Trees: Worship of Trees in Northern India*. New York: Oxford University Press.

Hiltebeitel, Alf. 2016. *Nonviolence in the Mahābhārata: Śiva's summa on Ṛṣidharma and the gleaners of Kurukṣetra*. London: Routledge.

Houben, Jan E.M. 1999. To Kill or Not to Kill the Sacrificial Animal (*yajña-paśu*)? In *Violence Denied: Violence, Non-Violence and the Rationalization of Violence in South Asian Cultural History*, ed. Jan E.M. Houben and Karel R. van Kooij, 105–183. Leiden–Boston–Köln: Brill (Brill's Indological Library 16).

Inden, Ronald. 1998. Ritual, Authority, and Cycle Time in Hindu Kingship. In *Kingship and Authority in South Asia*, ed. J.F. Richards, 41–91. New Delhi: Oxford University Press.

Jha, D.N. [2001] 2009. *The Myth of the Holy Cow*. New Delhi: Navayana.

King, Richard. 1999. *Orientalism and Religion: Post-Colonial Theory, India and the "Mystic East"*. London: Routledge.

Knipe, David M. 2015. *Vedic Voices: Intimate Narratives of a Living Andhra Tradition*. New York: Oxford University Press.

Lahariya, Khabar. 2018. Cattle-Skinners in Bandelkhand Are Looking for an Out. *The Wire*, April 18. https://thewire.in/caste/cattle-skinners-in-bundelkhand-are-looking-for-an-out. Accessed 13 November 2018.

Larson, Gerald James. 1995. *India's Agony over Religion*. Albany, NY: SUNY.

Leslie, Julia. 2003. *Authority and Meaning in Indian Religions: Hinduism and the Case of Vālmīki*. Aldershot, UK: Ashgate.

Lodha, G.M. (ed.). 2002. *Report of the National Commission on Cattle* (Chapter 1 Introduction). New Delhi: Department of Animal Husbandry, Ministry of

Agriculture and Farmers' Welfare, Government of India. http://dahd.nic.in/related-links/chapter-i-introduction. Accessed 25 September 2017.

McClymond, Kathryn. 2008. *Beyond Sacred Violence: A Comparative Study of Sacrifice*. Baltimore: Johns Hopkins University Press.

Mitra, Rajendralala. 1881. *Indo-Aryans: Contributions Towards the Elucidation of Their Ancient and Medieval History*, vol. 1. Calcutta: W. Newman & Co.

Monier-Williams, Monier. [1899] 1995. *A Sanskrit-English Dictionary*. New Delhi: Motilal Banarsidass.

Mukul, Akshaya. 2017. *Gita Press and the Making of Hindu India*. Noida: Harper-Collins.

N/A. [1971] 1983. *Review of 'Beef in Ancient India'*. Mathura, UP, India: Shri Krishna Janmasthan Seva-Sansthan.

Nagy, Kelsi. 2019. The Sacred and Mundane Cow: The History of India's Cattle Protection Movement. In *The Routledge Handbook of Religion and Animal Ethics*, ed. Andrew Linzey and Clair Linzey. London: Routledge.

Narayanan, Yamini. 2018. Cow Protection as 'Casteised Speciesism': Sacralisation, Commercialisation and Politicisation. *South Asia: Journal of South Asian Studies*. https://doi.org/10.1080/00856401.2018.1419794.

Olivelle, Patrick. 2005. *Manu's Code of Law: A Critical Edition and Translation of the Mānava-Dharmaśāstra*. New York: Oxford University Press.

Prabhupāda, A.C. Bhaktivedanta Swami. 2017. *The Complete Teachings of His Divine Grace A. C. Bhaktivedanta Swami Prabhupāda*. Vedabase CD-ROM Version 2017.2. Sandy Ridge, NC: Bhaktivedanta Archives.

Prabhupāda, A.C. Bhaktivedanta Swami. [1972] 1983. *Bhagavad-gītā as It Is*. Los Angeles: Bhaktivedanta Book Trust.

Ram-Prasad, C. 2003. Contemporary Political Hinduism. In *The Blackwell Companion to Hinduism*, ed. Gavin Flood, 526–550. Oxford: Blackwell.

Rocher, Ludo. 2003. The Dharmaśāstras. In *The Blackwell Companion to Hinduism*, ed. Gavin Flood, 102–115. Oxford: Blackwell.

Rogerson, J.W. 1998. What was the Meaning of Animal Sacrifice? In *Animals on the Agenda: Questions about Animals for Theology and Ethics*, ed. A. Linzey and D. Yamamoto. Urbana and Chicago: University of Illinois Press.

Rosen, Steven J. 2004. *Holy Cow: The Hare Krishna Contribution to Vegetarianism and Animal Rights*. New York: Lantern Books.

Safi, Michael. 2016. On Patrol with the Hindu Vigilantes Who Would Kill to Protect India's Cows. *The Guardian*, Thursday, October 27. https://www.theguardian.com/world/2016/oct/27/on-patrol-hindu-vigilantes-smuggling-protect-india-cows-kill. Accessed 13 August 2017.

Saraswati, Maharshi Dayanand. 1993, original Hindi 1881. *Gokaruṇānidhi* (In Defence of the Cow: With all Compassion). Translated by Khazan Singh. Ajmer: Paropkarini Sabha—Dayanand Ashram.

Schwab, Julius. [1886] n.d. *Das altindische Thieropfer, mit Benützung handschriftlicher Quellen.* Zürich: Zentralbibliothek Zürich. www.books2ebooks. eu.

Smith, Brian K. [1989] 1998. *Reflections on Resemblance, Ritual and Religion.* New Delhi: Motilal Banarsidass.

Smith, David. 2003. *Hinduism and Modernity.* Oxford: Blackwell.

Stewart, James. 2014. Violence and Nonviolence in Buddhist Animal Ethics. *Journal of Buddhist Ethics* 21. http://blogs.dickenson.edu/buddhistethics/.

Sutton, Nicholas. 2000. *Religious Doctrines in the Mahābhārata.* New Delhi: Motilal Banarsidass.

Thompson, Mark. 1993. *Gandhi and His Ashrams.* Mumbai: Popular Prakashan.

Valpey, Kenneth. 2004. Krishna in *Mleccha Desh:* ISKCON Temple Worship in Historical Perspective. In *The Hare Krishna Movement: The Postcharismatic Fate of a Religious Transplant.* New York: Columbia University Press.

Valpey, Kenneth. Forthcoming. In the Service of All that Lives: Gandhi's Vision of Engaged Nonviolent Animal Care. In *Animal Theologians,* ed. Andrew Linzey.

Valpey, Kenneth Russell. 2006. *Attending Kṛṣṇa's Image: Caitanya Vaiṣṇava mūrtisevā as devotional truth.* London: Routledge.

van der Veer, Peter. 1994. *Religious Nationalism: Hindus and Muslims in India.* Berkeley: University of California Press.

Wedemeyer, Christian K. 2007. Beef, Dog, and other Mythologies: Connotative Semiotics in Mahāyoga Tantra Ritual and Scripture. *Journal of the American Academy of Religion* 75 (2, June): 383–417.

4

Surveying the Cow Care Field

In this chapter, I look at current cow care practices in India. By "cow care" I mean, minimally, intentional arrangements for bovines to be protected for the duration of their natural lives. My primary aim is to provide an overview of issues that concern persons—in particular persons who identify more or less as Hindus—who are directly or indirectly engaged with cow care. Of course, the issues are centrally about the protection and well-being of the cows these persons are involved in caring for. Specifically, we want to consider what are the essential components of Hindu cow care. What makes this practice different, or similar, to any practice of cattle husbandry such as agribusiness dairy farming or ranching? What are the special challenges and constraints of Hindu cow care, and what are its rewards? Pursuing these questions, we will look at some specific cow care projects in India, and we will listen to some of the persons involved in these. It would be presumptuous to claim these vignettes to be fully representative of thought and practices in the wide scope of present-day Hindu cow care. Still, they show an important cross-section of mainly Vaishnava Hindu practice, especially in northern and western India.

© The Author(s) 2020
K. R. Valpey, *Cow Care in Hindu Animal Ethics,*
The Palgrave Macmillan Animal Ethics Series,
https://doi.org/10.1007/978-3-030-28408-4_4

The story this chapter tells is one of largely provisional measures to care for a relatively infinitesimal number of bovines in comparison with the number of those that become victim to the massive Indian dairy industry and therefore the meat and leather industries. It is a story of attempts, however small, to address India's increasingly festering condition of burgeoning cities and of human alienation from nature, a major symptom of which is seen in the pervasiveness of stray cows. This is the visible side of a dark reality—of dairy, meat, leather, and related industries' largely invisible operations that are legal, quasi-legal, or illegal but tolerated.

In contexts of cow care practices, what we will see are conscientious and sometimes self-conscious efforts to bring ideals to bear within the persistent realities of economic and related uncertainties. The broader reality, however, is a general public apathetic neglect of cows fueled by changing human diets attenuating a residual reverence for cows—a reverence that from time to time becomes sharply ignited in the political sphere.

One is inclined to point, above all, to ahimsa—nonviolence, as the most essential, emblematic ideal, from which other ideals of cow care follow. No doubt ahimsa is a central principle for cow care ethics and practice. And it is this ideal that brings the greatest challenge, for as understood by my informants, the irreducible requirement called for in *go-seva* and *go-raksha* (cow care and cow protection) is seeing to it that cows and bulls are maintained for their entire natural lives, whatever may be their "utility" or apparent liability. To what extent and how the attempt to uphold this ideal for cows—especially *deshi* (Indian indigenous) cows—may involve indirect or unintended violence in other spheres, or indeed, whether and to what extent the cow care practices described here can be regarded as truly nonviolent, will be questions to be kept in mind here and to be addressed more explicitly in Chapter 5. Here our main concern is with what are currently some practical means used in pursuit of the ahimsa ideal as lifelong cow care, and what further cultural resources—whether explicitly Hindu or otherwise (including modern organizational and technical resources)—are drawn upon to make contemporary cow care sustainably functionable and expandable.

Cows (Un)Sheltered

In 1970, the National Dairy Development Board of India launched a major project to increase dairy production, known as Operation Flood. The project involved initial financing from Europe to create Indian national milk processing facilities and transport infrastructure. The core principle of the project was empowerment of individual small farmers and dairy keepers, connecting them to large production and distribution facilities through a network of dairy cooperatives. Operation Flood (also known as the "White Revolution") proved to be an impressive success, such that before the year 2000 India's annual dairy production equaled or surpassed that of the United States (Scholten 2010, p. 1). Providing 18 million people (70% women) with employment, dairy became a major source of income for more than 27 million people (World Animal Protection 2014).[1]

What has been good for the Indian dairy industry and the Indian economy in general has not been good for either the dairy cows or their offspring. As with any Western dairy operation, aside from the several types of abuse imposed on cows to increase their milk yield—among them artificial insemination (especially in crossbreeding with Western cow breeds), hormonal manipulation, excessive confinement, and removal of calves from their mothers—is the shortened lifespan and destiny for slaughter of both male and female bovines.

For dairy farmers (who are Hindus in most areas), economic pressures to maintain their business give them generally three options what to do with a cow that no longer brings income. She can be set loose, leaving her to wander freely and forage as best she can; give her to a *goshala* or *pinjrapole* (a cow shelter or a Jain animal shelter) possibly paying for her care; or sell her to a dealer, who supplies cattle to slaughterhouses (Nagy 2019, p. 254;

---

[1]The award-winning 1976 Hindi film *Manthan* (The Churning; directed by Shyam Benegal, who wrote the story together with Verghese Kurien, Operation Flood's mastermind) portrays the beginnings of Operation Flood in Gujarat, focusing on village-level politics and the cultural inertia resisting state-sponsored cooperative dairy development. While representing well the struggle of Indian small dairy farmers (indeed, the film was, perhaps uniquely, funded by the 2-rupee contributions of 500,000 dairy farmers of Gujarat), no attention is given to the cooperative development's implications for the cows providing the milk.

Kennedy et al. 2018).[2] In the early years after Indian Independence, prior
to the launch of Operation Flood, the Indian Government set up cattle
sanctuaries called *gosadans*, where "old, infirm, or otherwise useless" cows
would be cared for. However, these proved to be financially unviable, and
the scheme was abandoned (Nagy 2019, p. 254).[3]

Conscientious Hindu farmers, not wanting to be instrumental in cow
slaughter, may be inclined to set loose their unprofitable cows, a practice
that follows a tradition called *anna-pratha*, literally "food practice" (Jha
2017). Presumably, this was based on earlier existence of extensive public
grazing lands, separated from farmlands.[4] But today, such grazing lands
have shrunk radically or are non-existent; instead, many cows seek their
fortune in the city, where they are more likely to meet with dire misfortune.

Some activists, such as Devi Chitralekha, work intensely to promote
awareness of this increasing problem. Devi Chitralekha is a young, popular
Bhagavata *kathakar* (public reciter of the Bhagavata Purana) in the Delhi
area. During one recitation to a sizeable crowd (plus a television audience),
while speaking of Krishna's cowherd activities as described in the Bhagavata
text, Devi paused her narration to deliver an impassioned admonishment
to her listeners. Knowing that many—perhaps most—of her listeners have
lapsed from the strict vegetarian dietary standard that would be expected

[2]Kennedy et al. suggest that farmers' fear of backlash from activists is as much a motivation for
not slaughtering or selling for slaughter as is farmers' veneration for cows. See also Baviskar (2016,
pp. 395–407) on dairies in Delhi and the complexities of conflicting interests with "bourgeois
environmentalists" to remove Delhi's 35,000 wandering dairy cows—and hence the dairies—from
the city's streets).

[3]Nagy (2019, p. 254), citing F. Simoons (1980), writes, "One study reported that it cost up to three
times more per animal at a *gosadan* than it cost per person for education. The failed state-sponsored
gosadan scheme influenced the Supreme Court to favor cow protection laws that 'allowed for the
slaughter of useless cattle and allowed for the protection of useful ones'." The economically viable
gosadan practice hinged on the hope that collected dung for fertilizer and leather from naturally
dying cattle would cover their maintenance costs. Whether the experiment was bound to fail or
whether mismanagement was involved may not be known.

[4]In his tract *Gaukaruṇānidhi* (referred to in the previous chapter), Swami Dayananda Saraswati
notes that in earlier, pre-Muslim times, kings would keep half of their land for animal grazing.
The current amount of grazing land in India is estimated to be 4% (Chakravarti 1985, p. 33). See
also Roy (2017, p. 167). Gadgil and Guha (1995, pp. 91–93) discuss a specific instance of the
grazing land issue with respect to ongoing conflicts between the "omnivores" (modern, non-tribal
Indians) and "ecosystem people" (tribals), whereby denial of cattle grazing land by the former (state
sanctioned) in the National Park at Bharatpur (Rajasthan) has had devastating results to the local
ecology.

for many Hindu castes, she urged them not to succumb to the social pressures of modern city life.[5] Connecting dietary choice with the fact that India currently has thousands of slaughterhouses (some legal and five times as many illegal),[6] she then appealed to them to consider the plight of the cows that are still alive but are seen wandering the streets in her listeners' neighborhoods.[7] She exhorted her audience:

> Please hear me out … Whatever garbage you collect in your homes and then throw in the bin, please don't wrap anything edible … in any kind of plastic or polyethylene and throw it away … Cows are attracted by the smell of food and consume the whole polyethylene together with the food and the garbage. And plastic in the stomach is such a frightening illness for the cows, which cannot be treated by any medicine but can only be removed by operation.[8]

A homeless cow that has become particularly bloated as a result of ingesting plastic may be noticed by a local resident who might—if conscientious

---

[5] See Biswas (2018), "The myth of the Indian vegetarian nation." For detailed discussions of Indian food semiotics, see several articles in Khare (1992).

[6] Maneka Gandhi insists that *all* slaughterhouses in India are illegal, because the so-called legal slaughterhouses slaughter many more times the number of animals they are officially permitted to slaughter (personal communication, 5 February 2019).

[7] Kelsi Nagy, who researched urban cattle practices in Mysore from 2015, writing to me (23 May 2018), notes that many urban cows have owners who let them out to wander in the morning and to whom they return, of themselves, in the evening. "In Mysore, almost all of the street cattle will be owned by an urban dairy farmer and a handful were kept as pets. Most farmers I spoke to told me that when their cows reached the end of their production cycle that they were either taken to a cattle fair where they were sold to a middleman (with the unspoken understanding that the middleman then sold them to the butcher) or they 'gave' or sold them to 'the Muslims' which also meant they would be butchered. A handful told me they gave their cattle to the Gaushala [goshala], although the director of Mysore's largest Gaushala told me this almost never happened and nearly all of the cattle they had in their Gaushala had been brought by the police that intercepted a truck taking cattle to Kerala for slaughter or were male calves that had been abandoned, often without even receiving their mother's first milk and these calves nearly always died. In Mysore urban dairy cattle were kept in a shed or tied up at night to protect from theft. I was told Muslims were stealing cattle at night and would also take strays."

[8] https://www.youtube.com/watch?v=nRdzQhoDmWQ (Translation from Hindi, accessed 21 May 2018).

and knowing of a nearby cow shelter (goshala)—phone the goshala and have the cow taken there for treatment.[9]

One shelter that accepts and treats such cows is Kamdhenu Dham Gaushala in Carterpuri, on the outskirts of Gurugram (Gurgaon), a one-million population satellite of Delhi. This goshala's manager, retired Brigadier S. S. Chohan, confirms Devi Chitralekha's account, adding that, along with forty to fifty kilograms of plastic,

> Every cow in Gurgaon has eaten … dirty material like nails, glass, detergent powder packets, blades, clips, even baby shoes. So, whatever we throw in the garbage in bags, she swallows it. She cannot open it, so she swallows it. And it is non-biodegradable. It ends up poisoning her and she dies.[10]

Kamdhenu Dham Gaushala has three veterinary doctors who live at the facility, taking in and treating cows that may be brought by the shelter's cow ambulance any time of day or night. A cow seen to have such foreign matter in her gut will be operated, after which, if all goes well, she can, in this particular goshala, expect to live out her life well attended by a trained and dedicated staff.

Chohan explains that the shelter's 3000 cows and bulls receive a more generous and richer diet than cows in most goshalas are likely to receive. Following the advice of a nutritionist, here the cows receive three meals per day, including some 15–20 kilograms of green fodder (per cow), 3–4 kilograms of a seven-grains mixture, 50 grams of rock salt (to increase the appetite), 30 grams of mineral mixture, and during the winter, 100–150 grams of jaggery (non-centrifugal cane sugar). Chohan's reasoning for giving such a good—and expensive[11]—diet to the cows is twofold. One is his concern that his goshala keeps its status as a model goshala for India, and second,

---

[9]Doron and Jeffrey (2018, pp. 43–44) note that plastic came to India in the 1970s, and the combination of a burgeoning middle-class and a population density of 445 persons per square kilometer, refuse processing, has become a major issue. This, despite a vast difference in the amount of waste produced by, for example, Americans, who create 150 times more waste than the average Indian.

[10]Interview with Brig. S. S. Chohan, 13 February 2018. See Doron and Jeffrey (2018, Chapter 2) on the waste problem in present-day India, a direct consequence of exploding economic growth.

[11]The current average cost of maintaining one cow at Kamdhenu Dham Gaushala is 80 rupees per day, or 2400 rupees (ca. $35) per month.

Because these are not ordinary cows. They have endured cruelties every day. Some of them, a loaded truck passes over them in the night, so you can imagine, their backbone and all their bones are crushed. They are disoriented … traumatized; and they cannot even stand, they are so weak [when they first arrive at the goshala].

Having been traumatized, rescued cows loathe to be approached by humans. Chohan explains that when newly arrived cows are brought to the goshala facility, he wants to approach them. However,

They seem to tell me, "Don't come near us!" I get this message from them: "You humans have tortured us, you are our greatest enemy; because of you we are on the roads; as long as we give milk, we are treated as 'divine mothers'—*go-mata*—and after we stop giving milk, you send us there—garbage dumps—for dying!?"

Thus, Chohan shows a sense of being able to hear these cows,[12] and the cows are, with his help, given voice, with which they express their sense of betrayal by humans. People's reverence for cows as "divine mothers" is, he suggests, a "conditional divinity" dependent on the flow of milk. Once a cow has passed her milk-giving age, the reverence may linger but the care will fade and then drop away.

As noted, Brigadier Chohan strives to maintain high standards of care in his goshala, which has been officially recognized as a model goshala by the Animal Welfare Board of India.[13] After describing the plight of the

---

[12]Chohan remarked, "First you must understand the cows' language, then they will understand your language."

[13]Chohan has produced a standard operating procedures document for goshalas, consisting of forty points. These include specifications of space required for the cow shed (120 × 40 feet, for 150 cows), size and height of feeding mangers, the need for proper ventilation and availability of sunlight, fans and heaters ("The cattle should feel comfortable and at ease at all times during all seasons in the cow sheds"), and space outside the shed for roaming, basking, and ruminating; a properly equipped hospital ("the nerve center of the goshala") with qualified, dedicated, resident veterinary staff, who perform regular vaccination and deworming as well as necessary treatments for sick and injured cows, including surgery; exacting details on feed standards, importance of proper inspection and storage of fodder, and importance of clean drinking water; the importance of daily cleaning and anti-bacterial spraying ("the cows are very fond of cleanliness"); the necessity of daily record-keeping of all aspects of the goshala and the cows' treatment; and cow dung management. His final stipulation is, "The Gaushala should be a place where people can experience peace and happiness in a serene

rescued cows and the special attention he and his eighty assistants give them, Chohan reports that after three months of such care, "the cows are laughing, healthy." Now the cows become approachable and, we are told, positively responsive to the show of human affection.[14]

It is late afternoon, the regular time when the cows at Kamdhenu Dham Gaushala have just returned to the metal-roofed open stall from their roofless corrals. Several local people, including children, are circumambulating the cow pens in clockwise direction—a way considered to both honor cows and to receive general physical and mental well-being from cows' proximity. In the stalls, the cows, although not tied up, are nonetheless quite crowded together. Chohan worries, because the goshala's capacity has already been overreached, and there are still many roaming cows in the Gurugram area needing shelter.[15]

To ease the pressure of increasing numbers, in previous years this goshala experimented with selling rehabilitated cows to carefully selected recipients—farmers who had to first show qualification according to written standards.[16] Most importantly, cows were not to be either further sold, given away, or let loose, but were to be maintained throughout their natural lives. But, Chohan says with disappointment, he decided to stop this practice because, despite promises and signed affidavits, some of the farmers, after a time, would again abandon the cow or bull they had previously

---

environment created by clean and green surroundings with soft and soothing devotional music filling the air."

[14]In a later interview, Chohan commented, "If you love the cows with intensity, the cows will love you with twice the intensity!".

[15]There is a similar situation of overcrowding in government goshalas in Delhi. The Times of India (Gandhiok 2019, 16 January 2019) reported, "The Shree Krishna Gaushala, located in Sultanpur Dabas, Bawana, is Delhi's biggest [goshala] and spread over 36 acres. It can accommodate up to 7740 cows. On some occasions, however, the gaushala has taken over 8500 cows, at which point it stops admissions and accepts only critical cases like injured animals. Lack of funds, however, hampers their functioning." The report further notes that a promised 40 rupees per cow per day from the government and a matching fund has not been received by this goshala since over a year. Turnbull (2017, p. 32) quotes a pseudonymous animal activist 'Smita': "[F]or the sheer number of animals, the number of *Gaushalas* [in India]…is grossly inadequate…In most *Gaushalas* you find they are concentration camps. You will find that the cows cannot even stand."

[16]The recipients of bovines had to sign an affidavit affirming their intention to follow twelve conditions of their care, including details on daily maintenance and shelter conditions, provision of medical needs, assurance that they will never be sold or slaughtered, and that the recipient will contact the goshala in the case he finds himself unable to continue caring for a bovine received from it.

purchased, and the animals would end up on the street where they had been before arriving at the goshala the first time. Chohan comments:

> It was the same story again. I found the same cows there on the road again, and they were cursing me. [The cows] were saying, "You have rescued us, you have made us healthy, and how the hell have you sent us again on the road? It is a great injustice!" They were talking to me like that. Those cows recognized me, I recognized them. So, I got them back, and I stopped selling cows.[17]

The problem of overcrowding in the goshala was not solved by selling cows to farmers and now, it seemed, some cows had been twice betrayed.

Today, cows in India are, as living beings with high symbolic significance, caught amidst contradictory forces. On one side is the ideology of reverence and care, coinciding with, and intertwined with, the traditional notions of dharma and bhakti. These complementary paradigms (dharma and bhakti) are seen as the force for human balance and relationship with nature's rhythms and the felicitous functioning of human beings within a higher order. Cows in particular are seen as embodying this force, and as such, they become a collective symbol of goodness. At the same time, real, living, individual cows are large, domesticated creatures requiring much care and attention by humans if they are to live well. Like any other creatures, they are prone to disease and as large animals they can, in some situations and depending on breed and other factors, be dangerous to humans. As such living beings, bovines are today subjected to a powerful contrary force which can be called the juggernaut of modernity (Smith 2003, p. 23).[18] This force is set in motion by the economics

---

[17]In a later interview, Chohan explained that one reason farmers abandon cows received from his goshala is that the prohibitive cost of paying off police extortions—as much as RS 10,000 (ca. $150) while (legally) transporting the cows from the goshala to their farms proves too much for them to bear on top of maintaining the cows.

[18]Smith calls attention to the origin of the word *juggernaut* as being the massive wooden festival chariot of the Hindu temple image named "Jagannath" (Lord of the Universe) in Puri, India. He continues, "While the original Jagannath car carried images of the gods that people worshipped, the modernity that is capitalism as it proceeds along its trajectory befuddles us with fetishisms, with factitious, fabricated images. The temple car characteristic of the lumbering, unmaneuverable, dangerous quality of Hinduism is transferred to its opposite, modernity, which is fast, unmaneuverable, and no less dangerous."

of consumerism and corporate rationalism, a massive vehicle careening out of control into an unpredictable future, determining cows' lives and deaths almost solely on the basis of economics. And their value while alive is limited by goods they produce which, once no longer supplied, renders them valuable only in death, to be slaughtered for final consumption.

To be sure, some cows are not killed but, left to their own resources as strays, they may die from consuming human waste; or fortunate cows may be rescued and cared for in goshalas, but generally in overly confined spaces. And if they are very lucky, they may find a place in goshalas where they are properly fed and cared for.[19] Our next task in sketching present-day cow care in India will be to get an idea of the economics of cow care projects—projects dedicated to caring for bovines throughout their natural lives. Similar to the dairy industry, some, but not all, of these cow care projects put importance on the cows' production of milk. But unlike dairies, which typically sell for slaughter the aging cows whose milk yields are diminished, cow care projects cannot (and of course are not intended to) maintain themselves in this way.

The Economics of Reverence and Care

There are different sorts of goshalas—institutions for maintenance or rescue and care for bovines in India, typically at least implicitly having a basis in Hindu identity.[20] Generally, these may be categorized as either temple-affiliated goshalas or as charity-based, or *vania* goshalas (Nagy 2019, pp. 255–256). Temple-affiliated goshalas are maintained and funded through temple organizations, of which there are various kinds and

---

[19] Stray bovines brought to goshalas can, if the goshala is poorly funded and managed, leave them worse off than if left to wander. Such has happened recently in Vrindavan, according to the text accompanying this video https://www.youtube.com/watch?feature=youtu.be&v=gAstcNBe5Cg& fbclid=IwAR12LUKadQhJ0O2eiWso5beIRtEouPNsreJqCHBbIOsiNt29N_j5uX20UtY&app= desktop (accessed 7 March 2019).

[20] The 2002 Indian Government Report of the National Commission on Cattle estimated 3000 *goshalas*, maintaining over 600,000 cattle (Kennedy et al. 2018, p. 4). Whether this refers only to officially registered goshalas is not clear. Devi Chitralekha quotes an estimate of 12,000 goshalas, contrasting this number with triple the number of abattoirs in India. Brig. Chohan mentions 6000 goshalas across India.

degrees of complexity, from very small and simple temples and organizations to the grandest of temples, such as that of Venkateswara at Tirupati, Andhra Pradesh, in South India. For most temple goshalas, funding is received by the temple as donations that are given as devotional offerings to the temple image(s) or directly for cow care (*go-seva*).[21] Vaniya goshalas are typically organized and funded by business people, often as caste-specific groups.[22] In both cases, the main source of maintenance is essentially charity, although to varying degrees the goshalas may also offset some expenses by selling cow-based products, including milk, ghee, cow dung- and cow urine-based products, especially traditional (Ayurveda) medicines.

Having noted these two major types of goshalas (of which there are sub-varieties), there are other types as well, one represented by the Kamdhenu Dham Gaushala in Gurugram, previously mentioned. This is a public–private partnership of the municipal government of Gurugram and Vishnu Charitable Trust, an NGO which is responsible for daily management of the goshala. Kamdhenu Dham Gaushala maintains no dairy, concentrating entirely on rescue and rehabilitation, so it receives no income from dairy products. Currently, it receives in donations roughly one lakh (100,000) rupees, or US$1400, per month, which is around 40 rupees or half a dollar per day for each cow, covering about half the goshala's running costs. It also produces and sells dung-based compost. But, with the help of the central and state governments, there is a plan to install a biogas unit. From the twenty tons of dung produced daily, this could bring 35,000 rupees *daily* income. However, with no prospect for obtaining more land, this goshala's prospects for expansion, even with such increased income, are severely limited.[23]

Another sort of cow shelter could be called a *sadhu goshala*. Sadhus are Hindu renunciants or monks, and it is not uncommon for them to

---

[21] Shocking as it may be, Yamini Narayanan (2017) reports that there are temples that, having received a calf or cow from a donor in good faith that the temple goshala will care for it, will then sell it for slaughter.

[22] Lodrick (1981) discusses four types of goshalas: temple, court, vaniya, and Gandhian; he also discusses Jain *pinjrapoles* and *gosadans*.

[23] One year after my first interview with Brig. Chohan, he reported that the biogas installation remains "on paper" (and he clarified that the idea is for a central biogas processing plant that would serve several goshalas in the area).

attract a following and, with followers' support, to undertake various pious projects such as the establishment and maintenance of goshalas. One such sadhu is Swami Datta Sharanananda, a tall, handsome, itinerant Hindu monk (*sannyasi*) who travels widely in India to propagate his message of cow protection and care. The goshala complex he has founded is a striking example of this type, the massive Shree Godham Mahatirth Anandvan in the Pathmeda district of southwest Rajasthan. In a several-hundred-acre area, some 44,000 cows and bulls are sheltered, though at one time there were more than 100,000 bovines.[24] Most of these are rescued animals, of local breeds (Kankrej and Tharparkar) as well as mixed breeds. Resident cowherd families each care for some 100 bulls or oxen, or of about 40 cows. There are also varying numbers of volunteers.[25] Financial support for daily operations and facility expansion comes from a broadly distributed donor base and from the sale of cow products—especially medicines, cosmetics, and other items from bovine dung and urine. Unlike the Gurugram goshala, the Pathmeda goshala has no land area constraints, with additional government land available for grazing.

As we have seen in the previous example of a rescue and rehabilitation goshala (the Gurugram goshala), here at Pathmeda also, donors play an essential role in the goshala economy. Thus, as with most goshalas, at Pathmeda there is no claim to having a simple self-sufficient economy, although the aspiration is to come to the point of growing sufficient fodder for a year-around supply. Lack of self-sufficiency can be viewed in two ways. From one side, it may be seen as a weakness that such institutions are dependent on constant outside charitable support. On the other side, the receiving of charitable assistance may be seen as a positive function of the institution, namely as a means by which (generally urban-dwelling) persons otherwise disconnected from cows are able to feel some connection with them and therefore blessed by them.

---

[24]The Shri Pathmeda Godham began in 1993, initially with eight cows. It is reported that in 2002–2003, during a "disturbed time" (*bhīṣaṇa-kāl meṇ*) 182 temporary and permanent centers for cow care were established, with a total of some 280,000 bovines (Dattaśaraṇānand, Saṁvat 2073). The Pathmeda Trust has three main goshala centers under its direct control, and some 64 smaller goshalas in the area are assisted by the Trust.

[25]The institute identifies three types of workers: (1) unmarried male student volunteers (*brahmacaris*), (2) older volunteers (*vanaprasthis*), and (3) paid workers.

Since charity is central to much goshala economics, to get a comprehensive picture of goshala functioning it is important to think about donors. To this end, I introduce two brothers, Arvind and Prabhav—Mumbai industrialists who have become closely involved in support of the Pathmeda goshala project.

When they first heard about the Pathmeda goshala in 2011, Arvind and Prabhav's mother was inspired to "adopt" ten of the goshala's cows. (Cow adoption is a scheme that is used in some goshalas as a means to ensure steady charity income.)[26] Eventually, they visited Pathmeda. Arvind explains,

> At Pathmeda we found *tan-man-dhan* [Hindi, literally "body, mind, wealth," namely, the opportunity to give service with these three capacities] … We asked the Swami [Swami Datta Sharanananda, founder of the goshala] if there is something we can do, and he kindly appointed me as the caretaker for all injured cows. So, we built a hospital there … that takes care of one thousand cows per day, treated by allopathy, Ayurveda, homeopathy and *raga-chikitsa* (music therapy).

The two brothers have also initiated a small enterprise intended to bring income for the goshala and, at the same time, give cow products' customers a sense of direct connection to the cows. The products are ritual items made with cow dung. So, for example, they produce small cow dung images of Ganesh, a divinity that is widely worshiped by Hindus, especially in Maharashtra (the state in which Mumbai is situated). They have also begun producing bovine fuel briquettes for cremation. Arvind explains his concept for using these briquettes to raise substantial funds for cow protection:

> [I thought,] can I write in my will, stipulating that my last rites (of cremation) shall be performed with these bull dung logs? If one percent of Hindus

---

[26]Typically, a person or family adopting a cow will commit to providing sufficient funds for maintaining a particular cow for life. The donors are encouraged to visit "their" particular cow or cows at the goshala, and they are kept informed about their welfare. At some goshalas, if it includes a dairy, the donor may receive regular "gifts" of dairy products. Especially, if it is a goshala connected to a temple, the donor may receive sweets made from the goshala milk that has been consecrated in offerings to the temple divinity.

would commit to this, and 250 kilograms [of these logs] are needed to cre-
mate one human corpse, we can save fifteen lakh [1.5 million] bulls [with
the money paid for the fuel]. Gurus can tell their followers to have this
written in their last will and testament.[27]

Such ideas are conceived on the basis of producing value-added products
that are directly from the cows that are being cared for—substances that
are then moderately processed, without addition of chemicals. Customers
(donors) can be expected to pay relatively high prices for such items, being
confident that the profit is going toward the care of cows throughout their
natural lives.[28] Thus, to purchase these products is to be also a patron of
the cows, through the institution that sees to their care. Broadly speaking,
it may be said that the value added to such products is the ideal of ahimsa,
the dharmic, ethical value of nonviolence, regarded as the highest form
of dharma. Yet for many customers the added value includes an element
of bhakti, devotion, in the sense that they see themselves contributing to
go-seva, service to cows.

While reckoning anticipated gain from their new enterprise, Arvind
and Prabhav emphasize the moral imperative that all profit from such cow
dung products must go exclusively for the care of cows:

> We don't do business with our mother, so how can we do business with
> go-mata [mother cow]? So, we have to be clear that everything we do, we
> do for free. There are two principles—honest earnings and selflessness.[29]

---

[27] A similar idea has been taken up by students in Delhi (IIT Delhi Students 2018).

[28] These Ganesh images (*murtis*) are actually made from the dung of calves, which is especially viscous,
making it possible to form the images without any additives. Ganesh worship is especially popular
in Maharashtra, and particularly on Ganesh Chaturthi, in August or September, when thousands of
temporary images of the "elephant god" are made and then, after the festival, submerged in the sea
or in a river, with considerable polluting effect. Such pollution is avoided with the Pathmeda cow
dung images.

[29] As may be expected, not all goshalas in India function on such a high level of ethical practice.
Nor is it always clear where the ideals of cow care give way to profit motive. The Gurugram goshala
is recognized as a model goshala for the country, and this suggests there are many that are far from
the ideal (Turnbull 2017). Further, standards in a given goshala may change over time, depending
on management changes and other factors.

And yet this sense of dharmic business ethics on behalf of cows is, for these industrialists, only a stop-gap intervention. From a broader perspective, such business arrangements are, at best, emergency adjustments to the demands of the modern globalized industrial economy. They serve to optimize conditions for cows within a system that is deeply inhospitable to the culture of cow care. What is urgently needed, they feel, is the recovery of a self-sustaining, cow-based agrarian economy, as has existed for untold centuries of India's past.

We begin to see that many sorts of people become involved in cow care, from founders of goshalas to managers, what to speak of workers (hired or volunteers), donors, and less directly, any number of persons involved in supply provision or doing business with or enabling wealth for donors. Yet for many Hindus engaged directly in cow care in India, there is another person involved in a crucial way, namely the Lord of the Cows, Krishna, or his divine consort Radha (known also as Radharani). This was explained to me by the manager of a moderate-sized goshala on the outskirts of Vrindavan, famous as the land of Krishna, as we discussed his donor base (see Fig. 4.1). Keshi Nisudan Das, the manager of Care For Cows,[30] first expresses appreciation for his workers:

> [Our workers] love the cows. When you love the cows—everybody is loving—the Lord is pleased. And when the Lord is pleased, there is no limit to what we can get. But it has to be sincere service. You must be able to sacrifice twenty-four hours a day and dirty your hands.

"What we can get" refers to support for maintenance of the goshala, pointing to Care For Cows' essential source of support, sympathetic donors. Strikingly, unlike most other Indian goshalas, Care For Cows is supported largely by an international community of people valuing their cause (hence the goshala's English name). Their financial contributions allow the onsite caretakers to continue their close attention to the cows. Conversely, the

---

[30]Care For Cows was founded in 1999 by Kurma Rupa Das, an American member of ISKCON (Hare Krishna Society) who had lived in Vrindavan for thirty years. In 2015, he breathed his last while staying with his cows at Kiki Nagla, Vrindavan. The CFC Newsletter, November 2015, a special in memoriam issue, quotes the Brahmanda Purana (21.93): "A place where cows stay is considered sanctified, and a person who dies there certainly attains liberation."

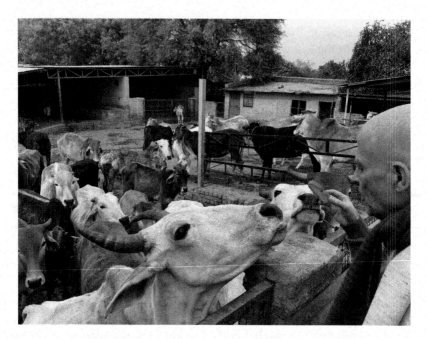

Fig. 4.1 The author offers a snack to rescued cows at Care For Cows, Vrindavan

international supporters feel encouraged that they are benefited by serving Krishna's cows, even if indirectly, from a distance.[31] As in Pathmeda, regular donors may "adopt" a specific cow, enabling them to experience a sense of connection with a particular bovine, to receive news about it, and when visiting Vrindavan, to directly meet and interact with their adoptees.[32] Donors have also been recognized in the (currently discontinued) monthly newsletter. However, a good number of visitors may give

---

[31]One striking example of a foreigner in India dedicating her life to cow rescue and care is Sudevi (Friederike Irina Bruning) from Germany. Since 1996, Sudevi runs Radha Surabhi Gaushala Niketan, near Radha Kunda (near Vrindavan), presently with 1800 cows. In 2019, in recognition of her dedication to this service, she received the Padma Shri award, the Central Indian Government's fourth highest civilian honor.

[32]Keshi reports that of more than 500 cows maintained in Care For Cows, some 250 are sponsored. Nine-tenths of monthly donations are spent on maintenance and the remainder goes into savings or for new construction. Keshi says, "For the monthly expenses, we somehow manage. It's tough, I have to work very hard. First thing in the morning, I come to my cows and say 'Hey, how much are we going to get today?' because we need such and such amount. We pay our staff well … and medicine last month took a big chunk. We feed our cows three times a day—we don't want to be stingy; we buy them enough, we feed them enough."

donations expecting no receipt or mention. Keshi likes to say that such donations are coming from Krishna's divine consort, Radharani (Radha).

From the bhakti perspective, this reference to Radha says that ultimately, because she is the divinity who oversees service to Krishna, especially in Vrindavan, it is by her grace that sufficient sponsorship comes to maintain what Krishna's devotees regard as Krishna's cows. According to Vaishnava theology, as the ultimate form of the divine feminine, it is she who "expands" as Lakshmi, who governs worldly wealth and opulence. Significantly, Lakshmi is associated with cows, and in delineations of the several divinities' specific locations in cows' bodies (as discussed in the beginning of Chapter 3), Lakshmi is located in the dung. Care For Cows generates a modest income for the goshala from the sale of dung to locals who use it for fertilizer. But Keshi emphasizes the goshala's focus on service as pleasing to Radha and therefore pleasing to Krishna, rather than on gain from the cows: "We don't want to go into business, because then our concentration on service becomes diverted. Then we will be thinking (only) of money. Money is essential, but then making money is a different, mundane activity."

While the spirit of service may dominate in cow care, there is no denying a strong emphasis on bovine products as affording multiple benefits for humans. Thus, invariably connected with goshala economics are considerations of these benefits. And although goshalas (such as Kamdhenu Dham in Gurugram) may not maintain dairies, others, such as the Pathmeda institution, do so as an essential practice. Beginning with cow milk, followed by the milk derivative ghee, and then dung, urine, and the mixture *panchagavya*, we can now consider how these products are regarded and used in India, keeping in mind the question whether, how, or to what extent it may be appropriate for humans to use bovine products. This question will occupy us on a theoretical level in Chapter 5. Here it bears brief mention that the ethical framework assumed for bovine product use is largely that articulated by M. K. Gandhi, who regarded India's predominantly rural civilization as "essentially non-violent" and "wrapped up with [its] animals" (quoted in Nagy 2019, p. 252). As "utilitarian protectionism," the view is that human utility can be accomplished with bovine well-being and benefit when well cared for throughout their natural lives (Nagy 2019, p. 255).[33]

Bovine Products as Added Value

Milk

As we saw in Chapter 2, cows (and the several words for "cow") in ancient India carried an extensive field of cultural meaning, and the same was true of cow products, especially milk and its derivatives, as indicated, for example, in the Mahabharata: "Kine by yielding milk, rescue all the worlds from calamity. It is kine, again, that produce the food upon which creatures subsist" (Ganguli 1991, vol. 11, p. 94; Mahabharata 13.71).

In the present day, along with multiple meanings of bovine dairy products, there are also multiple disagreements about their value and use. Some disagreements relate to human health and cow milk consumption, such as whether it is at all necessary for humans[34]; whether it is necessary to nourish specific bodily organs, such as for brain development; whether milk should be pasteurized or homogenized; and whether milk containing beta-casein protein A1 is a cause of certain diseases, in contrast to beta-casein A2 milk (an issue linked to the distinction between nonindigenous cows

---

[33] In contrast to this "rights without liberation" ethic of utilitarian protectionism, which we will consider more extensively in Chapter 5, Nagy (2019, p. 255) identifies two other ethical position types regarding bovine treatment, namely an "industrial animal-welfare science" ethic rooted in American agribusiness husbandry and an "abolitionist animal rights" ethic, which calls for the complete cessation of animal product use and the adoption of a vegan lifestyle.

[34] Lactose intolerance, a common condition, has been seen to arise naturally in humans as they grow out of infancy, as an indicator that it is no longer needed beyond infancy. Yet this intolerance can be overcome by boiling the milk—a standard practice in India to the present day, in which after boiling up, it is kept on a simmer for 5–10 minutes, allowing a molecular structural change to occur making it digestible (Velten 2010, pp. 21–22, 25). According to traditional Indian medicine (Ayurveda), milk can serve medicinal purposes, especially as a rejuvenator, but also as an aphrodisiac (Rastogi and Kaphle 2011). An Adventist Health Study project found that "Those drinking more dairy milk have lower rates of colon and rectal cancers (but preliminary findings suggest increased risk of breast and prostate cancers)" (Banta et al. 2018, p. 13; Jacob 2014, pp. 111–118). See also Marshall (2019) for a very brief overview of prehistoric to present-day use and attitudes toward animal milk.

and indigenous cows, the latter regarded as producing only A2 milk).[35] Also related to cow milk use in India is the issue whether buffalo milk is beneficial or detrimental for humans, and under what conditions.[36]

These are contemporary issues surfacing in post-industrial societies, including India.[37] Prior to this, in some but not all parts of India, bovine milk has been highly valued for rituals and for nourishment, especially of young children, often regarded as a necessity for their survival when mother's milk is inadequate. With a lack of refrigeration, milk was invariably turned to yoghurt if not immediately used or else immediately cooked (usually with grain). Processing milk to yoghurt and then to butter by

---

[35]See, for example, Sun et al. (2016), a study in China which concluded (p. 1 of 16, Abstract), "Consumption of milk containing A1 ß-casein was associated with increased gastrointestinal inflammation, worsening of PD3 symptoms, delayed transit, and decreased cognitive processing speed and accuracy. Because elimination of A1 ß-casein attenuated these effects, some symptoms of lactose intolerance may stem from inflammation it triggers, and can be avoided by consuming milk containing only the A2 type of beta-casein." Tangentially related, animal welfare activist and researcher Maneka Gandhi offers interesting advice, namely to drink camel milk, it being the most healthy in several ways, including being a "superfood" for diabetics. See "I never thought the day would come when I would recommend the drinking of milk!" at https://www.peopleforanimalsindia.org (accessed 7 February 2019). See also Pallavi (2015) for a brief overview of the A1-A2 discussion; the economic difficulties of Indian farmers, herders, and nomadic pastoralists who maintain indigenous cattle breeds; and research being done on milk properties of these breeds, particularly of the Gaolao breed, taking into account traditional knowledge thereof.

[36]On buffalo milk, see Sinha (2016), pp. 173–175. Sharma (1980, pp 175–181), discusses milk and ghee benefits in modern medicinal terms, citing Sateeshchandradas Gupta, *The Cow-in-India* vol. 1. Calcutta: Khadi Pratishthan, 1945. Also interesting if vague (given without specific reference) is Sharma's claim, that "[M. K.] Gandhiji [Gandhi] and S.C.D. Gupta collected experts' opinions and elaborately demonstrated and proved the superiority of cow milk to buffalo milk" (Sharma 1980, p. 8).

[37]Many cow care activists in India refer to scientific research to support various claims, especially about the benefits of cows' milk, bovine dung, and urine. A valuable discussion of modern science in the context of cow care would, if space would permit, consider how basic presuppositions of mainstream modern science lead to production of knowledge inherently opposed to traditional forms of knowledge whereby bovines are recognized to be integral to the maintenance of ecological balance in agriculture. See Shiva (2016, Chapter 1), "Agroecology Feeds the World, Not a Violent Knowledge Paradigm," and passim. This issue intersects with the broader theme of power/knowledge relationships with respect to the environment and the treatment of animals. For an extended analysis of the latter (animals and knowledge systems), see Johnson (2012). For a broad overview of the Hinduism and science discourse, see Dorman (2011).

churning has, as a common domestic activity, been enshrined in classical literature, as we saw in Chapter 2 with the story of Krishna breaking his mother's churning pot and stealing the butter (Mahias 1987, pp. 285–286).[38]

Of ethical concern for Hindu cow carers today—assuming that cows are cared for throughout their natural lives—is how much milk may appropriately be taken from cows in relation to how much milk should be reserved for their calves. The ancient Sanskrit guide to governmental management, the Arthashastra of Kautilya (ca. 4th c. CE) gives an interesting injunction that may be relevant: In the rainy season, autumn, and early winter, cows and she-buffaloes are to be milked twice per day; all other seasons, once per day (Tiwari, n.d.; Rangarajan 1992).[39] Some of the cow carers I interviewed emphasized that milk remaining after calves have their fill should be regarded as a "bonus" that is not to be expected, but rather graciously accepted along with the many other benefits of having and caring for bovines. They also point out that any restriction of milk imposed on a calf in its first months will effectively backfire, as the calf will be deprived of its full natural development and thus will be less productive in later life.[40] They expressed sadness that some cow carers breed bovines with the intention to increase milk yield. But then such breeders will say that they are not depriving calves of milk by intentional breeding for greater milk yield, and that this is not an improper imposition on cows. Rather, it is a response to an increasing demand—based on a genuine need—for pure milk from cows that are cared for throughout their natural lives.[41]

Interviewees who see themselves as sympathetic to cow protection typically expressed regard for milk from lifetime protected cows as "added

---

[38]The churning image has wide resonances in Indian literature, famously in this account, but also in the story of cosmic churning described in several early texts, including the Bhagavata Purana.

[39]Punishment for milking twice a day in the wrong season could be harsh for a cowherd of the king's cows, namely the loss of his thumb! Those tending the royal herd were paid in cash rather than in milk and ghee, to allay the possibility that they would otherwise limit the calves' milk to get a higher yield for themselves (Rangarajan 1992, pp. 88, 96–97).

[40]Dayal Mukunda Das interview, 10 January 2018; Sinha (2016, pp. 111–113).

[41]https://www.youtube.com/watch?v=um5Cj5B7LoQ&feature=youtu.be (ca. 5:30:00; accessed 26 November 2018). In this Cow Culture Conference talk, May 20, 2018 (Silicon Valley), Balabhadra Das, an American Vaishnava, gives pause for thought on milk production: "In Vedic times, cows were not bred for milk, they were bred for bulls, manure, and urine…Milk will come automatically, it is not our main concern. Our main concern is bulls."

value" milk that is especially healthful and nourishing. One reason given is that protected cows are surely aware of their protected condition, an awareness that plays out in unstressed body chemistry and in a relaxed sort of interaction of the cows with humans.[42] At the least, they point out, such milk is free from the several adverse substances imposed on industrial dairy cows, such as added hormones and antibiotics.

Most importantly, conscientious Hindus regard such milk to be infused with an ethical value enshrined in the principle of nonviolence, and they regard such "ahimsa milk" as therefore also having important medicinal properties.[43] Thus, milk and milk derivatives in general are most valued when obtained from protected cows.[44] This also explains why many of the larger Hindu temples in India (and, since more recently, elsewhere in the world) maintain goshalas with milking cows. For offerings of food preparations to temple images of Krishna, devotees favor preparations featuring milk and milk derivatives, thereby honoring his celebrated preference for these as a child. This understanding of Krishna's milk preference contributes to the sense that the temple cows are venerable as Krishna's cows, and that their daily care (*go-seva*) counts as service to Krishna, since the cows in his domain are especially dear to him (see Figs. 4.2 and 4.3).

Ghee

The derivative of milk—ghee (*ghṛta* in Sanskrit, clarified butter or anhydrous milk fat)—is the bovine product most specifically associated with Hindu culture. Some twenty-five liters of milk are required to make one

---

[42]Several cow carers interviewed pointed out cows in their care who were continuing to give milk years after their last calf—considered a clear indication that these cows are not only peaceful but happy to show their generosity in this way.

[43]Two Indian cow carer interviewees told of a tradition that, in earlier times, if a child in the household fell ill, the elders would whisper the nature of the illness in the ear of a family cow. This cow would then proceed, while grazing in open pasture or forest, to select certain herbs that could benefit the child, such that when the child would be fed the cow's milk from that evening's milking, it could be cured of the illness. This seems related to the tradition of wish-whispering in the ear of Shiva's bull image.

[44]Sitaram Das, who operates Ahimsa Milk dairy near Leicester, UK, says that he cannot keep up with the steadily rising demand for his products from fifteen cows. Despite his unavoidably high prices and membership fees, these products are valued specifically due to the "slaughter-free milk" standard. https://www.ahimsamilk.org/ (accessed 30 November 2018), and personal interviews.

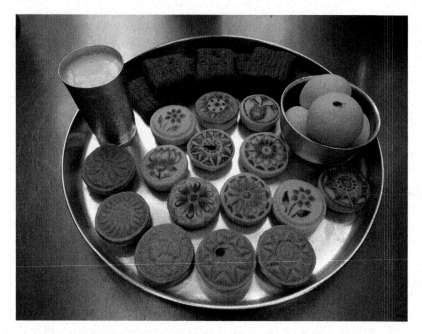

Fig. 4.2 Artfully prepared dairy sweets and hot milk for Krishna's daily early morning snack, at Bhaktivedanta Manor, near London

liter of high-quality ghee,[45] an indicator of how highly ghee is valued. Ghee is valued for three areas of use, namely for ritual purposes (especially for making ghee oblations into a sacred fire); for cooking—both for deep-frying and for sautéing; and for medical purposes, especially as a component of Ayurvedic medicines.[46] Because ghee can be stored for long periods and can be easily transported, it has long functioned in India as the main end-product of milk (Rangarajan 1992, p. 82).

Ritual use of ghee is invariably in relation to the performance of fire rites (*yajna*; *homa*), which we have already discussed as defining practices of the orthodox brahmanical tradition that later develops as the Hindu

---

[45] Damodar Dulal Das, Sri Surabhi Conference, https://www.youtube.com/watch?v=um5Cj5B7LoQ&feature=youtu.be (accessed 31 May 2018).

[46] On the use of ghee in Ayurvedic medicine (and a detailed explanation of the traditional Indian way of preparing it), see Malakoff (2005).

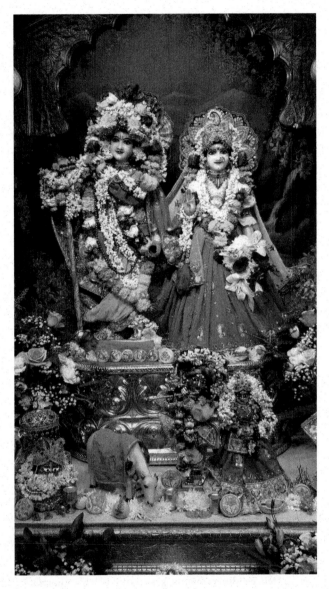

Fig. 4.3 Temple images (*murtis*) of Radha-Krishna at Bhaktivedanta Manor, rendered seven vegetarian food offerings daily

constellation of ideas and practices.[47] To be noted here is that ghee will be used in a variety of present-day Hindu rituals, including several rites of passage (*samskaras*) of which the wedding rite is central. Further to be seen as a ritual use of ghee is to give it in charity, an act much praised in the Mahabharata.[48] As for ghee in cooking, it is especially used on occasions of celebration, such as weddings, when abundance is particularly highlighted through the medium of rich vegetarian food. Further, ghee signifies food purity, especially of preparations that use it for deep-frying.[49] In Vaishnava bhakti traditions, ghee is generously used in temple cooking, as it is understood that Krishna is particularly pleased by food offerings prepared with ghee.[50]

In recent years, several proponents of cow care have been championing the medical benefits of cow ghee. But for ghee to have the desired medical benefits, as noted by Damodar Dulal Das, a leader of ISKCON-India's cow care projects,

> the cows (from which the milk has been taken, for making the ghee) have to be happy cows. First, we feed our calves with the full milk content from two of the mothers' four teats, so we don't deprive the calf of her milk. It is a

---

[47]Vedic texts prescribe ghee to be offered in the fire, as fire is the divinity Agni, who is "fed" in this way. Ghee is regarded as *virya*—potent—and as such purifying to the immediate ritual space of the fire rite, and purifying to the surrounding area. My thanks to Dr. Shalvapille Iyengar for this explanation. We may add that ghee's potency derives from its being the essence of an essence—the essence of milk, which is seen as the essence of the grass and other nourishment eaten by the cow.

[48]In the Anushasana Parva, Bhishma tells Yudhisthira, "Ghee is said to gratify the illustrious Vrihaspati, Pushan, Bhaga, the twin Aswins, and the deity of fire. Ghee is possessed of high medicinal virtues. It is a high requisite for sacrifice. It is the best of all liquids. The merit a gift of ghee produces is very superior. That man who is desirous of the reward of happiness in the next world, who wishes for fame and prosperity, should with a cleansed soul and having purified himself make gifts of ghee unto the Brahmanas. Upon that man who makes gifts of ghee unto the Brahmanas in the month of Aswin, the twin Aswins, gratified, confer personal beauty. Rakshasas [ogres] never invade the abode of that man who makes gifts unto the Brahmanas of Payasa [sweetened rice] mixed with ghee" (Ganguli 1991, vol. 11, p. 79; Mahabharata 13.65).

[49]Food categories may turn on whether something is prepared with water (usually boiling) or with ghee (typically deep-frying). Water, among other items, is considered disintegrating, whereas ghee is a preservative, making it especially fit for public (festival) events (Toomey 1994, pp. 49–50).

[50]There are two explicit mentions of ghee in the Bhagavata Purana. One (6.19.22) enjoins preparing rice cooked with ghee to offer as oblations in a ritual home fire, as part of a practice to prepare for having a child. The other verse (11.27.34) includes ghee in a list of preparations recommended for offering to a temple image of Krishna.

[function of] hormonal secretion. As much as the cow is happy, that much the hormone will be secreted by which she will give that much milk.[51]

The idea is that when cows are well treated and thus peaceful, and their calves are properly cared for and generously fed, the milk yielded by such cows will be of the best quality for producing high-quality ghee.

According to Damodar Dulal and another, widely known activist for cow care in India, Uttam Maheshwari, the medical benefits of high-quality ghee are numerous. While evidence of benefits tends to be anecdotal, ghee is recognized as an important healing agent in Ayurveda—a traditional Indian medical system—and some modern research has been done pursuant to verification of its efficacy.[52]

Some cow care institutions that have lactating cows and which have dairy facilities make ghee and offer it for sale to the public. Typically, such ghee will be sold at a considerably higher price than the same from an ordinary dairy, as a value-added product.[53] As noted regarding the value-added cow dung products of Pathmeda, what is understood to be the specific added value is the conscientious lifelong care for the cows from which the milk—and therefore the ghee—has come. And such conscientious care translates into a sense of ethical rightness for the ghee customers and a sense of quality—that the ghee, coming from cows that are contented, will be most efficacious in its various uses.

---

[51] Also considered essential by cow carers to ensure that milking cows are "happy" is that the milking of them is never to be done by a milking machine, but always by hand (although one interviewee, who found it necessary to use a milking machine because of having developed carpal tunnel syndrome, told me that his cows "did not object at all" when he began using it with them). Most importantly, several interviewees insisted that cows are aware if they are being given natural lifetime care or not. Thus, cows can only be "happy" if cared for to their natural end.

[52] Several Ayurvedic texts refer to ghee and its benefits; broadly, ghee serves as an "increaser" or tonic (*vardhaka*), in particular of the "seven essences" (*sapta-dhatu*) of the physical body. The Go Vigyan Anusandhan Kendra's publication "Research Activity Book" (pp. 65–73) includes lists of several preparations made with ghee including "household remedies" for several conditions. It also mentions some efforts to conduct studies of certain possible benefits, including the claim that regular ingestion of ghee can benefit intelligence. Anecdotal stories of remarkable cures of serious conditions with the help of ghee are told by some cow care activists in India. There are, for example, accounts of persons becoming free from epileptic seizures or waking from protracted comatose states as the apparent result of simply applying such ghee in one's nostrils. Such possibilities may be worth investigating.

[53] In India today, ghee is priced in a wide range, from ca. Rs. 300 to Rs. 1500 for 500 ml.

Dung and Urine

We recall the association of goddess Lakshmi with cow dung. Arguably, the most valuable products of bovines—female and male—are their body wastes. Throughout South Asia, one sees a standard type of village energy storage in the form of cow dung or buffalo dung patties drying on walls or, once dried, stacked neatly in large piles, ready for use as cooking and heating fuel. Dung may also be used to produce methane gas fuel, as we noted in connection with the Kamdhenu Dham Gaushala where, in addition, it is used in making compost.

At one project, the commercial Two Brothers Organic Farm (near Pune, Maharashtra), cows are maintained not for their milk, which is considered a "by-product," so much as for their dung and urine, from which fertilizers are prepared for their farm. The cows, which are of the northwestern Gir breed, graze freely on portions of the farm's land, otherwise receiving organic fodder from the farm's two acres reserved for this purpose. The dung and urine (which are swept together into a trough in the cow shed and then processed into slurry as a methane gas plant by-product) are used as an "inoculation" of healthy bacteria into the farm's soil. A guide explains that the Gir cows' ageless acclimatization to this area makes them ideal for generating a high density of healthy bacteria released into the dung.[54] The resulting fertilizer makes the soil exceptionally healthy, unlike chemical fertilizers, which destroy rather than fostering microbial life for healthy farm produce.[55]

As Lakshmi is understood to be present in bovine dung, Ganga Devi, the life-giving and preserving River Ganges divinity, is understood to be present in bovine urine. While cow urine may be used with dung to produce fertilizer, it can also be collected separately (from my observation, not without considerable patience of a person waiting behind the cows with a bucket in the very early morning!) for medicinal use. Its medicinal value

---

[54]The guide also notes that the Gir breed's intestines, being longer than the Western cows such as Jersey and Holstein, are better able to process the local fodder, thus producing richer dung from a thorough digestive process. Further, they have a very balanced pH of around 7, most favorable for good bacteria. https://twobrothersindiashop.com/ (accessed 15 March 2019).

[55]See Note 58 below.

is signaled in Ayurveda texts by its being referred to as *sanjivani* (comprehensive life-giving tonic) and *amrita* (elixir of immortality). Especially in distilled form, *go-mutra ark*—cow urine extract—is recognized for treatment of kidney disorders and diabetes mellitus (Somvanshi 2006). It is also considered beneficial against several other conditions, not least cancer, which we will discuss further in the next section (Mohanty et al. 2014).

Panchagavya

The three bovine products—milk, dung, and urine—are valued individually, and they are also valued in a mixture called *panchagavya* ("having five bovine substances") that includes two derivatives of milk, namely yoghurt and ghee. *Panchagavya* is especially valued both in traditional Ayurvedic medicine and in ritual, and also as a basis for soil fertilizer.[56] Today, medicinal properties of *panchagavya* are especially highlighted by cow carers and activists in India, who refer to Ayurvedic reference and to modern research studies. So, for example, the Go Vigyan Anusandhan Kendra in Nagpur (central India) credits *panchagavya* with aiding in the cure of numerous conditions, ranging from dandruff to rheumatoid arthritis to kidney stones and heart conditions (Research Activity Book, n.d., p. 2). And beyond these claims, there are claims and accounts of *panchagavya* cures for cancer.[57]

Several organizations in India, including for-profit businesses, produce medicines, and other products, use *panchagavya* (or one or more of its

---

[56]The ritual use is described in such texts as the Padma Samhita (from prior to eighth century CE), in particular as an important liquid substance to be poured on a temple image at the time of consecration or renewal. The text gives preference for all ingredients of *panchagavya* to be fresh and all from the same cow, which "should not be weak, old, pregnant, or without calf." Specific proportions of each ingredient are given, with increasing multiples from yoghurt to ghee, milk, urine, and finally (liquid squeezed from) dung. (Padma Samhita, Charyapada 8, vv. 118–130; Padmanabhan 1982, pp. 82–85; my thanks to Brahma Muhurta Das for this reference). Another ritual practice with *panchagavya* takes place after cremation rites, whereby ashes from the deceased are mixed with *panchagavya* prior to submerging the ashes in a sacred river. See Satyanarayana et al. (2012, pp. 62–63) for a detailed panchagavya preparation formula for fertilizer and a chart of its effect on micro-organisms. Another formula, from Dr. K. Natharanjan, is available here: http://www.newdelhitimes.com/the-utility-of-panchgavya/ (accessed 16 July 2018).
[57]Two examples of studies done on the efficacy of *panchagavya* or cow urine in cancer therapies are here, both cautiously indicating positive efficacy: Dhama et al. (2005) and Jain et al. (2010).

ingredients—especially cow urine) as a key ingredient. Such products are being widely marketed in India and in other countries.[58]

The common thread running through our discussion of bovine products is that the benefits of living bovines for humans and the environment cannot be measured with any one product, or even all combined, against supposed "benefits" of slaughtered bovines. Despite the difficulties of caring for cows, conscientious Hindus will say that care is far better than no care, and the fact that bovines yield products beneficial for humans is an added indicator of this. Brigadier Chohan, the manager of Kamdhenu Dham Gaushala (which does not run a dairy), put it this way, reflecting on the goshala's overcrowded condition in the face of a demand for more stray cows to be sheltered:

> If I say "no, I won't take [in more stray cows]," they will all be slaughtered. Which is the bigger crime, which my soul will not accept? At least their health is being looked after here. Their medicines are being given—they are very healthy. You will see [the cows] are laughing! So, it is a small price to pay [to avoid] their slaughter.

To be sure, one may object that the essentially anthropocentric character of such a care ethic is exposed as soon as there is any mention of bovines' benefits for humans. Yet arguably the ethical framework of cow care and protection is broadly dharmic, which is to say observant of regulation for human–animal coexistence in pursuit of the nonviolence ideal of ahimsa. How seriously and effectively this ideal is pursued will vary with different cow carers and organizations. Unfortunately, what goes under the name of cow care can, in some cases, look more like cow neglect or even cruelty.[59] Related to this issue, we must now proceed to another, possibly more

---

[58]The Go Vigyan Anusandhan Kendra (based near Nagpur, Maharashtra) is one prominent organization among several in India promoting cow products as medicine. Such products are fairly popular; yet one interviewee, a descendent of a several-generation family of Ayurvedic doctors, Sachi Kumar, expressed reservations about their value: First, traditionally, no bovine products were *sold*; second, benefits of these medicines are exaggerated, as much more benefit will come from eating organically grown produce that has been fertilized with cow dung and urine than from taking medicines containing these ingredients; and third, the claim that only *deshi* (indigenous) cows' products are medicinally beneficial may be exaggerated.

[59]See Nagy (2019, pp. 252–253) on Gandhi's sharp criticism of Hindu hypocrisy and "criminal negligence" with respect to bovines.

challenging, area of discussion, namely the keeping and engagement of male bovines for work.

Male Bovine Care and the Issue of Violence

India has been a land of subsistence farming throughout most of its history, and oxen, or bullocks, have done most of the ploughing, farm goods transport, and grain threshing that has made such farming possible. Since recent decades, in much of India, the same work is being done by tractors and other machines. Thus, where male bovines were once essential— even considered more important for agricultural economy than milk cows (Chakravarti 1985, p. 33)—they now become superfluous. And being so, unless kept as stud animals, bulls become the victims of early slaughter. That such profound change in India's agricultural landscape went initially unnoticed is suggested by Rudyard Kipling in his poem "What the People Said," at the time of Queen Victoria's Jubilee, in 1887:

BY THE well, where the bullocks go
Silent and blind and slow—
By the field where the young corn dies
In the face of the sultry skies,
They have heard, as the dull Earth hears
The voice of the wind of an hour,
The sound of the Great Queen's voice:
"My God hath given me years,
Hath granted dominion and power:
And I bid you, O Land, rejoice."

...

And the Ploughman settled the share
More deep in the sun-dried clod:
"Mogul Mahratta, and Mlech from the North,
And White Queen over the Seas—
God raiseth them up and driveth them forth
As the dust of the ploughshare flies in the breeze;

But the wheat and the cattle are all my care,
And the rest is the will of God."[60]

The Ploughman's dismissive comparison of rulers—local and foreign—that come and go like flying dust raised by his ploughshare (hinting at impending spiritual drought?) obscures the fact that such distant powers already had increasingly profound influence on the lives of humans and animals alike throughout India and the South Asian subcontinent. One of the most significant tangible changes for modern India would be brought by the introduction of the tractor. But prior to the tractor would be the railroad, which would provide fast transport of bovine meat to markets. The tractor would make it seem that there was no need for the live ("silent and blind and slow") bullock on the farm. Even less was bullocks' labor missed when, in the early 1960s, the "Green Revolution" took hold in North Indian agriculture. Nor with the impressively increased crop yields did it seem to matter that chemical fertilizers, pesticides, and over-irrigation would bring destruction of beneficial insects, soil degradation, and loss of biodiversity.[61]

We may recall from Chapter 3 how in the late 1960s and early 1970s (around the same time that the Green Revolution was expanding in northern India) Swami Prabhupāda began to inspire some of his followers to establish farm communities with cow care in Western countries, where agriculture should be conducted without depending on tractors. Prabhupāda was particularly concerned that bovine bulls be cared for, and integral to caring for bulls would be training them for draught work:

The Europeans have invented tractors, and the bull is a problem. Therefore [bulls] must be sent to the slaughterhouse. So, we cannot create that problem

---

[60] http://www.kiplingsociety.co.uk/poems_whatthepeople.htm (accessed 20 May 2018), the first and final of five strophes. "Mlech" refers to *mleccha* (Sanskrit), essentially "barbarian"—uncultured foreigner.

[61] As an example of tractor use, the number of tractors in Punjab state rose from 10,646 in 1962–1965 to 234,006 in 1990–1993. Fertilizer (NPK) increased in the same two periods from 30,060 tonnes to 1212,570 tonnes (Human Development Report 2004, Punjab, pp. 17–20).

[at our farm projects]. How the bull should be utilized? They should be used for transport, and ploughing.[62]

The connection Prabhupāda makes between the development and use of farm machinery and the resultant replacement of draught animals and hence their slaughter points again to the issue of industrialization and globalization as these have affected the human–bovine (and, more broadly, the human–nonhuman animal) relationship in India. But what is to be also noted here is that globalization's reach in India had additionally a sort of inverse effect, in that Hindu cow care practice has begun to find place outside India, in countries worldwide. Significantly, this practice outside India includes efforts to engage oxen in agriculture-related activities. In Chapter 6, we will look at current Western cow care practices; but first, in relation to experiences of oxen training and engagement, we can view briefly one ISKCON project in India, the Govardhan Eco Village (GEV) in northern Maharashtra, begun in 2003.

Govardhan Eco Village is situated some 100 kilometers north of Mumbai, in the foothills of the Sahyadri mountains. The project's 110-acre area is surrounded by small-holding indigenous (*adivasi*) farming families which GEV has been endeavoring to help overcome considerable economic and social challenges. GEV also functions as a retreat and conference center that caters largely to visitors from greater Mumbai and Ahmedabad. Moreover, it hosts yoga groups from the United States and visiting non-Indian Vaishnava Hindus from around the world. The project includes a cow care program, with currently some 104 bovines of the Gir and Tharparkar breeds (52 each of males and females, including 12 calves; 12 cows give milk at this writing). The GEV goshala has a specific educational function, namely to show visitors the virtues and spiritual rewards of cow care, while also showing the practicality of cow care, including the training and engagement of oxen.

The first ethical issue related to bulls and oxen is the matter of castration—the operation by which bulls become oxen, which is to say bovine eunuchs. The consensus at GEV is that it is an unavoidable, even if violent,

---

[62]Prabhupāda 2017, Vedabase: Room Conversation, December 10, 1976, Hyderabad. Quoted in *Cow Protection—Book 1*, ISKCON Ministry of Cow Protection and Agriculture, n.d., p. 38.

action if the bulls born into the community are to be positively cared for and engaged in labor that contributes to the community.[63] The castration process involves anaesthetization and is done by a veterinarian. If done properly, there is moderate, or no pain experienced.[64] Prahlada Bhakta, a former GEV goshala manager, explains:

> Here [at GEV] the veterinarian comes, the bull is laid down, the veterinarian gives an injection to make him semi-conscious, then he presses that nerve; then [the bull] comes back to consciousness and he is normal again. It is like that. So, it is done with minimum possible violence, I believe.

Present-day Vaishnava Hindus tend to feel ambivalent about bull castration. At Care For Cows in Vrindavan, some uncastrated bulls are kept on nearby land owned by a sadhu who stipulates that they are not to be castrated if they are to remain with him. Other bulls living at the Care for Cows' main facility are generally castrated, since they could otherwise not be sheltered in such proximity to the cows, as the limited space demands. As the Care For Cows manager told me, the founder, the late Kurma Rupa Das, had once commented in this regard, "We must be cruel in order to

---

[63] *Cow Protection—Book 1* (n.d.), the official manual for ISKCON cow care, states the following regarding bull castration: "Recommended: (1) Bull calves of European Taurean breeds should be castrated at 6 months to a year. Indian Zebu breeds should be castrated at 1 year to 2 years. (2) The method of castration should be by emasculation, specifically using the tool bordezio (bloodless castration) performed by a veterinarian, or experienced professional. Not Allowed: (1) Banding (using rubber bands around the testicles until they drop off). (2) Performing acceptable methods of castration by inexperienced cowherd." According to one standard Dharmashastra text, when *apaddharma* is applicable (irregular circumstances demanding adjustments to regular rules of *dharma*) if a brahmin takes up agriculture, using bulls for ploughing, they must be uncastrated (Bowles 2018, p. 249).

[64] In January 2015, the Indian Department of Animal Husbandry, Dairying and Fisheries (DADF) issued a circular that "cattle must be given anesthetics prior to castration." That this was announced with approval by PETA India indicates the organization's approval of the general practice of castrating bulls to enable engagement of oxen in labor. https://www.petaindia.com/media/taking-pain-cattle-castration-among-animal-welfare-reforms-now-required-india/ (accessed 29 November 2018). According to Maneka Gandhi, the best, most humane method of castration is "immuno-castration": injections given every six months, which reduce a bullock's testosterone production. ("Animal Cruelty and Ignorance," at https://www.peopleforanimalsindia.org [accessed 9 February 2019]).

be kind."[65] That is, in order to be able to shelter the rescued bulls, it was seen to be necessary for them to undergo this quick operation and thus deprive them of reproductive power.[66] On the other hand, it is reported that ISKCON's nearby Krishna Balaram Goshala in Vrindavan routinely engages uncastrated bulls in work (Dasa 1998, p. 71).

At GEV, engagement of oxen in work has been a priority of the project. But oxen training and engagement has been a learning process for the cow carers as much as for the oxen. In the early days of GEV, the oxen's noses were pierced so that they would be controlled with a rope through the nose, as is widely practiced throughout Asia.[67] Then, in 2011, the American Vaishnava, Radhanath Swami, the founder and spiritual leader of the community, requested the goshala managers to try to engage the oxen without the nose ropes. Initially, the men were skeptical. Prahlada Bhakta Das recalls,

> Radhanath Swami told us, "In Vrindavan we just walk by the bulls [in the streets] and they don't do anything [to disturb us], so why do we need to pierce [our oxen's] noses?" I said to him, "That is how it is done traditionally, and I think there is example in the Bhagavatam [the Bhagavata Purana] telling that just as the bulls are forced to move by a rope through the nose, so everyone is forced by the 'ropes' of maya [illusion] or destiny."[68]

---

[65] One interesting exception at CFC was the bull named "Baba," for whom Kurma Rupa devised a "chastity belt"! (CFC Newsletter, February 2006). I was informed by a CFC interviewee that actually the device fails to serve its function.

[66] Further regarding bull castration, Hindu sacred texts appear to be not univocal, similar to equivocal injunctions related to meat consumption we saw in Chapter 3. On one side, there are references (in the Shatapatha Brahmana, e.g., 2.2.3.28 and Taittiriya Samhita 1.8.17.1) indicating that an ox was to be given to a ritual priest as a sacrificial fee. But in Padma Purana, Bhumi-khanda 67.88, we find, "Those men who, being most sinful, strike the scrotum of bulls (i.e., castrate them) and they who harm cows' calves are residents of a great (i.e., very painful) hell." My thanks to Brijabhasi Das for providing these references.

[67] The recently produced manual for Indian goshalas (Khanna et al. 2017, pp. 70–71) speaks approvingly of bull castration and nose-ring insertion, noting that both should be done at one year of age. It also speaks approvingly of de-horning (within a few days of birth). This is strange, considering that one of manual's editors, Maneka Gandhi, writes strongly against these practices in her article "Animal Cruelty and Ignorance" https://www.peopleforanimalsindia.org (accessed 7 February 2019).

[68] BhP 6.3.12: Yama, the lord of death, compares the cosmic creation to a bull. "The world is controlled by Vishnu as [a bull is] controlled by a rope in its nose." Several more verses in the text employ the same analogy.

> Radhanath Swami said, "Yes, but if it is possible [to engage the oxen in work without nose ropes], why not do it?"[69]

By all reports (and my own observation), the experiment has proven successful, and now none of the oxen at GEV have nose ropes; rather, they work with a halter, without nose rope or ring.[70] However, as Jagannath Kripa Das, the present GEV goshala manager, points out, the goshala's concomitant challenge is to have enough engagement for the several resident oxen. Some ploughing and load-carrying (mainly transporting their fodder and dung) engage two pairs of oxen in a day, following a rotating system to keep all the oxen trained. Prahlada Bhakta Das observed,

> It is not difficult to drive oxen when they are well trained. I have taken them to the village to get fodder for the cows. Taking the cart, putting two oxen, and they are trained, they know the commands. ... So, it is not difficult to work with *trained* oxen, but it is difficult to train them.

Engagement of oxen requires training of those who engage them as well as training of the oxen. Prahlada Bhakta notes the problem of untrained trainers:

> There is a particular way to train the oxen, but because someone who does not have the knowledge [how to train them] wants to make them work, the oxen suffer, and you don't get any work done. So that knowledge is essential. We have to somehow train people to train oxen.

As an institution that has several start-up agricultural projects, ISKCON managers are sometimes faced with having inexperienced, if enthusiastic, herders and trainers. To address this problem, Syamasundara Dasa compiled a manual that anticipates this and all other, practical issues related to bovine care. Anticipating inexperienced oxen trainers, he writes,

---

[69] Interview with Prahlada Bhakta Das, 10 December 2017.

[70] Whether oxen can be engaged in work without the control of a nose rope or nose ring can depend on their breed. Gir and Tharparkar are relatively docile breeds in comparison with others. Large Western breeds of oxen need the control afforded by a nose ring, according to Antardvip Das (the oxen manager at the ISKCON-Hungary farm, which we will discuss presently).

At first the oxen will be quite nervous of many things, from putting on the yoke; the feeling of being trapped by it; the tugging on their noses; the closeness of another ox at the other end of the yoke (who may want to butt him); to the pulling of the load, etc. The trainer must be prepared for the oxen to be somewhat unpredictable and for this reason great patience and kindness should be shown towards them. They will undoubtedly make many mistakes at first, so one should be prepared and at the same time, willing to persevere. (Dasa 1998, p. 78)

An ox trainer must show "great patience and kindness" in leading new oxen into the habits they must have to perform the draught activities for which they are well suited. And the best and traditional way for a new ox trainer to learn the art is from an experienced trainer. In the absence of available personal guidance, in our Internet age, one long-experienced trainer, Balabhadra Das (William E. Dove), the founder of ISCOWP (International Society for Cow Protection), who has been training oxen over twenty-seven years, offers videos online in which he demonstrates the process in a step-by-step manner that involves the use of voice commands as the basis of gentle engagement of oxen.[71] Significantly, Balabhadra emphasizes that the first step in training oxen is making friends with them, which means spending time with them, addressing them by their names, and brushing and stroking them.

All of what has here been described in connection with bull castration, nose ropes or nose rings, and training of or working with oxen might be dismissed by some persons as clear affirmation that Hindu cow care is fraught with violent practices. Conscientious Hindus will acknowledge that there are aspects of cow care that have what some will label "violent" due to infliction of some temporary pain on bulls, and permanent denial of mating capacity. Yet Hindus will insist that, first, the dignity of bulls is not thereby compromised and, in fact, their lives are enhanced and valued more for the service they will give; thus, second, they remain protected and cared for throughout their natural lives—hardly the case for most bulls

---

[71] See, for example, "Training Oxen by Voice Commands." https://www.youtube.com/watch?v= aCJibJ4Axi8 (accessed 29 November 2018). ISCOWP's Web site has several videos: https://iscowp. org/videos/. Balabhadra's oxen are with halters, not pierced noses. ISCOWP is based in Gainesville, Florida.

that are killed soon after they are born or as soon as they reach "slaughter weight."[72] Further, they would say that one must view the composite practice as a whole—its context in the wider scheme of human living with nonhuman animals and the natural environment, as well as the spirit of those who directly engage with the cows. In my own visits to various goshalas in India, I found a variety of attitudes—some more and some less conducive to a sense that a serious effort to uphold dharmic principles is being observed. Yet in all cases and as a whole, what I saw was an important effort to demonstrate a positive alternative to the killing culture of modern agribusiness in all its pervasive forms of animal abuse and destruction.

Intangible Benefits of Bovine Care and Proximity

We have discussed bovine products—milk, dung, urine, and their derivatives—as tangible benefits from bovines. Similarly, labor of male bovines—drawing a plough or transporting goods and people—is a tangible bovine benefit. Yet as already noted, all these benefits do not add up to make the total sum of why cows are to be cared for, or why cow carers feel that all the challenges of cow care are worth the trouble. Here we will hear expressions of appreciation for cows' intangible, or non-quantifiable, benefits for humans and the environment.

Bovines as Purifying Agents

At Pathmeda I asked Swami Shri Datta Sharanananda Maharaja, the founder of this massive goshala complex in southwest Rajasthan and long-time India-wide itinerant cow care activist, how he might explain the benefits of lifelong care for cows, especially to persons unfamiliar with the ethos of Hindu cow care. Datta's extensive reply showed a deep conviction in the value of cows to render three sorts of benefit for human beings,

---

[72]Modern meat "production" functions in a globalized context with exacting calculations of "feed efficiency ratios" and the like, with the singular aim of bringing the animals up to the desired weight at which they can most profitably be slaughtered (Smil 2013, pp. 113–175).

namely benefits to *health*, to *prosperity*, and to *education*. A summary of his explanation will be useful to appreciate how a Hindu valuation of cows comprehends several aspects of human well-being.[73]

According to Datta, the general benefit of bovines resides in their power to favorably affect—to *purify*—natural elements, where "elements" are understood in terms of a classical Hindu analysis of nature.[74] According to the Bhagavad Gita (7.4), there are eight components ("elements") of gross and subtle matter, referred to as *ashtada-prakriti*. These eight components of matter, or temporal nature, are earth, water, fire, air, ether (*kham*), mind (*manas*), intelligence (*buddhi*), and ego (*ahamkara*). Considering that cows are known to favorably affect all these components of nature, Datta elaborates on how each of the three aspects of human well-being come about through human interaction with such favorably affected elements. Thus, maintenance and recovery of human health are based particularly on bovines' power to purify earth, water, and air. Earth, purified by the fertilizing dung of the cow, yields organically fertilized earth's nutrient-vegetation that we consume, contributing to the body's vigor. Water, purified by cow urine (as a disinfectant), contributes to the well-being of human bodily liquids, and air in the proximity of cows, purified by the cows' breath, ensures a healthy pulmonary system.[75]

Swami Datta next identifies properties of cows that help create and sustain prosperity. The main idea is that bovines' presence among humans fosters balance and moderation in human endeavor, specifically by their essential contribution to ritual procedures (*yajna*) for maintenance of cosmic order. As we discussed earlier, ghee produced from cows' milk, which is offered as oblation in the *yajna* fires, is understood to purify fire (one

---

[73] Interview with Swami Datta Sharanananda, 4 December 2018. For a similar appreciation of cows' positive effects on humans by Pandurang Shastri Athavale (1920–2003), founder of the Swadhyaya Parivar, see Jain (2011, pp. 39–41).

[74] The notion of "purity" and "purification" and their opposites, pollution and contamination, may signal the brahmanical ethos prevalent in Hindu discourse and, usually quite negatively valenced, in critical discourse about Hinduism. That cows and their high valuation are closely associated with brahmanical ethos seems to affirm this association. For further discussion of purity and pollution in Hindu thought and practice, focusing on bovine products, see Simoons (1974).

[75] Such understanding of cows' purifying powers and resultant human health benefits might be taken as "indigenous knowledge," to be dismissed as such. But several writers have argued strongly that such knowledge needs to be valued and recovered, as an integral feature of recovery from colonialist discourses of domination. See Henry (2015).

of the eight constituents of temporal nature). Moreover, even the lowing sound of cows purifies what is understood to be the basic medium of sound, namely "ether," or sky (*kham; akasha*).

A lack of regard for cows is directly related to the predominance of greed and avarice that characterize present-day economic enterprise—epitomized by fossil fuel extraction with the consequent environmental imbalances arising from its barely restricted use, including chemical fertilizer that poisons the earth. In terms of traditional Hindu analysis of cosmic dynamics called Samkhya (discussed in the Bhagavad Gita), the predominating present-day economic culture is permeated with nature's quality of passion (*rajo-guna*), the modality characterized by short-sighted and self-centered pursuit of ambition. In contrast, an economy rooted in due regard for cows such that they are cared for throughout their natural lives is sustainable and hence stable, thus upholding the sort of human order of prosperity characterized by the quality of illumination (*sattva-guna*).[76] In this latter case, greed and avarice can be subdued by cows' purifying—or stabilizing—effect on the mind, such that the human being's tendency to exercise oppressive control and exploitation of other beings and the environment is restrained. This effect complements cows' sobering effect on the subtlest of the eight components of nature, the "ego" (*ahamkara*) which is understood to be the sense of individuality that, in its negative aspect, is experienced as alienation, the locus of all human destructive impulses.

The third practical benefit of cows, according to Swami Datta, is their role in fostering the best conditions for human education. This aspect of human benefit arises from a dual function of giving and receiving in relation to cows. There are direct and indirect gifts of the cow that humans are able to receive. Milk and its derivatives, as well as dung and urine, are cows' direct gifts, as we have already discussed; and indirect gifts are the produce from agricultural processes in which cows are involved. That is

---

[76]We will discuss the Samkhya system of thought further in Chapter 6. Suffice to note here that it may be roughly compared to the Chinese Taoist notion of *yin/yang*, though in the Indic system there are three, rather than two, constituents, and these three are generally graded in preference from *tamas* (darkness, ignorance) to *rajas* (energy, passion) up to *sattva* (illumination, true-being) in terms of conduciveness to attain spiritual fulfillment.

to say, cows benefit education by building a character and value system of people and community engaged in their care, as integral to agricultural life.

All of these benefits foster illuminated intelligence (*sattvika-buddhi*) when received gratefully. But such benefits can only come when the cows that bestow these gifts are given proper and affectionate care in return. Such care includes providing all the necessities of maintaining them in a healthy and peaceful condition, free from anxiety. Moreover, Swami Datta emphasizes, to properly reciprocate with cows for their gifts that benefit the world, they are to be shown special regard through formal practices of veneration (*upasana*), the appropriate spirit of which is to be nourished by regular cultivation of faith (*shraddha*) that comes from hearing sacred texts—including those that extol cows—as well as hearing from and assisting persons dedicated to these texts, the *sadhus* and learned brahmins.

Learning Lessons from Cows

In thinking about intangible benefits of cow care, tangible challenges cannot be ignored. On one side, there are considerations of cow product values, including both physical products with their economic valuation and the value of intangibles, such as the sense of well-being experienced when cows are properly cared for. And still there are the costs that invariably come with proper care of cows (including costs of land, buildings, fodder, and medical costs; hired labor costs, including their needs (including proper training); and the costs for any equipment such as for milk processing).[77] For a private person who cannot expect the kind of donor support that institutional goshalas typically receive, economics becomes a major issue. The commitment required for maintaining cows in a healthy and happy condition throughout their natural lives is certainly high, and some who feel that they would otherwise want to care for cows may conclude that it is more of a commitment than they could realistically make. As we have seen, for many, the only commitment they can make for cow care is to give

---

[77]Whether or not there is hired labor, whoever takes part in the cow care activities must also be nicely maintained, with all the expenses this will involve.

regular donations to a goshala or similar institution. And yet there are also individuals for whom the personal rewards of direct cow care are worth all the trouble and expense. Of this sort of person here is one vignette. Aside from the theme of intangible bovine values, this vignette affords us a look into a very small-scale project, quite the opposite of Pathmeda with its thousands of cows.

Janmastami Das, an Indian native from a several-generations family of Krishna-*bhaktas*, cares for his 105 bovines on his three-acre farm amidst a jungle, just off the Mumbai–Ahmedabad highway a few kilometers north of Mumbai. Recalling the multiple hardships that he and his wife and son endured in establishing their project, Janmastami admits that at one time he wanted to give up and return to his former life in the city. But his wife said to him, "You can go if you like; I will stay here with the cows." Inspired by his wife's resolve, Janmastami mustered his own determination, and now, since several years, he sees his cows as his instructors, teaching him essential lessons in the culture of bhakti.

One lesson he reports to me involves the Vaishnava tradition's exhortation to cultivate humility. "By regarding oneself as lower than the straw on the ground … one can always glorify the Lord, chanting his names."[78] Janmastami explains,

> It is one thing to think oneself lower than the straw, and it is quite another thing to realize it. One day I was washing down the cowshed, hosing out the straw. There was one small piece of straw that just wouldn't move, however much I blasted it with high water pressure. Then it dawned on me: the cows, pressing the straw down repeatedly with their hooves, are showing me that if I would become *actually* humble like this straw, then the heavy forces of lust, anger, greed, envy, and so on, cannot overwhelm me.

Janmastami ties this lesson in humility to a second lesson he credits the cows with helping him to understand:

---

[78]This is from stanza 3 of the 8-stanza Shikshashtakam attributed to Sri Chaitanya (1486–1533): "By regarding oneself as lower than the straw, by being tolerant like a tree, by expecting no honor (for oneself) and offering honor to all others, one can always glorify the Lord, chanting his names" (Prabhupāda 2005 [1974], p. 1442; Chaitanya Charitamrita, Antya 20.21, my translation).

We should remember that Krishna is known as Govinda, a name that reminds us of his relationship to cows. We daily chant this name in the mantra that also includes the word *svaha* which—so we usually think—means "oblation," as one would pronounce when offering ghee in a ritual fire. In a fire ritual (*yajna*), we keep many things with us, we are not really giving up everything. But Govinda—the Lord of the cows—teaches us how to give *everything* and take full refuge in him.

Janmastami insists that taking full refuge in Krishna as Govinda is essential for one to be able to take proper care of cows. Recalling Keshi's comment on how everything necessary for cow care (at Care For Cows) is made available by the grace of Krishna's consort Radharani, we may also appreciate Janmastami's observation that if one takes refuge in Govinda, "Mother cow gives everything I need. I'm seeing now that I'm the richest person: I am able to do *seva* [service] to my parents, my guru, Krishna, and mother cow—four types of *seva*, so I am the richest person in the world."[79]

The expression *go-seva* was often used in conversations I held with cow carers and cow activists; indeed, a preferred term for themselves is *go-sevak*—one who serves cows. The idea of *serving* cows, as opposed to being served by them or being the beneficiary of cows' products, is a common theme among these Hindus. From this perspective, cow care may be regarded as an ethics of service, whereby "relational humility" (Dalmiya 2016) fructifies with a sense of inner and outer abundance.

"Keeping Cows, You Keep Your Sanity"

Another striking example of a dedicated single-family cow care project in India is that of Hrimati Dasi, a German native who lives since 1996 near the Hooghly River, a Ganges tributary, 130 kilometers upstream from Kolkata in West Bengal. As a follower of Swami Prabhupāda, for most of the twenty-two years she has lived in this area she has kept cows. Presently, she has ten–eight cows, one bull and one ox. Hrimati gives credit to the cows for her well-being—for maintaining her "sanity," as she puts it—while also expressing concern about future conditions for herself and the

---

[79] Interview with Janmastami Das, 28 November 2017.

cows. It was the milk of her first cow that, she says, sustained her and her four children when, for a time, she was without income and without the help of her husband, from whom she had separated.

> [My children and I] were living on milk, spinach, and donations of rice; the cow was giving one and a half liters' milk. Then we had a bull, and one boy came and gave a donation to make a bullock cart. After a few days, within a week, the cow was giving five liters per day. We were drinking two liters [of milk] and I could sell three liters.

Supplementing her minimal income from milk with the sale of home-made cloth dolls—forms of Krishna and his various associates—Hrimati gradually learned by trial and error how to care for her cows. She learned a key lesson from working with her first cow, Vishnupriya, a mixed reddish Sahiwal breed she had received from the nearby goshala of ISKCON, Mayapur, in the year 2000. As one of the several dozen cows in that goshala, Vishnupriya had been receiving minimal attention. Hrimati says that thereafter, under her direct care, the marked increase in attention inspired Vishnupriya to more-than-triple her daily milk yield.

Giving ample attention to individual cows is good and important for cow carers, but of course cows also need substantial daily nourishment, a constant challenge for Hrimati with the one acre of her neighbor's land she is allowed to use for growing fodder. Twenty-five to thirty kilograms of green grass fodder per cow is required, plus one and a half kilograms of grain mixture (including flax seeds, soaked chickpeas, a mineral mixture, and wheat bran or crushed maze). Keeping the cows well fed keeps them stress-free, minimizing the chance of becoming diseased. Hrimati now hires two men to assist her in feeding the cows (three times a day, plus two times a day they are led out for grazing), but their wages, plus the cost of fodder that is supplementary to what she can grow, are becoming a strain. All the children have grown up and left home, and Hrimati's own health issues give her further worries.

Yet despite the challenges, this hardy woman from the West, who now speaks fluent Bengali, considers her cows to be her family, in a place where she finds a cultural climate in which she sees at least some respect for cows.

For her, such respect and care for cows are the very substance and foundation for what she calls "living simply and depending on Krishna," a principle drawn from a motto often expressed by her guru, Swami Prabhupāda, as "plain living and high thinking."[80] Such a minimalist lifestyle ideal grounded in a sense of dependence on divine grace is, Hrimati feels, seriously compromised by high reliance on modern technology. She expresses concern about the overly convenience-dependent lifestyle of present-day Vaishnavas (both Indian and non-Indian), those who should be more closely embodying the ideal they propound:

> Prabhupada said [that Vaishnavas, devotees of Krishna, must learn] to depend on Krishna. But are we actually depending on Krishna? What are we doing different from the *karmis* [persons absorbed in self-centered activities], actually?[81]

On several occasions, Swami Prabhupāda assured his followers that if they would live on the land and take care of cows, all their needs would be fulfilled.[82] Hrimati Dasi, although continually challenged by material conditions, goes on caring for her cows, bolstered by faith in her guru's words and in Krishna.

Go-seva and Bhakti

Indeed, in the practice of Krishna-bhakti, according to the sacred texts, the initial step on this path is to have at least a minimal sense of faith (*shraddha*) that the practice of bhakti and the object of bhakti (Krishna) are true and real. Such initial faith is then nourished by regular practice,

---

[80] For example, in a letter to his student Hayagriva Das (June 1968), referring to a newly acquired farm in West Virginia that would become New Vrindavan, Swami Prabhupāda wrote: "It may be an ideal village where the residents will have plain living and high thinking. For plain living we must have sufficient land for raising crops and pasturing grounds for the cows. If there is sufficient grains and production of milk, then the whole economic problem is solved" (Prabhupāda 2017, Vedabase: Letter to Hayagriva—Montreal 14 June, 1968).

[81] Interview with Hrimati Devi, Mayapur, West Bengal, 22 January 2018.

[82] Swami Prabhupāda writes in his Bhagavata Purāṇa commentary (to v. 9.15.25): "The whole world must learn from Kṛṣṇa how to live happily without scarcity simply by producing food grains (*annād bhavanti bhūtāni* [Bhagavad-gita 3.14]) and giving protection to the cows (*go-rakṣya*)."

essential to which is menial service for one's preceptor, the guru. We may recall the story of the student of the guru in the Upanishad (Chapter 2) caring for the guru's cows. This same tradition continues today.

One Vrindavan *sadhu*, Satya Narayan Das Baba, remembers how his own guru, the late Shri Haridas Shastri, a highly learned Sanskrit sacred text scholar and author, would, despite study and teaching duties, spend most of his day with the cows in his goshala. He would say to his Vaishnava theology students,

> We are worshipers of Krishna, who is Gopal [the divine cowherd], and Krishna himself took personally care of the cows. Krishna has the *abhiman* [the mood] of a cowherd boy. That is his identity, and if we want to be with him, then we have to get into that mood. … If you attain perfection and go to [the eternal atemporal realm] Vrindavan, what will you be doing there? If you are a cowherd boy [in your eternal, spiritual identity] you will be taking care of cows; if you are a *gopi* [cowherdess, as your eternal identity] you will still be taking care of the cows. So, we better start practicing, doing it here [in this world]!

The "practice" being referred to in this exhortation is a regimen of devotional activities (*sadhana-bhakti*) that dedicated Krishna devotees, *bhaktas*, daily perform. This practice is designed to maximize one's attention to the service and remembrance of Krishna as both the supreme person, or God (*bhagavan*), and the absolute reality (*satyam param*). Such practice, rooted in teachings of the Bhagavad Gita and Bhagavata Purana, aims at constantly endeavoring to absorb one's consciousness in Krishna in the course of one's life. Thus, one can look forward to attaining Krishna's eternal realm, there to be ever freed from the repetition of death and rebirth and to participate perpetually in Krishna's ever-new "pastimes," or divine play (*lila*).[83] As such practice necessarily involves activity with

---

[83]The details of how *sadhana-bhakti* is to be practiced are extensively elaborated in the two texts mentioned, as well as in commentaries to these and in later works composed by practitioner-preceptors. The Bhagavad-gita provides basic instructions for the practice of devotional, Krishna-directed activities, indicating that the result of successful practice is to attain, after death, Krishna's "state of being; of this there is no doubt" (Bhagavad-gita 8.5; Goswami 2015 trans.). For a study of bhakti practices in the Vaishnava Hindu tradition (including meditation on Krishna as he is situated in Vraja with the cows), see Holdrege (2015, especially Chapters 5 and 6).

one's physical body and mind, and since care for cows necessarily involves the practitioner with the world and bodily necessities, this practice is seen as an ideal way to position oneself in this world so as to connect with the atemporal realm to which the atemporal self (*atman*) permanently belongs.

Clearly, such an understanding of cow care, as a Vaishnava Hindu spiritual practice, partakes in what today is a quite rarefied and rarely seen sphere of human cultural values.[84] Yet it is arguably from such an ideational locus of bhakti practice that we can best appreciate what it is that drives Hindu cow care that is connected with the practice of Krishna-bhakti. Put simply, for Krishna-*bhaktas*, by caring for cows they regard as belonging to Krishna, the cows reciprocate in such ways that the *bhaktas'* devotion to Krishna is enriched and strengthened.[85]

Ritual Bovine Veneration: Creating and Affirming Community

In Chapter 2, we encountered a Sanskrit ritual manual, the *Gavārcanaprayoga*, "Procedure for the Worship of Cows," and we noted that it includes rituals both for the benefit of cows and benefit for humans from the cows, including a mantra for protection *by* cows. What is not

---

[84]According to the Pathmeda goshala organization, they have succeeded in helping "thousands" of people to become free from addictions by doing *go-seva*, service to cows (Dattasharanananda 2017, back cover). Whatever truth there is to the claim, it points to a general notion I heard several times from cow carers—that cows have a calming and "purifying" effect on the mind when one engages in their service.

[85]One striking story of dedication to the service of Krishna's cows was told to me by Raju, a resident of Govardhan (in the area of Vraja) and cowherd for the thirty cows of one Ukrainian resident, Arca Murti Dasi. Raju suffered an accident while servicing an electrical inverter when the device's liquid acid exploded onto his body and face, completely blinding him. While being cared for by his family at home after returning from the hospital (where he had been informed that he would never see again), at night he dreamt that Surabhi, the senior cow of the herd he had been taking care of, appeared and spoke to him, complaining of his neglect. In the dream, he explained to her what had happened to him, saying, "If you bless me with eyesight, I can again care for you." Within a few days his eyesight was fully restored, a recovery that he fully credits this cow for giving him, inspiring him to vow that he would always, for the rest of his life, serve Krishna's cows (interview with Arca Murti and Raju, 14 February 2019).

stated explicitly in this manual, but is nonetheless significant, is that cows create community, in particular by way of ritual performance dedicated to cows.

Among nine types of activities practiced and promoted in relation to cows at the Gaudham Mahatirtha Anandvan goshala complex at Pathmeda, three activities stress the importance given to ritual practices in relation to cows. It bears emphasizing that these practices are understood to be essential for affirming the proper place and function of human beings in relation to the cosmic order in the broadest sense.[86] This is the order expressed by the term dharma, which, in turn, is upheld when cows are served and, on occasion, formally honored in a hospitality ritual known as *puja*.[87] Important to note is that these rituals—much simplified today from the ancient rituals indicated in Chapters 2 and 3—are most often public events that constitute focal points of spiritual retreats attended by guests—typically urban people who are regular donors and who identify with the mission of the project.[88] Such a ritual of *go-puja*—honoring of cows—was underway when I visited there in late 2017. Each of some fifty guests was simultaneously presenting the prescribed auspicious items to a respective cow standing opposite them, while a priest guided them through the actions and chanted the appropriate mantras, all in the duration of well over an hour. As one might expect, the venerated cows showed little interest in the proceedings, except toward the end as they were offered delectable snacks! For us to note is that the event brought the guests together in a common ritual activity, in effect creating a temporary community that had as its identity the veneration of bovines, thereby transforming the cows, for a time, into a sort of collective "bovinity," or bovine-divinity.

---

[86]These three rituals refer to acts that acknowledge three out of five congenital debts. See Chapter 5, "Dharma as settled duty" and Chapter 5 footnote 6 for an explanation. *Sattva-puja* responds to the debt to divinities; *srishthi-yajna* responds to the debt to ancestors; and *svadhyaya* responds to the debt to the sages (*rishis*). The ritual veneration of cows is, according to the tradition followed by Pathmeda, integral to the complex of these rites.

[87]For a survey of *puja* theory and practice in Hindu traditions, see Valpey (2010).

[88]At the Pathmeda event I observed in 2017, some 200 guests had assembled, of whom around 50 participated in the *go-puja*. There prevailed a lighthearted atmosphere of jovial camaradarie among the guests, blended with a sense of earnestness in showing reverence to the cows, particularly in the presence of the highly respected Swami Datta Sharanananda.

Up to now, I have a few times invoked the term "bovinity" to call attention to Hindu regard for bovines as sharing in and embodying divinity in animal form. As we look at the ritual dimension of Hindu cow care, we do well to pause and look more closely at the theological reasoning in this notion. I draw again from Swami Datta Sharanananda, quoting from his preface to *Gavārcanaprayoga*, the previously mentioned ritual manual for venerating cows. Swami Datta begins by explaining why specifically *cows* are venerable.

> In every hair of the universal mother, *go-mata*, reside the countless divinities. By venerating *go-mata*, the celestials, sages, ancestors, and all beings— moving and non-moving, conscious and non-conscious—are satisfied. Go- mata alone in the form of earth shelters all moving and non-moving beings in her lap, and thus in both forms [as cow and as earth] she provides them nourishment. … If there is just one cow in the home that is served daily, it is as if all the celestials, sages, ancestors, Vedas, sacred rites, and so on, being attended, are all kept satisfied. By using the substances from cows for sacred rites (*yajna*) and so on, the basis of protection for bovines and their servants is at hand.

Swami Datta goes on to explain that of five major divinities, four of which are male in gender, the one feminine Maha-Shakti is most important, as all benefits coming from the male divinities' worship come about only by her grace. He then explains that there are varieties of veneration, depending on the motivation of the worshiper. The highest form, which is very rare, is extremely secret (*gopaniya*), bringing benefit for all beings. Further, there are two types of worship, depending on the object of worship—either a physical form made of earth (or earth-based, that is, stone or metal) or else a living form. Of the latter, the only form that is authorized (*svikrita*) is that of Shri Surabhi Go-Mata—mother cow, who is the blessed divine Surabhi.

The identification of cows in general with the divine Surabhi (includ- ing males—one hears the term *go-vamsh*, an inclusive term for male and female cows) locates cows as representative of the divine feminine which, in turn, is identified with the earth as the source of sustenance for all beings and, more abstractly, with *prakriti*, nature as a whole. Thus, cows manifest the divine-and-natural feminine, over against the divine-and-human male principle, *purusha*, which is present in all humans (but in fact in all living beings, according to Samkhya philosophy) whether the body is male or female. According to Swami Datta, the rare persons who comprehend these identities will naturally venerate cows, knowing that by doing so all of nature will be venerated and all beings (*purushas*), being supported and sheltered by venerated nature, will be satisfied and peaceful. The rarity of this understanding, Swami Datta implies, is due to the fact that the vast majority of people seek satisfaction for themselves and their immediate circle of friends and family. Such persons are likely to venerate predominant male divinities—Brahma, Shiva, Vishnu, or Ganesh—thus missing the opportunity to be instrumental in benefiting the whole world through veneration of Surabhi.

There is a sense, then, that cow veneration serves to affirm and celebrate the existence of an all-inclusive community of living beings. As ritual action, cow veneration as conceived here partakes of the broader cosmic cycle of which Krishna speaks in the Bhagavad Gita, centered on the practice of sacrificial rites (*yajna*). One may regard *puja* as a simplified and democratized form of *yajna*, whereby humans act as agents for cosmic regeneration by performing ritual offerings to invisible divinities. In the case of cow veneration, cows are very much visible and alive, their tangible presence offsetting the intangibles they represent.

In contrast to the *go-puja* at Pathmeda just described, which created a temporary sense of community among the congregants, here is a brief description of a similar, but much smaller-scale cow veneration rite observed at GEV. The point of contrast is not just the scale, but the fact that this is a residential community. Prahlad Bhakta tells how, through one particularly inspiring occasion of celebration involving veneration of the cows, he came to realize just how uplifting such a community can be when serving the cows together:

> To conclude the Govardhan Puja festival, we brought two cows and an old ox from the *goshala*. We decorated them with colored cloth on their backs, flower garlands, and sindhur [red powder] hand prints on their sides. While everyone gathered around and sang *kirtan*, the *brahmacharis* [student monks] were offering the standard sixteen items [to the bovines], and

I recited the appropriate Sanskrit mantras, reading from a book I had, containing directions for *go-puja*.[89] We felt so nice; after the festival everyone was commenting, "We feel so happy in our hearts right now. It is such a joyful environment, we can feel the change."

From the perspective of Hindu cow care tradition, the sense of a "joyful environment" could be explained as affirmation that the proper relationship between humans and animals is being manifested, whereby humans show (day by day, and occasionally through ritual) their gratitude to the animals for their gifts; and that such joyfulness is indicative that cosmic order, dharma, is being upheld.

As a summary of the varieties of ways that cows are seen as benefiting the human world, we may recall the Rigveda verse from Chapter 2 (RV 6.28.6):

> You fatten even the thin man, o cows. You make even one without beauty to have a lovely face. You make the house blessed, o you of blessed speech. Your vigor is declared loftily in the assemblies.

Cows can bring well-being to all, and significantly, they are represented here as possessing "blessed speech," suggesting that language is somehow involved in their having beneficent power. Cows "speak" to humans in such ways that humans feel compelled to respond—to care—about and for them.

Concluding Reflections

This chapter began with accounts of urban cows in India as victims of modernization and industrialization and of how organizations and individuals respond with cow shelters, efforts at attentive Care For Cows' welfare, and

---

[89]As described in Chapter 2, Krishna lifts Mount Govardhan in defiance of Indra. Krishna had advised the Vrindavan residents to offer a feast to Govardhan rather than to Indra, and to venerate the cows. This episode is celebrated annually by Vaishnava Hindus in autumn. *Kirtan* is typically congregational singing of Krishna's names, in call-and-response fashion. Sixteen items of worship include waving of ghee-soaked cotton wick lamps before the cows, and giving them pleasing food, such as bananas and jaggery.

various attempts to raise public awareness and involvement. As cows are left to scavenge human refuse, they ingest "foreign" matter,[90] themselves having become literal outcasts as if they had been made members of social "outcaste" groups. Yet at the same time, paradoxically, these same cows—in particular *deshi* (indigenous breed) cows—are revered as *go-mata* (or *gau-mata*)—mother cow—and as such, many Hindus sympathetic to Hindu nationalist ideology identify cows (again, in particular those of indigenous breeds) metonymically with the land of India as sacred land. With such identifications, cows' bodies have become the sites of multiple battles in India.[91] The contours of these battles may be conceived variously. In a broad sense, for some Hindus, they take on the bigger-than-life dimension of a civilizational struggle—of a quickly degrading land struggling to recover what is regarded as pristine tradition. On the well-intentioned side of this narrative, there are people—not only Hindus—who want to see that cows are protected in a protective culture that resonates with the sense of dignity for all beings implicit in the notion of *sanatana-dharma*, enduring cosmic order. But on the dark side of what appears to be the same narrative is an increase—rather than a decrease—in violence, when "cow vigilantes" or Islamophobic Hindu villagers engage in lynching of (typically Muslim) cow butchers or beef eaters. Thus, the cow, "a poem of pity," as we have seen M. K. Gandhi referred to them (Gandhi 1999, vol. 24, p. 373), continues to be highly politicized in India, as we saw in the previous chapter. Simultaneously, they are objects of benumbed indifference at worse or of tolerance at best, as cows roam cities and towns, causing the occasional traffic jam if not getting hit or killed by reckless drivers.

Here our concern has been with the connections between the routine practices of cow care, the economics of such care, engagement with cow products, and what may be called a "missionizing orientation" to these practices, tethered to an ideology of modern Hindu thought, with its wide variety of inflections. Bovine utility rates high in the calculus of cow

---

[90]The play on the word "foreign" is intentional: The inorganic products of industry ingested by cows can be seen as having their origin in the globalized industrial complex of which India has become increasingly a part (since at least the eighteenth century).

[91]In the West, cows have also been the object of intense struggle over ownership, grazing rights, and questions of disease causes and proliferation. See Carlson (2002).

care values that range from physical, economic, and ritual value of living bovine products—milk, dung, urine, and traction—to intangibles such as purity and social upliftment. And all these are tied to, or in tension with, ethical values, especially nonviolence (ahimsa), animal welfare, animal rights, and human rights. By focusing on cow care practices especially at cow shelters (goshalas), this chapter serves to locate attempts to bring these values into balance in specific sites of human organization set apart from the sites of agribusiness and dairy industry. I have purposefully dwelt on specifics of living bovine utility, since all of these—tangible and intangible goods—are greatly emphasized by most if not all Hindu cow carers and activists.

"To bring these values into balance" is a way of expressing the notion of dharma, which I have mentioned a few times in this and the previous chapters. Here we can anticipate a point to be treated further in the next chapter: In classical Sanskrit texts such as the Mahabharata, dharma is sometimes designated as one of four "human aims" (*purusha arthas*), and the other three being satisfaction of desire (*kama*); pursuit of wealth (*artha*); and pursuit of freedom (*moksha*). The point to note here is simply that cow care as the pursuit of right action (dharma), when linked to valuing of living bovine tangible utility, can be viewed as ethics oriented toward the pursuit of desire and wealth. When linked with bovine intangible utility, dharma can be seen as ethics oriented toward the pursuit of freedom. Yet even if dharma serves to balance these pursuits by facilitating all of them in harmony with higher order, these aims remain in the realm of selfish interest (rooted, according to Samkhya thought, in *ahamkara* or "ego") and hence are the stuff of anthropocentrism, or the sense that all values are rooted in human interests. "Anthropocentrism" is another name for human alienation from nature. Thus, according to Vaishnavas, cow care that is divorced from the devotional principle, or the bhakti paradigm, even if practiced for the sake of dharma, is sure to perpetuate a sense of alienation. As a result, the principle of dharma that is so highly valued, nonviolence, remains imperfectly achieved. This is why I have selected each of the goshala projects briefly examined in this chapter. What they all have in common is, in my perception, a strong bhakti ethos, such that there prevails a sense that the cows are cared for as vulnerable, and very wonderful, creatures—*beings* in their own right, rather than objects of ownership (Johnson 2012, pp. 100–122).

This and the previous chapters serve as background for Chapter 5. This background is essential to appreciate the literary, historical, and current living context in which one major sphere of Hindu animal ethics concern—that of cows—has unfolded. In the next chapter, we step back for a more theoretical and wide-angle view of Hindu animal ethics, keeping in mind the specific concern of cow care. Then, in Chapter 6, we refocus on bovines to explore possible futures for their care.

References

Ahimsa Milk Dairy. n.d. https://www.ahimsamilk.org/. Accessed 30 November 2018.

Banta, Jim E., J. W. Lee, G. Hodgkin, Z. Yi, A. Fanica, and J. Sabate. 2018. The Global Influence of the Seventh-Day Adventists on Diet. *Religions* 9(251). https://doi.org/10.3390/rel9090251.

Baviskar, Amita. 2016. Cows, Cars and Cycle-Rickshaws: Bourgeois Environmentalists and the Battle for Delhi's Streets. In *Elite and Everyman: The Cultural Politics of the Indian Middle Classes*, ed. Amita Baviskar and Raka Ray, 392–418. London: Routledge.

Biswas, Soutik. 2018. The Myth of the Indian Vegetarian Nation. BBC News, 4 April. https://www.bbc.com/news/world-asia-india-43581122. Accessed 7 February 2019.

Bowles, Allen. 2018. Law During Emergencies: *Appaddharma*. In *Oxford History of Hinduism—Hindu Law: A New History of Dharmaśāstra*, ed. Patrick Olivelle and Donald R. Davis, Jr. Oxford: Oxford University Press.

Carlson, Laurie Winn. 2002. *Cattle: An Informal Social History*. Chicago: Ivan R. Dee Publisher.

Chakravarti, A.K. 1985. Cattle Development Problems and Programs in India: A Regional Analysis. *GeoJournal* 10 (1): 21–45.

Dalmiya, Vrinda. 2016. *Caring to Know: Comparative Care Ethics, Feminist Epistemology, and the Mahābhārata*. New Delhi: Oxford University Press.

Dasa, Syamasundara, and Stuart Coyle. 1998. *Protecting Cows: A Handbook of the Principles & Practices of Vegetarian Cow Husbandry*. Hove, Sussex, UK: HATAGRA.

Dattaśaraṇānand, S. Saṁvat 2073/2017. *Kāmadhenu Kṛpā Prasād* (The Merciful Blessings of the Wish-Fulfilling Cow). Pathmeḍā, Rajasthan, India: Shri Kamdhenu Prakashan Samiti.

Dhama, K., R.S. Chauhan, and L. Singhal. 2005. Anti-Cancer Activity of Cow Urine: Current Status and Future Directions. *International Journal of Cow Science* 1 (2): 1–25.

Dorman, Eric R. 2011. Hinduism and Science: The State of the South Asian Science and Religion Discourse. *Zygon* 46 (3): 593–619.

Doron, A., and R. Jeffrey. 2018. *Waste of a Nation: Garbage and Growth in India.* Cambridge, MA: Harvard University Press.

Gadgil, Madhav, and Ramachandra Guha. 1995. *Ecology and Equity: The Use and Abuse of Nature in Contemporary India.* London: Routledge.

Gandhi, Mohandas K. 1999. *The Collected Works of Mahatma Gandhi (CWMG).* New Delhi: Publications Division Government of India.

Gandhiok, Jasjeev. 2019. Gaushalas Haven't Got Promised Delhi Government, Corporation Funds for a Year. *Times of India*, 16 January. https://timesofindia.indiatimes.com/city/delhi/gaushalas-havent-got-promised-delhi-government-corporation-funds-for-a-year/articleshow/67548865.cms?fbclid=Iw%E2%80%A6. Accessed 12 February 2019.

Ganguli, Kisari Mohan, trans. 1991 [1970]. *The Mahabharata of Krishna-Dwaipayana Vyasa.* New Delhi: Motilal Banarsidass.

Goswami, H.D. 2015. *A Comprehensive Guide to Bhagavad-Gītā with Literal Translation.* Gainesville, FL: Krishna West.

Henry, Paget. 2015. Indigenous Knowledge: An Engagement with George Sefa Dei. *Confluence: Online Journal of World Philosophies* 2. https://scholarworks.iu.edu/iupjournals/index.php/confluence/issue/view/26.

Holdrege, Barbara A. 2015. *Bhakti and Embodiment: Fashioning Divine Bodies and Devotional Bodies in Kṛṣṇa Bhakti.* London: Routledge.

Human Development Report. 2004. Punjab. Government of Punjab.

IIT Delhi Students Fight Air Pollution By Replacing Wood With Cow Dung Logs For Cremating Dead, 21 October 2018. https://amp.indiatimes.com/news/india/iit-delhi-students-fight-air-pollution-by-replacing-wood-with-cow-dung-logs-for-cremating-dead-355168.html?fbclid=IwAR0GWQRsPvdQE_bE5HPpmJKl43cM9EDhsC1S-iajw2hHxxliW0AES_AmI5M. Accessed 6 December 2018.

Jacob, Ludwig M. 2014. *Dr. Jacobs Weg des genussvollen Verzichts: Die effektivsten Maßnahmen zur Prävention und Therapie von Zivilisationskrankheiten.* Heidesheim am Rhein: NutricaMEDia.

Jain, Pankaj. 2011. *Dharma and Ecology of Hindu Communities: Sustenance and Sustainability*. Farnham, UK: Ashgate.

Jain, N.P., V.B. Gupta, R. Garg, N. Silawat. 2010. Efficacy of Cow Urine Therapy on Various Cancer Patients in Mandsaur District, India—A Survey. *International Journal of Green Pharmacy* (January–March). https://doi.org/10.4103/0973-8251.62163.

Jha, Shiv Pujan. 2017. Uttar Pradesh: Here's Why People Abandon Cows in Bundelkhand. https://www.indiatoday.in/india/story/abandoned-cows-bundelkhand-anna-pratha-vigilante-groups-972987-2017-04-22#close-overlay. Accessed 30 November 2018.

Johnson, Lisa. 2012. *Power, Knowledge, Animals*. New York: Palgrave Macmillan.

Kennedy, Uttara, Arvind Sharma, and Clive J. C. Phillips. 2018. The Sheltering of Unwanted Cattle, Experiences in India and Implications for Cattle Industries Elsewhere. *Animals* 8(64). https://doi.org/10.3390/ani8050064.

Khanna, Sujoy Dr., Maneka Sanjay Gandhi, and Meenakshi Awasthi. 2017. *Gaushala*. New Delhi: People for Animals.

Khare, R.S. (ed.). 1992. *The Eternal Food: Gastronomic Ideas and Experience of Hindus and Buddhists*. Albany, NY: State University of New York Press.

Lodrick, Deryck O. 1981. *Sacred Cows, Sacred Places: Origins and Survivals of Animal Homes in India*. Berkeley: University of California Press.

Mahias, Marie-Claude. 1987. Milk and Its Transmutations in Indian Society. *Food and Foodways* 2 (1): 265–288. https://doi.org/10.1080/07409710.1987.9961921.

'Maithilaḥ' Paṇḍita Gaṅgādharapāṭhakaḥ. Vikram S. 2068/2011. *Gavārcanaprayogaḥ–Saṭīka-tippaṇī-vibhūṣita-gosambandhi-vividhānuṣṭhāna-samanvitaḥ*. Pathmeḍa, Rajasthan: Śrī Kāmadhenu Prakāśana Samitiḥ.

Malakoff, Peter. 2005. Ghee: A Short Consideration from an Ayurvedic Perspective. http://www.ancientorganics.com/ghee-a-short-consideration-from-an-ayurvedic-perspective/. Accessed 8 June 2019.

Marshall, Michael. 2019. Why Humans Have Evolved to Drink Milk. http://www.bbc.com/future/story/20190218-when-did-humans-start-drinking-cows-milk. Accessed 21 February 2019.

Mohanty, Ipsita, M.R. Senapati, D. Jena, and S. Palai. 2014. Diversified Uses of Cow Urine. *International Journal of Pharmacy and Pharmaceutical Sciences* 6 (3): 20–22.

NA. n.d. *Cow Protection—Book 1*. Moundsville, WV: ISKCON Ministry of Cow Protection and Agriculture.

NA. n.d. *Guidelines on Animal Traction*. Pretoria: Directorate, Animal and Aquaculture Production.

NA. n.d. *Kāmadhenu Kṛṣi Tantra Kisān Praśikṣaṇ Śibir Pustikā* (Kamadhenu Farming Techniques Farmer Training Camp Pamphlet). Nagpur, India: Go Vigyan Anusandhan Kendra.

NA. n.d. *Research Activity Book*. Nagpur, India: Go Vigyan Anusandhan Kendra & Gorakshan Sabha.

Nagy, Kelsi. 2019. The Sacred and Mundane Cow: The History of India's Cattle Protection Movement. In *The Routledge Handbook of Religion and Animal Ethics*, ed. Andrew Linzey and Clair Linzey. London: Routledge.

Narayanan, Yamini. 2017. Cow Protectionism and Indian Animal Advocacy: The Fracturing and Fusing of Social Movements, 14 July 2017. https://archive.org/details/YaminiN. Accessed 6 December 2018.

Padmanabhan, Seetha, and V. Varadachari (eds.). 1982. *Padma Saṁhitā*. Chennai: Pancaratra Parisodhana Parisad.

Pallavi, Aparna. 2015. The Deshi Cow Milk Jinx. *Down to Earth*, 7 June 2015. https://www.downtoearth.org.in/blog/the-deshi-cow-milk-jinx-45095. Accessed 17 February 2019.

Prabhupāda, A.C. Bhaktivedanta Swami. 2005. *Śrī Caitanya-Caritāmṛta of Kṛṣṇadāsa Kavirāja Gosvāmī* (One Volume Edition). Los Angeles: Bhaktivedanta Book Trust.

Prabhupāda, A.C. Bhaktivedanta Swami. 2017. *The Complete Teachings of His Divine Grace A. C. Bhaktivedanta Swami Prabhupāda*. Vedabase CD-ROM Version 2017.2. Sandy Ridge, NC: Bhaktivedanta Archives.

Rangarajan, L.N. (ed.). 1992. *Kautilya: The Arthashastra*. New Delhi: Penguin.

Rastogi, Sanjeev, and Krishna Kaphle. 2011. Sustainable Traditional Medicine: Taking the Inspirations from Ancient Veterinary Science. *Evidence-Based Complementary and Alternative Medicine*. http://dx.doi.org/10.1093/ecam/nen071.

Roy, Tirthankar. 2017. Land Quality, Carrying Capacity and Sustainable Agricultural Change in Twentieth-Century India. In *Economic Development and Environmental History in the Anthropocene: Perspectives on Asia and Africa*, 159–178. London: Bloomsbury Academic.

Satyanarayana, T., B.N. Johri, and A. Prakash (eds.). 2012. *Microorganisms in Sustainable Agriculture and Biotechnology*. Dordrecht: Springer.

Schmidt, Ron. 2009. *The Untold Story of Milk*. Revised ed. Washington, DC: New Trends Publishing.

Scholten, Bruce A. 2010. *Operation Flood, Food Aid, and Development*. London: I.B. Tauris.

Sharma, B.V.V.S.R. 1980. *The Study of Cow in Sanskrit Literature*. Delhi: GDK Publications.

Shiva, Vandana. 2016. *Who Really Feeds the World? The Failures of Agribusiness and the Promise of Agroecology*. Berkeley, CA: North Atlantic Books.

Simoons, Frederick J. 1974. The Purificatory Role of the Five Products of the Cow in Hinduism. *Ecology of Food and Nutrition* 3(1), 21–34. http://dx.doi.org/10.1080/03670244.1974.9990358. Accessed 8 August 2017.

Sinha, S.N. (ed.). 2016. *Cow Keeping in India*. 5th ed. (1st ed. 1891, I.S.A. Tweed). New Delhi: Biotech Books.

Smil, Vaclav. 2013. *Should We Eat Meat? Evolution and Consequences of Modern Carnivory*. Oxford: Wiley-Blackwell.

Smith, David. 2003. *Hinduism and Modernity*. Oxford: Blackwell.

Somvanshi, R. 2006. Veterinary Medicine and Animal Keeping in Ancient India. *Asian Agri-History* 10 (2): 133–146.

Sun Jianxin, Xu, Xia Lu Leiming, Gregory W. Yelland, Jiayi Ni, and Andrew J. Clarke. 2016. Effects of Milk Containing Only A2 Beta Casein Versus Milk Containing Both A1 and A2 Beta Casein Proteins on Gastrointestinal Physiology, Symptoms of Discomfort, and Cognitive Behavior of People with Self-Reported Intolerance to Traditional Cows' Milk. *Nutrition Journal* 15: 35. https://doi.org/10.1186/s12937-016-0147-z.

Taking Pain Out of Cattle Castration is Among Animal Welfare Reforms Now Required in India. n.d. https://www.petaindia.com/media/taking-pain-cattle-castration-among-animal-welfare-reforms-now-required-india/. Accessed 29 November 2018.

Tiwari, Lalit. n.d. Animal Husbandry and Cattle Management in Arthashastra. http://www.indianscience.org/essays/t_es_arthasastra_husbandry.shtml. Accessed 24 August 2017.

Toomey, Paul M. 1994. *Food from the Mouth of Krishna: Feasts and Festivals in a North Indian Pilgrimage Centre*. Delhi: Hindustan Publishing Corporation.

Turnbull, Jonathan. 2017. Got Milk? Material Biopolitics and More-Than-Human Health at the *Gaushala*. Unpublished MSc. dissertation, University of Oxford.

Valpey, Kenneth. 2010. Pūjā and Darśana. In *The Brill Encyclopedia of Hinduism*, vol. 2. Amsterdam: Brill.

Velten, Hannah. 2010. *Milk: A Global History*. London: Reaktion Books.

World Animal Protection. 2014. A Case Study of High Welfare Milk Production in India. https://www.worldanimalprotection.org.in/sites/default/files/in_files/high-welfare-milk-production-india.pdf. Accessed 23 November 2018.

5

Cow Care and the Ethics of Care

My aims in this chapter are, first, to show a way of approaching animal ethics broadly speaking through the lens of Hindu thought, while keeping the focus on cow care as a value to be pursued and realized. Here the question can be phrased, how can Hindu thought contribute to a general discourse on animal ethics? The second aim is to bring non-Indian (Western) animal ethics thought to bear on Hindu animal ethics (including the pursuit of cow care). What elements of Western animal ethics discourse can complement and make more comprehensive, persuasive, and comprehensible, the traditional Hindu (or Indic) discourse, leading toward a more inclusive and comprehensive vision of nonhuman animal care while also giving appropriate place for cow care in particular?

Our discussion will revolve largely around three key terms found in Hindu traditions, two of which we already encountered in Chapter 2, namely *dharma* and *bhakti*. A third term, *yoga* (briefly alluded to in that chapter), will also be important. These terms, each with their respective (and overlapping) semantic fields, are central to early brahmanical Hindu texts (also already introduced in Chapter 2) including the Mahabharata

© The Author(s) 2020
K. R. Valpey, *Cow Care in Hindu Animal Ethics*,
The Palgrave Macmillan Animal Ethics Series,
https://doi.org/10.1007/978-3-030-28408-4_5

(with its important dialogue on ethics, the Bhagavad Gita) and the Bhagavata Purana. An additional relevant classical text to be introduced here is Patanjali's Yoga Sutras (YS), a highly influential work on the philosophy and practice of yoga. Yoga, an important current in Hindu thought and practice since ancient times, may be seen as a conceptual and practical link in the "polarity of value" identified in Chapter 2, serving to integrate dharma and bhakti into a comprehensive worldview from which ethical thought and action unfold. Because each of the terms—dharma, yoga, and bhakti—carry significance characteristic of conceptual "patterns," we will have occasion to refer to each as *paradigms*—the *dharma paradigm*, the *yoga paradigm*, and the *bhakti paradigm* (Long 2013).

From the Western perspective, we will give attention mainly to the recently developed *ethics of care* discourse, particularly as applied to animals. We will also consider *animal rights* discourse, particularly as reconceived in terms of (domestic) animals-as-citizens, a notion that will lead us into a brief discussion concerning the politics of cow care, especially in light of *anticipatory communities* (Rasmussen 2013) as locations of a *dharma-based communitarian* political theory to support animal care. In the course of this discussion, I consider *abolitionist* objections to animal citizenship in relation to Hindu cow care to argue, in part, that while a reduction of dairy consumption by humans may be appropriately called for, rather than complete elimination of dairy consumption (and thereby the ultimate abolition of bovine domestication), a positive dharmic, yogic, and bhakti ethic of cow care best serves the higher ideal of freedom and felicity for all beings. Ultimately what is aimed for is a sense of devotional *service* (*seva*), as both means and goal of realizing the good.

Dharma and Animal Ethics

Dharma is a major sphere of Hindu thought and practice that necessarily contributes to any discussion of animal ethics. This may be obvious, since it is generally regarded as that sphere of Hindu thought particularly concerned with duty, law, and the sustaining of social and cosmic order. Along with the normative dimension of dharma is its equally important descriptive aspect. As description, dharma can mean nature, character, peculiar condition, essential quality, or property. We might call it the *is* aspect of the *is* versus *ought* distinction in ethical discourse. Dharma as normativity corresponds to the *ought* dimension, whereby the term approximates notions of "good works, practice, customary observance or prescribed conduct" (Monier-Williams [1899] 1995, pp. 510–511). These two dimensions combined point to dharma as the sphere of human culture that aims to bridge (or close) the gap between *is* and *ought*.[1] In other words, dharma aims to effectively address the reality of an ever-contingent world of fault, danger, and disorder (all implied in the term *adharma*, the lack of or opposition to dharma)[2] with the appropriate vision and means to realize what ought to be (the good).

Considering animal ethics in terms of dharma, we must note two different yet overlapping aspects of dharma's normativity. The first aspect comprehends act-centered, moral obligational, deontic (duty-based) ethics, in terms of both deontology and consequentialism (Fink 2013, pp. 669–670), in what we may refer to respectively as *dharma as settled duty* and *dharma as deliberation on duty*. Dharma as settled duty is typically based on what are considered clear and fixed identities, such as one's *varna* (brahmin, kshatriya, and so on).[3] Dharma as deliberation is

---

[1]Thus, a modern Western parallel can be found in Immanuel Kant, with his project to "maintain a balance between the actual and the possible" (see Neiman 2008, p. 137). Frazier (2017, p. 154), discussing structuring practices in Hindu traditions and referring to anthropologist Clifford Geertz, notes: "Like Geertz's model of a worldview, the various structuring practices of Hinduism thus have two dimensions in that they are both *descriptive*, highlighting the potential for order in the world, and also *prescriptive*, encouraging human beings to help create and sustain that order."

Sanskrit texts concerned with dharma also emphasize that it is *humans* who practice, or observe, or uphold dharma, whereas nonhuman animals—though doubtless pursuing their purposes in wonderful ways (Nussbaum 2011, pp. 239–240)—cannot be said to pursue dharma in its normative sense. A well-known Sanskrit proverb in the *Hitopadeśa* of Narayaṇa states (0.30), "Eating, sleeping, feeling afraid and copulating—these things men have in common with animals. But man distinguishes himself by doing his duties [dharma]; those who neglect them are like beasts" (Törzsök 2007, p. 67). This distinction in no way gives license for humans to exploit animals, and neither does it forbid humans to engage with animals in non-exploitative ways.

[2]See Glucklich (1994, pp. 7–10) and *passim* for a phenomenological study of dharma and *adharma*. Here, I focus mainly on textual expressions of these terms.

[3]The modern term "caste" refers generally to what in India is called *jati*—one's clan-related identity associated more or less with occupation and assumed to be determined by birth. Some 3000 *jatis* have been identified in modern India. *Varna*, on the other hand, is a broad, fourfold categorization that, according to the Bhagavad-gita, is *not* based on birth; rather, it is determined by *guna* (quality) and *karma* (activity) (Bg. 4.13). The four *varnas* are the brahmins (*brahmaṇas*—priests, teachers);

foregrounded when, for example, identities or circumstances are ambiguous or in situations of moral dilemmas. The second aspect comprehends virtue ethics and may be called *dharma as virtue*—the sphere of ethical reflection and practice that locates the basis of right action in the cultivation and exercise of one or more virtues, qualities, or dispositions.[4]

Dharma as Settled Duty

Dharma as settled duty recognizes that humans live amid what Jessica Frazier calls "layers of embodiment," a condition involving complex relations of an individual human being not only with other humans, but also with other beings, both visible and invisible. At the heart of these relations is the fact of dependency and interdependency, which points, first and foremost, to obligations. But the dharmic sensibility also recognizes that we humans have agency, choice, and indeed creative power by which we seek to access hidden possibilities and bring them under our control (Frazier 2017, pp. 195–198).

Frazier's suggestive phrase "hidden possibilities" calls our attention to a further basic feature of dharmic sensibility, namely, that the real is inclusive of dimensions that are (generally) beyond human perceptions of time and space.[5] As we noted in Chapter 2, in Hindu traditions the universe is understood to be populated with powerful beings—gods (*devas*) or divinities and lesser beings that have agency and influence in the world, and to whom humans, as beneficiaries of godly power and order, are

---

kshatriyas (*kṣatriyas*—administrators, rulers); vaishyas (*vaiśyas*—farmers, bankers, business people); and shudras (*śūdras*—laborers, artisans).

[4]We may take Alexander's and Moore's (2016) brief definition of deontological ethics as a good reference point in relation to consequentialism and virtue ethics: "[D]eontology falls within the domain of moral theories that guide and assess our choices of what we ought to do (deontic theories), in contrast to those that guide and assess what kind of person we are and should be (aretaic [virtue] theories). And within the domain of moral theories that assess our choices, deontologists—those who subscribe to deontological theories of morality—stand in opposition to *consequentialists*."

[5]If we think of normative dharma as a legal discourse, it clearly displays a theological dimension. Speaking of law in general, Donald Davis notes how law is the product of theological reflection about the mundane world. "The act of reflection converts a mere act, a movement of the body, into an obligation. This kind of reflection, focused as it is on the ordinary world and ordinary actions, is theological because it is a reflective attempt to impart meaning and purpose to quotidian acts" (Davis 2010, p. 3).

expected to offer due respect. Humans thereby also are understood to fulfill their specific role in the maintenance of cosmic order.

Classical brahmanical Hindu tradition expresses this sensibility of obligation particularly in the practice of the *fivefold sacrifice* (*pancha-yajna*). This is a daily practice enjoined for brahmin householders to acknowledge and repay debts that are congenital or existential (not contractual but nonetheless existing).

> [A] person is indebted to the *deva-s*, the managers of the forces of nature, for supplying the means to sustain his or her body (*deva-rinam*); to the seers of yore, the *rishi-s*, and the teachers who received and then passed on the knowledge about the ultimate meaning of life and the means to attain it … (*rishi-rinam*); to the *pitri-s*, or former generations who helped him or her to be what and where s/he is now (*pitri-rinam*); to the goodwill and support of his and her fellow humans (*nri-rinam*) and to all living beings who help that person to sustain him- or herself (*bhu-rinam*). (Stamm 2015, p. 94)

The Dharmashastra texts prescribe methods for addressing each of the five debts, involving, for example, daily ritual oblations for the *devas*, of uncooked grains and clarified butter into the home's perpetually burning sacred fire. Hospitality is strongly enjoined for the householder; hence, the debt to humanity is absolved especially through hosting strangers in the home and by providing the needy with food, clothing, and land. The debt to nonhuman living beings is addressed by making feed available to both domesticated and non-domesticated creatures.[6]

To be sure, this fivefold sacrifice of orthodox brahmins reflects and affirms the conservative worldview that these persons embody. In this worldview, human life is to be well but austerely lived so that the good is accomplished in widening spheres of rule-bound life. Personal and direct family good is accomplished as the rule-bound tradition is preserved and

---

[6]The Manusmriti (3.70) refers to the fivefold sacrifices as *maha-yajnas*, or "great sacrifices," indicating their centrality in the ritual life of the brahmin householder. Davis suggests a connection between this system and the triple debt enjoined in the relatively early (c.800–600 BC) Taittiriya Samhita: "A Brahmin, at his very birth, is born with a triple debt—of studentship to the seers, of sacrifice to the gods, of offspring to the fathers. He is, indeed, free from debt who has a son, is a sacrificer, and who has lived as a student" (Davis 2010, pp. 71–72).

perpetuated, with the reward of eventual rebirth into the same tradition and possibly into the same family. These same rules uphold the sense of continuity that is valued as a social good, and the sense of cooperation and participation sustained by prescribed actions yields a confirmation of cosmic good.

Yet embedded in this world of rules is also an important lesson for the householder: He must not become subject to possessiveness. Rather, he (and the texts do privilege the male householder) is to be generous, functioning within a cosmic system of exchange that is conducive to fostering a sense of honoring all beings appropriately according to position and needs.[7] As Donald Davis notes, in this worldview, the notion of debt functions as a metaphor for law in general, as a "vision [suggesting] an ethics of the controlled self-emptying of one's personal character and substance into the world as a way of pursuing religious salvation" (Davis 2010, p. 71). By such "controlled self-emptying," the brahmin aims at going beyond the boundaries of worldly existence to become a knower of brahman, the unbounded ultimate reality of *being*.

Dharma as Deliberation on Right Action

Dharma can also be construed as the practice of ethical deliberation, making choices for right action responsive to ever-changing contingencies, based on the resources of dharma tradition, injunctive dharma texts, and sagely guidance. Such deliberation may involve careful interpretation of dharma texts, a practice that developed into a veritable philosophical school from early centuries of the Common Era, the Mimamsa (literally, "deliberation") school. A noteworthy example of the Mimamsa way

---

[7]See Frazier (2017, pp. 141–147) for a summary of modern scholarly interpretations of Hindu brahmanical ritual, which she broadly classifies as functionalist theories of social constraint versus emphasis on elements of creativity and self-determination that shows "a participatory, innovative and expressive dimension in many practices" (p. 145). She further summarizes her summary: "These various theories of ritual action thus reflect the open, malleable character of the Hindu cosmos: embodiment is naturally active, but this means that it is volatile, dynamic and must be constrained—nevertheless it can be controlled in order to reshape (both outer and inner) reality and gain the highest levels of the universe for the practitioner. The self…embodied in the physical and mental materials of the universe can be controlled through special practices, but it can also be trained to use its powers creatively, in order to become or interact with higher levels of the cosmos" (pp. 146–147).

of reasoning is one particular analysis of a dharma text passage we already considered in Chapter 3, namely the Manusmriti's seemingly contradictory injunctions on eating or abstaining from animal flesh. In his discussion of this oddly incongruous passage, the tenth-century Mimamsa commentator Medhatithi argues for its consistency. To do so, he draws on a common Mimamsa interpretive technique, namely the distinction between a rule and an explanation or exhortation, concluding that it is (as a rule) indeed legally *permissible* to eat certain types of meat, *and* there is (as an exhortation) a "legal and moral enticement to abstain from it." For Medhatithi, Donald Davis explains,

> [K]illing and eating meat in specified contexts is legally permissible, but the law does not stop there. Instead, a fully hermeneutic understanding of law demonstrates that the law calls on us to abstain from the actions for the "great rewards" that abstention brings. Both are the law, *dharma*, but the *dharma* that produces higher reward is to be preferred over that of mere acceptability. (Davis 2010, pp. 57–58 and n. 19)

Important to note from this example is the acknowledgment of choice: While the act of meat-eating is understood to be permitted, human beings can—and do well to—choose not to do so. Further, although the non-meat option involves an enticement of "great rewards," there is an implied invitation to awaken awareness that higher rewards must indicate a superior moral position, rooted in a superior understanding of the value of life.

As we saw in Chapter 2, dharma as deliberation is also dealt with extensively in narrative fashion in the Sanskrit textual tradition, famously in the Mahabharata, in which problems portrayed as moral dilemmas highlight the difficulty of deliberating to a satisfactory decision how to act.[8] And as we saw, in the case of the king who is forced to suffer despite having no ill

---

[8] A well-known case in point in the Mahabharata is the attempted disrobing and humiliation of Draupadi, the five Pandavas' wife in common, in the dice match assembly. Yudhishthira, the paragon of dharma, in a gambling stupor, loses all his possessions and brothers and then himself, and even their wife, to the Kauravas. Draupadi's sharp-witted challenge to these proceedings is met with silence by the seniors present. It is in the *silences*, notes Vrinda Dalmiya, that can be heard the message of questioning dharma's adequacy to resolve ethical quandaries and thereby the "crying needs of a vulnerable subject" (Dalmiya 2016, pp. 50–52).

intentions in donating a cow that he was unaware was not his to donate, the Mahabharata also raises the question whether it is at all possible to perfectly uphold dharma, even with the best of intentions.

The issue of dharma's place in guiding human right living is related, in the Mahabharata, with a debate on the position of dharma as one of four broad spheres of human aspiration (*purusha arthas*, mentioned in Chapter 4). Which one of the four spheres is foundational to the others, namely *kama*—the pursuit of bodily sense satisfaction; *artha*—the pursuit of wealth, possessions, and self-centered well-being; and *moksha*—the pursuit of freedom from all forms of bondage, ultimately from the cycle of death and rebirth? Depending on which one of these four is accepted as foundational to the others, radically different ethical approaches unfold. Arguably, the Mahabharata favors the conclusion that dharma holds the foundational position in relation to the other three human aims, which is to say that it considers dharma as an intrinsic value, essential for the realization of any other aims.[9] But when dharma is pursued only instrumentally for worldly pleasure and gain, to realize *kama* and *artha*, rather than as an end in itself and to the neglect of *moksha* (including the affirmation and protection of others' freedom and dignity), dharma's purpose and power as a process of ethical deliberation become obscured.[10] Recognizing this danger, the Mahabharata famously asserts that the true path of dharma, while involving deliberation, also calls for guidance from "great persons" (*mahajana*).[11] With such enlightened guidance, dharma can be appropriately re-visioned and applied in response to changing circumstances (Dalmiya 2016, p. 49).

---

[9] Vyasa, the traditional compiler of the Mahabharata, has himself quoted in its final stanzas, saying "I am without pleasure and have raised my arms, but no one is listening to me. If dharma and kama result from artha, why should one not pursue artha? For the sake of kama, fear or avarice, and even for the sake of preserving one's life, one should not give up dharma. Dharma is eternal. Happiness and unhappiness are transient. The atman is eternal, but other reasons are transient" (Debroy 2015, vol. 10, p. 682).

[10] There is a sense in which all four *purusha arthas* complement each other, such that a conscientious Hindu seeks a balance among them. Such balance relates to cow care, whereby appropriate and effective care is sustained when it is understood how all four human aims are enhanced by properly caring for cows (Interview with Shrivatsa Goswami, 15 February 2018).

[11] Although widely quoted, the Mahabharata Critical Edition (Sukthankar 1942, vol. 4, p. 1089) places this stanza in an appendix, not recognizing it as part of the text proper.

A fitting example of re-visioned dharma comes in a narrative near the end of the Mahabharata. As King Yudhisthira (son of Yama, considered personified Dharma) prepares for death during his Himalaya ascent accompanied by a dog, Indra, chief of the celestials, invites the king to take his place in heaven. Yudhisthira is pleased to oblige, but not without his faithful and dependent dog. Indra's insistence that no dogs can reside in heaven confronts Yudhisthira's firm resolve not to leave his canine companion behind. The impasse dissolves when the dog reveals himself to be the celestial personification of Dharma.[12] As Vrinda Dalmiya notes, this story shows Yudhisthira "finding his relational self" (Dalmiya 2016, p. 63), suggesting that dharma's deeper purpose, beyond regulative normativity, is self-transformation. This idea leads to the second major conceptualization of dharma, namely as cultivation of virtue or as virtue-nourishing practice.

Dharma as Cultivation of Virtue

The identification of dharma with deontological and consequentialist ethics would not, by itself, give a full sense of dharma's substance and meaning in Hindu tradition. What Western traditions call "virtue ethics" plays a major role in Hindu tradition in the form of extensive praise for a wide variety of virtues and praise for persons who show these virtues. Further, we can find substantial exhortation for individuals to consciously cultivate within themselves either specific virtues or a virtuous disposition. Particularly in this context, dharma is characterized by its didactic function, instilling a sense of humility, obligation, and responsiveness to contingencies of worldly conditions. Learning to nurture such virtues is

---

[12]From the ethics of care perspective (which we will discuss shortly), Dalmiya (2016, p. 63) suggests that this episode highlights how Yudhisthira "finds his relational self," a self that is fundamentally related with, and therefore impelled to respond to, the needs of other beings. In discussing another Mahabharata story of animals—in this case a dove and a hawk—involving a king's resolve to protect the vulnerable dove, Veena Howard (2018, p. 130) writes, "The animal parables [in the MBh] using the tropes of disguised gods invite us to listen to animal voices for understanding the deeper messages embedded in the tales, messages that disrupt speciesism and address ethical concern for animals themselves."

understood to render a favorable mentality for conducting right action according to context.

From Chapter 2, we recall the Bhagavata Purana's allegory of the bull, Dharma personified: Three legs—compassion, austerity, and purity—have been wounded or destroyed by Kali—the embodiment of time's cycle of degradation—and the remaining leg—truth—barely functions. As a bull stands and moves on four legs, the bull that is dharma—righteous action engendering and sustaining well-being that can lead to liberation—is supported by four "legs," each of which can be regarded as a *virtue-nurturing practice*. Each practice supports and enhances the other three, and together, if conscientiously pursued, they support a life characterized by "illumination" (*sattva*).[13] Specifically, compassion fosters right action toward the weak and vulnerable; austerity fosters self-restraint in relation to one's own desires; purity fosters respect for sexual boundaries; and truth can be construed, in this context, as the practice that fosters higher self-awareness in comprehending the reality of personhood constituting all beings and right action arising from such awareness in relation to the environment.

In the debilitation or absence of the first three (compassion, austerity, and purity), the power to discern objective truth becomes crippled and truthfulness is compromised, degenerating into cultures of half-truth and untruth, devolving yet further into individual and collective illusion and delusion. Hence, the Bhagavata Purana claims that in the present age, the purpose of dharma—realizing the good—becomes severely compromised, and dharma is largely neglected as a viable means for establishing appropriate ethical guidance of human relations with nonhuman animals.[14] In this condition, humans tend to neglect illuminating (*sattva*) values and become driven by passion (*rajas*) and covered by darkness (*tamas*). These latter two qualities of living (*gunas*) severely limit the ability to uphold

---

[13]Here, a distinction should be made between this sense of virtue as an intrinsic moral value and virtue as "pious credit" (*punya*), a sort of positive karmic capital that is a reward for pious action. Rather, by virtue-nurturing practice I point to the cultivation and habituation to a disposition characterized in the Bhagavad-gita as *sattvika* or the mode of goodness and illumination.

[14]The Bhagavata Purana (12.2) paints a dark picture of the present age (Kali-yuga), in the future tense. Among several signs of degradation listed are these: "Dharma is observed only for the sake of reputation"; people's occupations are characterized by "theft, lying, and needless violence"; and (oddly), "cows will be like goats" (12.2.6, 13–14).

dignity, freedom, and harmonious attunement of human aspirations with the natural environment and its creatures.

A further reason Hindu dharma suffers neglect and even scorn in the current age is the perception that it is deeply rooted in a hierarchical social paradigm that indulges privileged strata and oppresses the marginalized. Especially dharma texts concerned with rules and law, such as the Dharmashastras, are indeed typically concerned with ranked identities, especially social ranking in the "system" of fourfold occupational divisions (*varna*). Less known is that such texts are also concerned with dharma principles that apply to everyone, in what is known as "general" dharma (*sadharana-dharma*). The recognition of commonality indicated by *sadharana-dharma*—general duties to be followed by all human beings—points to a deeper understanding, whereby differences in qualifications are acknowledged only to empower all persons to realize ontic equality (Sutton 2000, pp. 303–304).[15] In turn, this deeper aim of dharma points to another key term for Hindu animal ethics, namely yoga—an important paradigm of thought and practice wherein recognizing the ontic equality of all living beings is a vital principle.

From Dharma to Yoga

Classical yoga serves importantly to further illuminate Hindu animal ethics. In Chapter 2, we suggested that the literature of India of which the Hindu "bovine imaginaire" is derived can be conceptualized in terms of polarities, one of which we called a "values polarity" that stretches between the notions of dharma (as maintenance of cosmic order) and bhakti (as devotion toward an ideal being). Now I want to suggest that this conception will also serve our attempt to understand Hindu animal ethics. Further, I suggest that we can regard the classical yoga tradition as the link that ties dharma and bhakti together, especially as articulated in the Yoga Sutras of Patanjali and as expressed with a strong bhakti inflection

---

[15] *Sadharana-dharma* can be understood as directives intended for all human beings at all times and which, much more than injunctions for specific groups (*sva-dharma*), can be identified as injunctions toward the pursuit of morality and the cultivation of virtue.

in the Bhagavad Gita. Somewhat in contrast to the dharma paradigm, yoga is typically represented as a "path" (*marga*) of systematic, purposeful practice that enables individuals to realize ultimate freedom (*moksha*) as life's highest aim. Whereas dharma looks in two directions—outward to worldly well-being (*kama*, pursuit of pleasure, and *artha*, pursuit of wealth) and inward to ultimate freedom—yoga seeks to bring one fully beyond the impediments of worldly attachments, which invariably draw one into relationships of domination and exploitation, characterized by tendencies toward violation of and violence against other beings. On the other side, in contrast to bhakti's strong emphasis on realizing a divine ideal, a supreme person, as the perfection to be pursued, yoga's emphasis is on rigorous practices to free the mind from all false and illusory conceptions and "afflictions" (*klesha*), to reach perfect concentration (*samadhi*) and freedom (*kaivalya*).[16]

Despite important differences between dharma and yoga paradigms, there are also striking overlaps in some elements of practice, especially elements impacting ethics. In particular, similar to dharma as cultivation of virtue, yoga also demands careful attention to specific practices conducive to fostering virtue. Patanjali's Yoga Sutras, the celebrated summary of classical yoga, includes a description of yoga as an eightfold process (*ashtanga-yoga*). The first two processes—restraints (*yama*) and observances (*niyama*)—each stipulate five components as prerequisites for further progress.[17] The first of the five *yama* practices—ahimsa, nonviolence—is already familiar to us from Chapter 3. Yet we do well to linger on this practice in the context of yoga for the particular treatment it receives by classical commentators on Patanjali's Yoga Sutras.

After listing the eight yoga "limbs" (YS 2.29), Patanjali lists five components of restraint, beginning with ahimsa, which the traditional commentator to the text, Vyasa, identifies as the "root" of the remaining four

---

[16] Both *moksha* and *kaivalya* have similar meanings, with shades of difference. Patanjali's Yoga Sutras uses *kaivalya*, whereas *moksha* is found in texts such as the Mahabharata.

[17] The five yoga restraints (*yama*) are listed by Patanjali as "nonviolence, truthfulness, refrainment from stealing, celibacy, and renunciation of [unnecessary] possessions" (Bryant 2009, p. 243; YS 2.30).

restraints (Bryant 2009, p. 243).[18] The next aphorism (YS 2.31) makes clear that the "great vow" to observe the five restraints is meant for everyone, without exception, regardless of social position, place, or time (much like the notion of "general dharma" mentioned previously). As Bryant points out, Patanjali is "being as emphatic here as the straightforward and plain use of human language allows" (Bryant 2009, p. 249).

After listing the five observances (*niyama*: cleanliness, contentment, austerity, study [of scripture], and devotion to God, YS 2.32), Patanjali offers simple but powerful advice on how to progress in adhering to the restraints and observances: "Upon being harassed by negative thoughts, one should cultivate counteracting thoughts" (YS 2.33). What constitute negative thoughts? The next aphorism explains:

> Negative thoughts are violence (*himsa*), etc. They may be [personally] performed, performed on one's behalf by another, or authorized by oneself; they may be triggered by greed, anger, or delusion; and they may be slight, moderate, or extreme in intensity. One should cultivate counteracting thoughts, namely, that the end results [of negative thoughts] are ongoing suffering and ignorance. (Bryant 2009, p. 257; YS 2.34)

Since the specific example given of negative thought is violence, traditional commentators give special attention to it. As Bryant notes, the eleventh-century commentator Bhoja Raja highlights Patanjali's explicit reference to performance of an act (of violence, such as killing an animal) "on one's behalf by another" as a warning to the "dull wit" consumer of meat who thinks he or she can avoid karmic responsibilities by having others do the slaughtering. The fifteenth-century commentator Vijnanabhikshu goes further, saying that even scripturally condoned violence (as in the killing of animals in ritual sacrifices, as we saw in Manusmriti) is herewith rejected (Bryant 2009, p. 258). We should also note Vijnanabhikshu's explicitly theistic reasoning. Bryant summarizes:

---

[18]The restraints are called by Shyam Ranganathan the "five political ideals" in Yoga (2017b, p. 189). Strikingly, he proposes, "Putting non-harmfulness first is to privilege objectivity over truth: when we do not harm, we allow for the objectivity of things in our environment, including ourselves and other people, as self-determining objects in the world. The *truths* of the world change, from one of tyranny to social freedom. We are hence free to endorse the following ideals of respecting people's property, their sexual boundaries, and not being encumbered by stuff" (p. 190).

Ultimately, all creatures are parts of *Īśvara*, God, explains Vijñānabhikṣu, like sons to the father and sparks to the fire. Therefore, violence against others is violence against God. He quotes the [Bhagavad-] *Gītā*: "Envious people act hatefully towards me [Krishna] in their own and in others' bodies. I continually hurl such cruel hateful people, the lowest of mankind, into *samsāric* [repeated death and rebirth] existence, into only the impure wombs of demons" (XVI.19). (Bryant 2009, pp. 259–260)

As we noted, nonviolence is regarded as the "root" of all the restraints and observances, all of which together build the ethical foundation for successful yoga practice. And it is noteworthy that Vijnanabhiksu makes an explicit connection between nonviolence and theism, particularly when we consider the last of Patanjali's five observances, namely *ishvara-pranidhana*—devotion to God. For, according to Patanjali, successful practice of yoga culminates in *samadhi*—singular absorption of one's awareness in the reality of one's non-physical identity. And, says Patanjali, the specific practice that, when perfected, brings about *samadhi* is *ishvara-pranidhana*: "From submission to God comes the perfection of *samādhi*" (Bryant 2009, p. 279; YS 2.45). This idea confirms the link of classical yoga to bhakti, and we might view it as the Bhagavad Gita's point of departure. There Krishna assures Arjuna (Bg. 6.46–47), "A *yogī* surpasses ascetics, and is even held to surpass the learned. A *yogī* surpasses ritualists. Therefore be a *yogī*, Arjuna. And of all *yogīs*, I consider as most linked in *yoga* one whose inner self has gone to Me, who faithfully reveres Me" (Goswami 2015, p. 175).

Through the disciplines of yoga, one may well become largely free from the tendency to commit violence on other beings, and this goes hand in hand with progressive comprehension of ontic equality among all living creatures. Yet yoga's importance for animal ethics is not limited to negative virtue—the avoidance of harming other beings. Just as important is the freedom of action that yoga affords practitioners, including freedom from habitual response to predictable circumstances, thus addressing the problem of dharma as deliberation in the face of unexpected situations (Perrett 1998, pp. 22–23). This freedom, referred to in the Yoga Sutras as *kaivalya*, is sometimes translated as "aloneness," which Ian Whicher construes as "*puruṣa's* [*purusha*, the living being's] innate capacity for pure, unbroken, nonattached seeing/perceiving, observing or 'knowing' of the content of the mind (*citta*)" (Whicher 1998, p. 276). Such freedom is, very significantly, also enjoyed by the objective world that the yogi perceives. Whicher (p. 278) notes that, although *purusha* is, from the enlightened perspective, in fact ever free,

> it would not be inappropriate to suggest that, figuratively speaking, in the state of "aloneness" (*kaivalya*) *puruṣa* [spirit] and *prakṛti* [the phenomenal world] are simultaneously liberated in that, all ignorance having been removed, *they are both "known," included, and are therefore free to be what they are.* (emphasis in original)

This has the intriguing implication that it is by virtue of yogic freedom achieved by the *yogi* that true freedom of other beings can be conceived. In other words, it is within the auspices of yogic perception in the state of freedom that the freedom of beings in general can be properly conceived. Further, because the perfected *yogi* does *not* (as is usually interpreted) lose his or her personhood, it is such a person who can properly be considered fit to relate with all creatures in appropriate ways, which means acknowledging *their* personhood.[19]

Thus far I have suggested that dharma, in the broad sense of injunctive statements and deliberative practices, may be correlated with normative ethics in its two directions—deontic and consequential grounding of action. In its second feature, dharma as cultivation of virtue, dharma shows points of commonality with the two initial components of yoga, the practice of five restraints and five observances. In all these cases, points of relevance to animal ethics lean strongly on the side of prohibition or negative ethics. The sense of responsibility that humans may have toward nonhuman animals, as might be derived from these texts and their interpretive traditions, is largely one of providing minimally for certain animals and otherwise refraining from intentionally harming them. In more positive terms, the dharma and yoga paradigms of thought and action unsettle

---

[19]Whicher (1998, p. 277) writes, "[I]t can be stated that *kaivalya* in no way presupposes the destruction or negation of the personality of the yogin, but is an unconditional state in which all the obstacles or distractions preventing an immanent and purified relationship or engagement of person with nature and spirit (*puruṣa*) have been removed." For a detailed discussion on the meaning of *kaivalya* in YS, see Whicher (1998, pp. 275–294).

anthropocentric presuppositions, locating the value of human existence in the facility it gives for realizing an ultimate cosmic order (through dharma) and for realizing atemporal selfhood, free from self-serving action (through yoga).

A third dimension to this picture of Hindu animal ethics is to be found in the bhakti current, or paradigm, which we have touched on briefly in previous chapters. Now we revisit this theme as we consider how it may contribute to a positive vision and practice of animal ethics, especially as articulated in a relatively recent development in Western ethics discourse, the ethics of care.

From Yoga to Bhakti

Turning toward the bhakti end of the dharma-bhakti polarity of value, we keep in mind the linking function of yoga between dharma and bhakti. The term "bhakti"—typically translated as "devotion"—is often linked to the term "yoga" in the bhakti literature (Bryant 2017).[20] Thus, *bhakti-yoga* is the regular and intentional practice of devotion, pursued with an aim to realize the self as essentially relational. Whereas classical yoga regards desire (*raga*) as an obstacle to be overcome for making progress, in the domain of bhakti, the aim is to channel one's desires and love toward the supreme person, as the ultimate object of relationship and love (Bryant 2017, p. 66). To do so constitutes the perfection of practice, leading to further devotional activity rather than to any sort of cessation. In terms of moral theory, as Shyam Ranganathan explains, bhakti can be seen as a fourth, distinctly Indian, theory apart from the three commonly accepted categories, namely virtue, deontic, and consequentialist theories. Distinctive of bhakti as a moral theory is that engagement in bhakti practice ("doing the right") is *itself* "the good" outcome, whereas with the other three theories, there is a necessary distinction between the right and the good (Ranganathan 2017a, pp. 26–27).[21]

---

[20] For a summary of Chaitanya Vaishnava texts (especially Bhagavata Purana) linking yoga and bhakti, see Sinha (1983, pp. 39–43).

[21] The distinctiveness of bhakti as the culmination of Hindu thought has been carefully articulated by Jarava Lal Mehta (1912–1988). Ellis (2013, pp. 126–128) elaborates on Mehta's analysis of the

To channel one's desires and love toward the supreme person is to simultaneously cultivate a deep sense of relationality with all creatures. An extended episode in the Bhagavata Purana (5.8–13) illustrates how yoga imbued with bhakti becomes the basis for deep relationality between human and nonhuman animals, and how this sensibility can have the power to transform the heart of one initially blind to the value of such relationality. In this episode, an ascetic sage, Bharata, formerly a king who renounced his kingdom to seek yogic perfection, is intently practicing yogic meditation alone in a forest. One day, he becomes suddenly distracted by the roaring sound of a lion. Seeing that a pregnant deer, in her fear of the lion, has given birth to a fawn before expiring, Bharata takes the orphaned fawn to his hermitage. There he raises the fawn with tender care, but in doing so he becomes increasingly drawn away from his yoga meditation practice. Indeed, his care for the fawn becomes so absorbing that, as he meets with an accident and loses his life, because his thoughts at the moment of death were on the young deer, Bharata's immediate next birth is as a deer. Remembering his previous life of yoga practice, deer Bharata finds shelter in the hermitage of other sages until his life in this form comes to a natural end.[22] The Bhagavata Purana continues the story, with Bharata's subsequent birth occurring in a brahmin family where, because now his determination to reach yogic perfection has become so intense, in order to avoid the distractions of brahmin social life, from earliest childhood he feigns as a deafmute (*jada*). This serves his purpose of keeping his attention fully on the practice of bhakti-yoga, although he thereby suffers considerable abuses from relatives.

Having grown to adulthood, because he is well built, Jada Bharata, as he is now known, is conscripted into service as a palanquin bearer for

---

"logic of the Hindu tradition" as having a trajectory with three hermeneutical focal points, namely the Rigveda, including the Upanishads; the epic tradition, especially the Mahabharata; and finally, the Bhagavata Purana. It is the latter text that brings forth the tradition's culmination in *viraha-bhakti*, love-in-separation, the most intense mode of love for the other. It is this mode of love that is seen as the *good* that is realized, even if incompletely in early stages of practice, by the *right* practice of bhakti.

[22]The text does not explicitly indicate it, but the implication is that Bharata, in the deer body, would have benefitted from hearing the discussions on spiritual culture conducted by the sages. A similar notion is found in Buddhist literature and among present-day Buddhist monks of Sri Lanka, both of which indicate a belief that "passively listening to dharma preaching, whether it is understood or not, has spiritually productive consequences" for animals (Stewart 2017).

the provincial ruler, Rahugana. But Jada Bharata fails to keep pace with the other bearers, being preoccupied in avoiding harm to ants as he steps forward. The resulting shaking of the palanquin precipitates the king's anger and abusive words. Jada Bharata now breaks his lifelong silence. In the course of the ensuing dialogue between him and the king, it becomes clear to the king (and to us, the readers or listeners) that Bharata is profoundly wise. Rahugana is deeply humbled, submitting himself to this unlikely sage for spiritual guidance.[23] And what Rahugana learns from him is what Bharata had learned by direct experience through the practice of devotional yoga that led him through the life of a nonhuman animal—as a deer—while retaining the previously developed consciousness of a *yogi*. He experienced directly that the transmigratory mechanism of nature (*prakriti*) can, depending on the actions (*karma*) and disposition (*guna*) of living beings, bring a human being into a nonhuman body and vice versa. He also learned that all bodies of living beings are only superficially different, their physical elements all coming from the same source, the earth. Further, he learned that the living beings, all of the same non-material quality, are each accompanied by the one higher self (*paramatman*) and, says Bharata, it was by virtue of his resolute devotion to this higher self, whom he identifies as Krishna, that he has come to this comprehension of reality (BhP 5.12.8–15).

In contrast to Jada Bharata's heightened sensitivity to living beings' conditions is the initial insensitivity of the king, whom the devotional *yogi* chides for arrogantly posing as the citizens' protector. Although not explicitly charged with harming animals, Rahugana displays a materialistic disposition as a ruler implicated in a life of violence and thus in the crippling bondage of retributive karma. But now, having met and heard from Jada Bharata, all this has changed. As a conversion story, this episode represents a major theme of the Bhagavata Purana, namely, that encounters

---

[23] In contrast to the dharma-bull, to whom the Bhagavata Purana gives voice, the deer cared for by Bharata and then the deer that Bharata becomes are both silent. Yet as the silent, apparently deafmute Jada Bharata is challenged by the proud king, he speaks forth the Bhagavata's *bhakti* message, indicating that the higher truth of right action is often voiced best by those who are socially marginalized and who have an affinity with nonhuman animals.

with spiritually enlightened and caring sages can be profoundly transformative.[24] By such good fortune, one can undergo the sort of change of heart that sets one on the devotional path of care, radically dislodging the embodied being's false sense of identity and possessiveness (*ahamkara*—literally "*I* do"; *mamata*, "mine-ness"). Such a devotional (bhakti) path is the attentive practice previously mentioned, whereby the ultimate good of all living beings becomes the measure of right action, in a spirit of service.[25] All beings are seen as eternal, infinitesimal in size and power, and unique instances of the one all-sentient, relational being, *bhagavan* (the same as *paramatman*), characterized by infinite qualities and virtues and having an exquisite, atemporal form with three core features—eternity, cognizance, and felicity (*sat, cit,* and *ananda*). Jada Bharata's transformative outreach to the benighted king thus indicates a political dimension, namely, that by virtue of higher vision with respect to living beings, the truth that devotional yoga yields for its practitioner can positively affect the world and stands to prevail over blind, ignorant worldly coercive power, since the devotional *yogi* participates in a higher spiritual order that governs the universe.

A final implication of the story for us to note has to do with a deeper dimension of bhakti-yoga, namely the sense of absence and loss as a wellspring of intense devotional emotion. Bharata's initial care for the young deer points toward this notion. The text indicates that whenever the fawn would venture away from the sage's hermitage, Bharata would be stricken with anxiety for her well-being. His expressions of longing in "separation" anticipate the later full elaboration, in the Bhagavata's Book 10, of Krishna's beloveds in Vraja pining for him in his absence. Bhakti in this tradition is particularly characterized by the sense of intense devotional longing that Krishna-*bhaktas* experience for Krishna when he seems to be absent from his land of cows, Vraja (Holdrege 2013; Schweig 2013). Vaishnavas regard

---

[24]This theme is also present in the Mahabharata, typically in the context of dharma-as-virtue; at times, it is represented such that a sage—already advanced in spiritual knowledge—learns an essential lesson from a socially marginal person. See Dalmiya's (2016, pp. 108–114) summary and analysis of the Mahabharata's story of sage Kaushika, who learns "relational humility" from a housewife and then a butcher.

[25]The Bhagavad-gita (3.25) also features bhakti as a practice aiming toward benefitting all beings, through "detached action," contrasting this with the attached action of the "nonlearned." Thus, *right* action is identified with an attitude, namely detachment from the results of action.

Vraja as the place where all creatures are absorbed (being situated in the state of *samadhi*, the goal of yoga) in relational care for Krishna—and thus care for each other—and Krishna is equally absorbed in relational care for all creatures.

Reverence in the Bhakti Paradigm

To further appreciate the bhakti paradigm for animal ethics, let us consider the notion of *reverence*. We recall that the final component of the fivefold yoga observances (*niyama*) is *ishvara-pranidhana*, devotion or submission to God, a practice that leads to samadhi, which we defined as "singular absorption of one's awareness in the reality of one's non-physical identity."[26] But unlike classical yoga, wherein the emphasis is on emotional restraint to realize samadhi, bhakti celebrates salvific emotional awakening to non-temporal being and to divinity as both the means and the goal of devotional life. In its most developed form, such devotionally emotional awakening is also regarded as samadhi that goes beyond mere awareness of one's non-physical identity to absorption in love and service to God.[27]

With such theistic orientation, Hindu bhakti tradition apparently runs counter to a strong current in the contemporary Western zeitgeist—one of suspicion, if not outright rejection, of theistic grounding for ethical deliberation and practice. As moderns, we tend to dismiss the notion that the discernment of right action and the good should proceed from divine revelation. In the West, the questioning of divine authority in moral issues goes back to at least the Euthyphro dialogue of Plato, with its portrayal of divine command theory and its dilemma over the locus of the good. Is an act good because it is commanded by God (or gods), or is good commanded by God (or gods) because it is good? Later Christian reflection

---

[26]"A practice that leads to samadhi" is an important understanding indicated in Patanjali's Yoga Sutras. Yet the text also makes clear that *ishvara-pranidhana* is not merely instrumental to higher yogic accomplishment, for it is also itself the goal. In other words, *ishvara-pranidhana* is *itself* the state of *samadhi*, as becomes thoroughly clear in the Bhagavata Purana. I am grateful to Graham Schweig (personal conversation) for clarifying this point.

[27]In the Bhagavata Purana (11.12.12), Krishna uses the term *samadhi* to describe the intense devotional absorption of his beloveds, the Vraja cowherdess, in thinking of him, "as sages enter into samadhi, like rivers flowing into the ocean."

on this issue will speak of *voluntarism* (the creation of morality out of God's free will) and *intellectualism* (God's discernment of eternal moral truths, valid for both God and creatures). For us to note here is that the bhakti paradigm foregrounds not so much God's will as God's *preference* in matters of moral decision-making, leaving human beings free choice to act or not to act in pursuit of, or in harmony with, this preference. This understanding resonates with a third alternative to voluntarism and intellectualism, namely, that God is essential to morality because morality flows from his *motives*, which are components of his virtues, which in turn point to his personhood (Zagzebski 2004, pp. 185–206). This understanding preserves, and indeed celebrates, free choice as the basis for authentic love for God-as-person.[28]

This third option, expressed in terms of divine motive and preference, may point a way toward appreciating and recovering a core value of the European Enlightenment, namely *reverence*. As Susan Neiman (2008, p. 112) points out, contra popular opinion that Enlightenment thinkers were religion bashers, "The Enlightenment took aim not at reverence, but at idolatry and superstition." In a similar spirit, Indian bhakti traditions, especially from the sixteenth century onward, tended to question meaningless observance of prescribed rituals (excesses in the name of dharma observance) and valued reason as a support for cultivating a sense of valuing and revering the world as divine creation.[29]

---

[28]Taking the Bhagavad-gita as a point of departure for elaboration on this point, there *are* statements suggesting both sides of the dilemma. On the one hand, out of his free will God creates the world (e.g., 9.7; 10.8), and on the other, out of a sense of duty he acts in this world to give example for human behavior in the world (3.22–24). I would suggest, however, that divine preference is indicated early in the Gita, when Krishna emphasizes the value of *yajna* as the means for becoming free from the bondage of karma (3.9). A key phrase here is *tad-artham karma...samācara*—"perform action well, for that purpose," where "that" refers to *yajna*, which Vaishnava Hindus identify as an embodiment of Vishnu. The *artham*—"purpose"—is the key term suggesting divine preference, "Vishnu's purpose." Krishna also indicates that he does not resent those who ignore him; rather, he simply gives them what they want and deserve (7.21; Goswami 2015, p. 36) Further, in relation to divine motives, we may note the Gita's reference to "higher nature" and "own nature," *param bhavam; sva-bhava* (7.24; 9.11; 8.3), as its way of expressing this notion, along with several statements indicating divine wish for alienated souls to take final refuge in him.

[29]See Prentiss (1999, especially pp. 25–42), for a discussion of differing historiographies and theories of bhakti as a movement. My generalizations here are intended only to highlight bhakti in contrast with dharma and yoga. One identifier for bhakti literature is its use of vernacular languages rather than Sanskrit; yet there is also a rich body of bhakti literature in Sanskrit as well, among which

Yet already in the ancient Bhagavad Gita, Krishna famously questions ritualism, valuing instead simplicity rooted in devotion. A particularly telling statement relevant to this and our general subject can be seen as Krishna's broad invitation for all to practice bhakti, engaging with the simplest of ingredients provided by nature: "When one dedicates to Me with devotion a leaf, flower, fruit or water, I accept that devoted gift from a dedicated soul" (Goswami 2015, p. 182; Bg. 9.26). Thus, the theistic framework of bhakti ethics, while holding human beings responsible for their actions, emphasizes open opportunity—as an invitation—to serve divinity. Such divinity is comprehended as the supreme person who, as "superself" or "oversoul" (*paramatman*) within the constraints of the temporal realm, bestows sanction and power to act. Such divinity guides creatures toward freedom in action that is grounded in a progressive unfolding of value and meaning rooted in love.

Just how the relationship between choice and divine guidance in the bhakti paradigm unfolds is shown in an eighteenth-century devotional song from the Chaitanya Vaishnava tradition. In his *Prema-bhakti-chandrika* (10), Narottamdas writes (in Bengali) *sadhu-shastra-guru-vakya chittete koriya aikya, satatam bhasibo prema-majhe.* "Bringing the words of the devotees, of the scriptures, and of the preceptor into a single understanding in my heart, I will float amidst love" (Babaji 2010, p. 115). This suggests that devotees (*bhaktas*) come to understand how best to act after consulting with fellow practitioners as well as with their spiritual guides and relevant sacred texts. These resources combined are considered effective in attuning oneself to guidance from *paramatman* within the "heart" or core of one's being. Further, and importantly, such attunement affirms the rightness of action in relation to living beings through the recognition that all life, being not reducible to matter, calls for attentive reverence and appropriate care. Thus, the Enlightenment project of recovering reverence—which turned particularly to nature as the objective manifestation of divine order and perfection—may be seen as enhanced by the bhakti paradigm, in such a way that reverence is appropriately extended to all living beings.

---

the Bhagavad-gita and Bhagavata Purana have enjoyed prominence and continue to do so in the present.

Ethics of Care and Hindu Animal Ethics

With the foregoing discussion of the three paradigms—dharma, yoga, and bhakti—in relation to ethical thought, we can return now to our central question of this chapter: In what ways may Hindu animal ethics be best understood in relation to Western animal ethics discourse, particularly in connection with cow care, a major concern of many Hindus? Contemporary animal ethics discourse has, with greater or lesser persuasiveness, over recent decades, drawn points of argument from general ethics (including varieties of deontic and virtue ethics) to establish compelling, reasoned grounds for nonhuman animal protection, with special concern to establish nonhuman animals as rightly possessing moral status. However, some ethicists have argued that standard forms of normative ethics discourse (deontic, consequentialist, virtue) have proven inadequate to the task of bringing significant and lasting reform to behavior within human society. Similarly, persons concerned with animals have been dismayed by the lack of substantial positive change with respect to human–nonhuman animal relations despite the high volume of animal ethics discursivity in recent decades (Donovan and Adams 2007, pp. 1–20; Donaldson and Kymlicka 2013, pp. 1–11).

One response to these disappointments has been the rise of the "ethics of care" from the early 1980s and, in relation to animal ethics, from the late 1990s. Both currents share an identification with feminist concerns, characterized by pioneer author Carol Gilligan as articulating and practicing a "morality of responsibility," contrasted with the masculine inflected "morality of rights" (Donovan and Adams 2007, p. 2). Vrinda Dalmiya (2016, pp. 4–5) identifies five themes characterizing the metaethical framing of care ethics, namely (1) *relationality* (acknowledgment of the embodied condition of all subjects of moral action); (2) recognition of *needs* (addressing often conflicting needs of corporeal and hence vulnerable, selves); (3) *affectivity* (the recognition that emotions have an important place in moral decision-making); (4) *contextualism* (the awareness that moral judgments always take place in specific relational contexts); and, finally, (5) *responsibility* (the recognition of "moral remainders"—of feelings such as guilt and uncertainty regarding inevitable limits to one's capacity to respond). More specifically referring to the ethics of care in relation to animals, Donovan and Adams (2007, pp. 3–4) identify *attention* as a "key word in feminist ethic-of-care theorizing about animals." Along with the importance of attention to individual suffering animals, attention is necessary also to "the political and economic systems that are causing the suffering."

To gain a sense of how these themes might unfold in the context of Hindu animal ethics, I return briefly to the Mahabharata episode mentioned earlier, in which King Yudhishthira insists on having a companion dog accompany him to heaven. In this account, the king acknowledges a *relationship* with the dog such that he does not regard embodiment as a dog as an impediment to sustaining the relationship, despite traditional Indian (especially brahmanical) disdain for dogs. He therefore answers to the dog's *need*, which is to be in the king's protection. Further, the king acknowledges his own *feelings* for the dog as a result of the dog's demonstration of unwavering loyalty; the king takes account of the situation's *context* to the extent that he is willing to forego entrance into the heavenly realm, in favor of preserving the caring relationship with the dog. Finally, King Yudhishthira takes *responsibility* for his decision, whatever faults might arise as a result. As for *attention*, we can appreciate that it is present in all these five themes, in such a way that Yudhishthira is attentive to the individual dog and, at the same time, he is resistant to the political current that would reject his act of care.

For us to note in particular from this king-and-canine story is how a broad care ethics perspective—initially limited to moral concerns among human beings, exemplified in the mother–child relationship—may be appropriately applied to human–nonhuman animal relationships. And the key to this extension is the simple, common awareness that humans can and do have relationships with specific animals, relationships involving various sorts of reciprocity and, typically, active caring on the part of humans for such animals. Such relationships are usually seen in human interaction with companion animals—pets or horses—but they can and do extend to other animals as well.

Yet an important issue arises in consideration of animals in the context of care ethics. Whereas care ethics in the human sphere is (generally) free from notions of ownership on the part of moral agents regarding their subjects of care, animals are mostly regarded as *owned*—in the possession of—their carers or of persons for whom carers work. This applies especially (but not only) to animals we denote as "domestic" or "domesticated" and to farm animals, which are generally confined to particular human-demarcated spaces. However, returning once more to Yudhishthira, the story suggests that the king's purpose is not to remain the dog's master and controller; rather, it is to bring him to a state of freedom (represented in the Mahabharata context as "heaven"). Thus, the implication is that the king, embodying dharma in its deepest sense, aims to acknowledge the non-material reality of the dog as a conscious, non-temporal being with inherent value and pursuing its need for freedom.

Going a step further, we may imagine Yudhishthira, as he ascends the mountain with the dog, aspiring for the yogic state of freedom (*kaivalya*). As we discussed earlier, in its deepest sense, *kaivalya* of classical yoga means facilitating not only one's own freedom but also the freedom of other beings, such that relationality is enriched among all. In fact, the term *kaivalya* is also employed within the bhakti paradigm, wherein it refers to selfless devotion to the supreme person, *bhagavan*, who is the very embodiment of complete freedom.[30] Also, in the Bhagavata Purana, King Yudhishthira is celebrated as such a selfless devotee, suggesting that his actions are entirely oriented toward responding favorably to divine preference.[31] By virtue of his identity as king, with responsibilities to all citizens of the kingdom, his engagement with the dog may be seen as conforming to the didactic function of leaders that Krishna refers to in the Bhagavad Gita: "Whatever the greatest one does, common people do just the same, following the standard he sets" (Goswami 2015, p. 162; Bg. 3.21). In this case, the king teaches not only that people should respect and appropriately care for animals. Arguably, he also teaches that animals—in particular domestic animals—are appropriately regarded in important ways—though not in all ways assumed in common usage today—as *citizens*, or as citizens-in-the-making. As citizens or aspiring citizens, at least certain animals can be regarded as members of the moral community such

---

[30] Krishna instructs his friend Uddhava on the nature of the supreme person in the Bhagavata Purana's Book Eleven, including that he is *kevalānubhavānanda-sandoha*—"the aggregate of the experience of the bliss of kaivalya" (Bhagavata Purana 11.9.18).

[31] For example, Bhagavata Purana 1.8.5 refers to Yudhisthira as *ajāta-śatru*—"he whose enemy is not born" (he who has no enemies).

that a central principle of bhakti can be realized with maximum inclusiveness, namely *seva*—attentively caring devotional service as an integral feature of bhakti practice (*sadhana*). By such devotional service, "relational humility" (Dalmiya 2016, pp. 2–3)—the disposition that makes effective caring and its resultant knowing possible—is realized.

Animal Citizenship, Community, and Bhakti

We have encountered a possible problem in applying the ethics of care to human–nonhuman animal relations as opposed to human–human relations, namely the issue of ownership. It is clearly the case that present-day rampant and pervasive abuse and slaughter of farm animals for human use and consumption are deeply rooted in the supposition of ownership. Recognition that animal ownership drives and sustains animal abuse has led to a sharp distinction between "welfarist" and "basic rights" approaches to animal advocacy.[32] According to prominent animal rights advocates, any apparent success in raising animal welfare standards of treatment serves only to legitimate and intrench the system of animal exploitation, reaffirming the status quo of animal ownership for human use and consumption.[33] By this reasoning, from an animal rights perspective, the objection may be raised that even if animals are not subject to slaughter and consumption and they are provided ideal living conditions, the very fact that such animals are held as property (and are even only minimally confined) means that their care is compromised. The "owner" of an animal, no matter how caring she or he may be, remains always in a position of power over the animal, ultimately the power of life and death. Such an "owner" may decide—even despite feelings of affection toward, say, his or her family cow—to sell her for slaughter, pleading inability to continue financially

---

[32]As noted by Donaldson and Kymlicka (2013, pp. 3–4), a third, "ecological holism" approach is similarly inadequate for effectively protecting animals. "In this case, the interests may be less trivial [than those that limit the scope of welfarism]. Nevertheless, ecologists elevate a particular view of what constitutes a healthy, natural, authentic, or sustainable ecosystem, and are willing to sacrifice individual animal lives in order to achieve this holistic vision."

[33]See Francione (2004), quoted in Kansal (2016). See the latter for a relevant legal discussion on animals as property in the context of animal welfare law in India.

maintaining the non-productive cow.[34] Such cases (which are more the rule than the exception) lead into the question, what can be said about Hindu animal ethics as an inflection of care ethics? Is the welfare/rights distinction appropriate and, if so, where would Hindus locate themselves on this map? To consider these questions, it will be helpful to return to our main subject in relation to Hindu animal ethics, namely care of cows.

From a responsible Hindu perspective, there is no doubt that present-day animal "husbandry" (mal)practices with bovines exceed all boundaries of decency and morality. Neither is there a question of animal welfare (even if legal welfare standards are met) in animal husbandry establishments, what to speak of there being any consideration of rights for the cows. As we have noted in Chapter 4, the massive dairy industry in India functions only on the basis of either releasing dry cows to fend for themselves (*anna pratha*), giving them to a cow shelter, or sending them for slaughter. Conditions for bulls are almost always worse, invariably destined for slaughter at a very early age (unless kept for reproduction). What, then, might be appropriate criteria for identifying a model of care for cows according to Hindu understanding, and would such criteria withstand the insistence of some animal activists—abolitionists—that the only proper relationship of humans with animals can be one in which humans make no use whatsoever of bovine products?

To this last question, the answer from the position of abolitionist and animal rights activism may well be, "Whatever criteria Hindus may set will surely be unacceptable. The criteria of care for cows by Hindus will surely allow for taking the cows' milk (even if only excess milk) and castrating the bulls (even if under anaesthesia) to work them as oxen, both of which involve various forms and degrees of violence. None of these could pass as acceptable ethical behavior, because any such use is unnecessary and exploitative." Cow care rejection would be rooted in the rejection of animal ownership and the concern that bovines are involuntarily confined, cows are involuntarily milked, bulls are involuntarily engaged in work, and bovines are subjected to controlled and forced breeding by artificial means.

---

[34] See Govindrajan (2018, pp. 65–66, 84–87) for a detailed description of such a case she witnessed in an Indian Himalayan village community. In this case, it was a "Jersey" (non-indigenous cow) for which, although the owner felt it was probably "not a sin to let it go," she had felt strong affection to the point of tears when the cow was taken away (for slaughter) after being sold.

Indeed, from this abolitionist perspective, the practices of cow care, however much care, attention, and affection would be given to cows, is fundamentally exploitative and is, therefore, appropriately compared with human slavery (Clark 2011; Wise 2011, p. 20; Schuster 2016, p. 218). In this understanding, cow care—however conscientiously practiced it may be—partakes in moral discrimination on the basis of species, which is rooted in anthropocentrism. It is akin to discrimination on the basis of race, sex, gender, class, ethnicity, or sexual preference. This is a position that stands firmly for radical human lifestyle change, to a strictly vegan diet (in particular for people of the Global North with their greater choice of diet and necessary economic means).[35]

Although Hindus would generally question the notion that cow care is inherently exploitative, important features of the vegan stance can be appreciated by conscientious Hindus—in particular, veganism's commitment to foreswearing all unnecessary violence. Practices that minimize violence, especially practices related to food production and consumption, are certainly praiseworthy and desirable. The abolitionist position gives good reason for Hindus to reconsider their consumption of cow milk, even from cows that are well cared for throughout their natural lives. Could it be that the *amount* of milk one has become habituated to consume is disproportionate to need, assuming there is a need? Could it be that one is unnecessarily subjecting cows and bulls to one's own purposes, thus violating these beings-in-animal-bodies and thereby violating the principle of nonviolence as the highest dharma (as per Mahabharata 13.117.37–38)? Further, from the perspective of the bhakti paradigm (which, as we saw, values responsiveness to divine preference), does it not happen that, in the name of pleasing Krishna with lavish dairy-based food offerings, one may be overindulging one's own predilection for these? If misconstrued,

---

[35]For one representation of what he calls the "vegan imperative," see Steiner (2013, especially pp. 195–215). He defines ethical veganism as "the principle that we ought as far as possible to eschew the use of animals as sources of food, labor, entertainment, and the like, inasmuch as eating, enslaving, or otherwise doing avoidable violence to one's kin is fundamentally wrong" (p. 206). Responding to the argument that the taking of milk and eggs for human consumption "need not take the form that it currently takes," Steiner concedes that this is technically correct. "But it misses the larger point that using animals as delivery devices for food (and clothing, etc.) to be consumed by humans, viewed from the standpoint of cosmic holism and in the light of felt kinship, is a perverse idea" (p. 213). This view may be contrasted with that of Cochrane, quoted later in this chapter.

the bhakti orientation can spawn excesses on the side of veneration that results in "extreme transcendentalism" that can obstruct clear thinking and action for genuine care of cows.[36]

The analogy of cow care with slavery also calls for consideration. In its favor, the slavery analogy calls attention to what may be understood as an absence of "consent" on the part of bovines—consent of cows to being milked or consent of bulls to being worked. At the same time, it may be right to consider in what sense consent might be applicable to nonhuman animals (and what are the indicators of consent or lack of consent for bovines).[37] While it is true that human slavery and the condition of animals have been compared since ancient times (Clark 2011), as with all analogies, there are limits to this one. So, for example, enslaved humans have been intentionally prevented from becoming literate as a key means of keeping them in bondage. But unlike enslaved human beings, there is no reason to suppose that bovines—as long as they are in bovine bodies—would ever be able to use human language and thus adopt the life of full human citizenship as is understood today. Put differently, it is not necessarily "speciesist" to recognize differences among species while making ethical judgments with respect to treatment and care thereof.[38]

---

[36] In another, related context, David Haberman (2006, p. 135) identifies as "extreme transcendentalism" a tendency of some Hindus to ignore the polluted condition of sacred rivers, claiming that their sacrality cannot be compromised by temporal conditions. In the name of care for bovines considered "sacred," I have seen some shelters in which cows are clearly underfed or unduly tethered.

[37] In her Kantian account of human interaction with animals, Korsgaard (2011) argues that in the absence of the ability to perceive consent to various treatments by animals, the *plausibility* of consent must be accepted where animals are well treated and not subjected either to experimentation or early death. Donaldson and Kymlicka (2013, pp. 111–112) share an interesting account of "dependent agency" among cows at the family farm of Rosamund Young (in Worcestershire, UK) (Young 2003, pp. 10, 52) that emphasizes the individuality of the cows in their choices regarding diet and movement.

[38] For a discussion of speciesism, anthropocentrism, and questions of similarity and difference between/among human and nonhuman animals, see Freeman (2010). Freeman identifies two "natural" moral principles of humans, namely *cooperation* to garner social support and *moderation* for bringing ecological balance. She urges that moderation should be "based on the idea of taking only what we need for our basic survival, complementing the principles of deep ecology, with any excess acts of harm constituting exploitation and a breach of ethics" (p. 22). This has a striking parallel in the ancient Ishopanishad statement (v. 1), albeit without the latter's strongly theistic orientation: "This visible world, and whatever exists beyond perception, is under the control of the Lord. Because of this you should enjoy only what is allotted to you by the Lord through *karma*. Do not hanker for more than that. Whose property is it?" (Swāmī 2006, p. 13, trans. of the eighteenth century Vaishnava commentator Baladeva Vidyabhūṣaṇa's rendering of the text).

This is *not* to endorse a premise of moral hierarchy that invites speculation on "acceptable levels of animal exploitation" (Donaldson and Kymlicka 2013, p. 4). Rather, it challenges us to recognize that we live with multiple differences (not "higher" and "lower," but having *difference*) among species, and these differences may be morally relevant for ethical behavior of humans in relation to nonhuman animals. As Alasdair Cochrane (2012, p. 11) points out, recognizing differences between species and their capacities impels us to consider that,

> some practices that are objectionable when done to humans are not objectionable when done to animals: keeping an animal as a pet is quite different from keeping a human as a slave; use animals to undertake certain kinds of work is quite unlike coercing human beings to labor; buying and selling animals is quite unlike trading human beings, and so on.

One distinction is particularly relevant for our discussion, namely among domestic, wild, and "liminal" animals—those that are brought into human community, those that are quite independent of humans, and those that live in partial relation to humans (Donaldson and Kymlicka 2013). Indeed, making these distinctions may lead us to entertain a reconceptualization of domestic animal political identity to better accomplish proper care. As we tend to locate citizenship and slavery on opposite ends of a polarity of civic freedom and bondage, let us consider Sue Donaldson's and Will Kymlicka's (2013) novel proposal, namely, to extend the concept of citizenship to be inclusive of domestic animals.[39] Donaldson's and Kymlicka's point of departure is that animal rights theory, while valid and important, has focused exclusively on negative rights—basically the right of animals not to be harmed. While this thinking has driven important advances in animal advocacy, "[t]he animal advocacy movement has nibbled at the edges of this [global] system of animal exploitation, but the system itself endures, and indeed expands and deepens all the time, with remarkably little public discussion" (pp. 1–2). Drawing inspiration from

---

[39] As they propose "citizenship" for domestic animals, Donaldson and Kymlicka propose "sovereignty" for wild animals and "denizenship" for liminal animals. Such categories and designations of community membership are intended to recognize animals "not just as individual subjects entitled to respect of their basic rights, but as members of communities—both ours and theirs—woven together in relations of interdependency, mutuality, and responsibility" (2013, p. 255).

the disability movement, the authors argue that a conceptual framework of citizenship can and should be conceived for inclusion of domesticated animals and that this is possible if one sets aside the arbitrary limitations imposed on citizenship by a cognitivist interpretation of required capacities for citizenship. This involves a change in the conception of citizenship that "recognizes that we are all interdependent, and experience varying forms and degrees of agency according to context, and over the life-course" (p. 108). It then becomes possible to recognize that domestic animals (including bovines) possess, in their own ways, the three capacities specified as required for citizenship. Domestic animals demonstrate (1) the capacity to have a subjective good and the ability to communicate it; (2) the capacity to participate (specifically, by sheer presence in human settlement, as opposed to being made invisible, as in the modern meat industry); and (3) the capacity for cooperation, self-regulation, and reciprocity (pp. 103, 108–122).[40] Among nine specific areas of presupposition for citizenship discussed by the authors, we can give attention to four, with respect to cow care[41]: (1) mobility and the sharing of public space; (2) use of animal products; (3) use of animal labor; and (4) sex and reproduction (p. 123).

Regarding *mobility and sharing of public space*, the authors conclude that animals, like humans, need "sufficient mobility, not unlimited mobility. This need may be met with large fenced ranges and pastures, and parks," and restrictions on mobility would be justified by the need for protection of the animals and/or humans. Yet justifiable restrictions would, in such a vision of citizenship, "always have a provisional status—open to appeal, negotiation, and ongoing evolution. We simply don't know what human-animal society might eventually look like under these conditions" (p. 130). Bovines *should* have large areas of open space for grazing, but as we have

---

[40]So, for example, domestic (including farm) animals (1) show preference, interests, and desires, through vocalizations, gestures, movements, and signals—communications that humans can and should attend to; (2) can, by their sheer presence, be advocates and agents of change or show resistance to work; and (3) can experience a wide range of emotions, including empathy, trust, altruism, reciprocity, and a sense of fair play (Donaldson and Kymlicka 2013, pp. 108–117).

[41]The other five areas are: (1) basic socialization; (2) duties of protection; (3) medical care; (4) predation/diet; and (5) political representation.

seen in the previous chapter, in India such conditions have become the exception. And yet, the fact that cows are seen freely roaming the streets of village, town, and urban areas is a striking indicator of how human-animal society could be imagined if these cows would be properly cared for (see Fig. 5.1).[42]

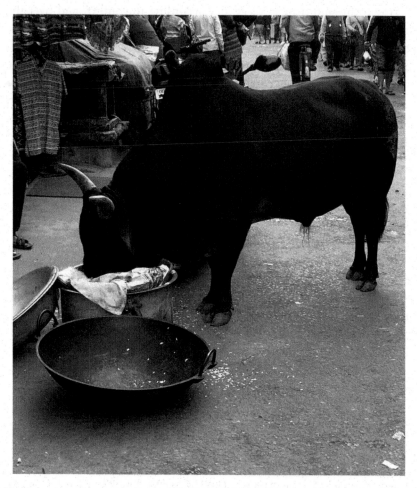

Fig. 5.1   A street-wandering ox in Puri is given a full pot of rice by a shopkeeper

Use of animal products. The *Zoopolis* authors argue that to distinguish between (legitimate) *use* of animals and their (illegitimate) *exploitation* is comparable to seeing what forms of use of humans are "consistent with full membership in society, and what forms of use condemn people to the status of a permanently subordinated caste or class" (p. 134). They reject the idea that any use is necessarily exploitative or that use inevitably leads "down a slippery slope to exploitation." Rather, they suggest that "a refusal to use others—effectively to prevent them from contributing to the general social good—can itself be a form of denying them full citizenship" that is as problematic as it is for one group to be kept as a permanently subordinated caste. Significantly, the authors give as example the careful sheering and collection of wool from sheep that due to domestication and breeding can no longer shed their wool naturally: To not (carefully) sheer them in timely fashion would be a form of abuse and to not make use of their wool "begins to look perverse" (pp. 136–137).

What particularly increases the danger of exploitation is commercialization of the product or products in question, and this is certainly a major—arguably *the*—issue with respect to cow milk. The ideal is for there to be village culture wherein cow milk that is truly surplus over calf feeding would be highly valued by the human village members and, in accordance with the bhakti paradigm, would offer it (and the other dairy products and derivative preparations) as delicacies to temple or home images, especially of Lord Krishna, the thus sanctified offering (*prasada*) to be subsequently given mainly to human children. The *Zoopolis* authors point out that the considerable difficulties involved in maintaining cows in a non-exploitative way would result in a highly reduced bovine population (p. 139). In fact, if this were to happen, it could be a blessing for the global natural environment that currently suffers acutely from excessive animal—especially bovine—husbandry for commercial purposes. Further,

---

[42] It could be argued that when bovines become strays, they are forced out of the category of domestic animals to become liminal animals. Yet strays must be distinguished from what might be called "day wanderers"—bovines with human owners who are set out during the day to wander (usually in village or semi-urban areas in India) and return to their owners in the evening. One can often see such "day wanderers" being provided some food by particular neighbors of their owners, and they are known to quickly learn which homes they can expect to receive food and will then stop at those homes each day.

for Hindus, rarity of cows could serve to enhance the sense of their venerability and therefore be conducive to their proper care.

Use of Animal Labor. Certain animals, such as certain dogs and donkeys, can with little training perform such activities as shepherding and protection. Donaldson and Kymlicka invite readers to imagine non-exploitative arrangements for involving such animals in types of labor that come naturally to them. At the same time, they call attention to the danger of animals' "adaptive preference" being misread as behavior that is accepting or welcoming of their labor, when it is actually the result of training that is thinly disguised coercion (p. 141). As we saw in Chapter 4, oxen trained for work have been perceived by their trainers as showing eagerness to exert themselves in drawing a plow or a cart. Whether this would be regarded as adaptive preference would be a matter of debate, but it is clearly the case that bovines, both male and female, need to be given opportunity for sufficient regular bodily movement and exercise, an opportunity usually denied in cow shelters.[43]

Sex and Reproduction: Domestication is fundamentally involved in reproduction control, usually with the aim to increase certain traits in animals considered favorable or useful for humans and to reduce or eliminate traits considered unfavorable. That humans see such practices to be morally acceptable is deeply ingrained; one could argue that such practices fundamentally counter any notion of nonhuman animals being seriously regarded as co-citizens with humans. However, the *Zoopolis* authors point out that regulation of sex and reproduction occurs in several ways both within human society and wild animal societies and, of course, is also regulated by external factors in all cases. Also, to allow unrestricted breeding among domestic animals such as bovines would be against their own interests, as it would lead to a breakdown of the conditions in which they can live. With bovines, an important starting point for reproduction regulation in a Hindu care ethics milieu would be a *reduction* of reproduction for cows, unburdening them of forced pregnancy in the interest of increased milk production. Related to this could be to abandon crossbreeding for

---

[43]That bulls and oxen should be treated gently is indicated (in a rather curious way) in the Mahabharata, wherein the only exception to the rule that they should not be driven with goad or whip is when engaged in plowing the ground in preparation for a ritual sacrifice (Ganguli 1991, p. 88; Mahabharata 13.69).

increased milk production. This is a major issue in contemporary India where, as we saw in Chapter 4, there is growing concern to preserve and recover indigenous bovine breeds to counter the practice of crossbreeding indigenous with non-indigenous—especially European—bovines.

Dharma-Based Communitarianism

Surely from this very brief sketch of four areas of presupposition for citizenship, we can only begin to picture a citizenship framework that is inclusive of animals, particularly of cows. And while this framework is predicated on an animal rights orientation to animal activism, my proposal is that the ethics of care approach, with its positive attention to relationship, needs, feelings, context, and responsibility, can serve to better comprehend how animal citizenship can become a reality among individual humans and communities. Yet citizenship, as we understand it today, has no meaning without the existence of a state, the modern locus of political activity and political background of community. We may ask what sort of political theory would best respond to and complement a Hindu—especially a dharma, yoga, and bhakti-based—animal ethics. Here I will put forth *communitarianism* as a starting point for our purposes, hastening to add that "communitarianism" is not to be confused with "communalism," the term used in contemporary India to describe the divisive socio-political and religious force seen as cause and perpetuator of conflict in India, especially between Hindus and Muslims or between Hindus and Christians.

As a political theory, communitarianism is typically contrasted with utilitarianism and with liberalism. Unlike utilitarianism, communitarianism derives the common good from the shared norms of *particular* societies, and unlike liberalism, communitarianism urges active involvement by the *state* in promoting what is determined to be the common good, over the rights and liberties of individuals (Cochrane 2010, p. 91). In applying communitarian political theory to questions of animal care, a standard formulation of communitarian thought can be problematic in several ways. Broadly speaking, to establish principles for determining what constitutes just negative regulation (regulations preventing injustice and abuse of animals) can face knotty questions regarding human rights (Cochrane 2010, pp. 76–91).[44]

I propose, rather, a *dharma-based communitarianism* as an alternative approach, one that is necessarily inflected with the devotional vision of the Bhagavata Purana text and the culture it represents.[45] Bhagavata-dharma-based communitarianism would have as its basis for deliberation and decision-making the discernment of applicable principles rooted in the three paradigms previously sketched, namely dharma, yoga, and bhakti. Application of such principles may not be possible in entire states, but in particular communities within states application could occur with the guidance of persons who are recognized by such communities as qualified to do so. We recall (from Chapter 2) the Bhagavad Gita's statement (3.21), "Whatever the greatest one does, common people do just the same, following the standard he sets," and we recall that King Yudhishthira, by his care for the dog, proves to be an exemplar of such a "greatest one," as does Bharata in his concern for ants (discussed earlier in this chapter). The Bhagavata Purana offers several such model practitioners of bhagavata dharma (including Yudhisthira), elaborating extensively on their qualities and qualifications as leaders of society.[46]

---

[44]Cochrane (2010, p. 91) summarizes the challenges that communitarianism faces with respect to animal care: "Firstly, any attempt to promote the shared values and norms of a community raises the question of whose values and norms are to be promoted. For as we have seen, states contain a number of different communities. Secondly, this is important in the case of animals because often states contain communities which have quite different attitudes and practices relating to animals when compared to those of wider society. Thirdly, one option for communitarian thinkers is to advocate 'multiculturalist' policies which allow communities to be exempt from general animal welfare standards. This allows for the goals and values of a range of communities to be respected and promoted. Finally, however, such policies are extremely controversial and have been objected to on the grounds that such practices cause real harm to individual animals, and because it is often unclear just which types of group warrant such exemptions and why."

[45]As noted in Chapter 2, the Bhagavata Purana, an early Sanskrit text of the Purana genre of sacred lore, thrives in popularity in the present day and is highly esteemed in learned Hindu circles. It is therefore, as well as for reasons of its intrinsic value, most appropriate to bring it to bear in this discussion of ethics in relation to animals in the context of political philosophy.

[46]One epithet of Krishna mentioned by Queen Kunti (the mother of Yudhishthira and the other Pandava brothers) is *akinchana-gochara*—"he who is accessible to persons who have no material claims" (BhP 1.8.26). Noteworthy in relation to cow care is that *gochara* (accessible) literally means "cow pasture." As in English, a cow pasture is also a "range," spiritually progressive persons, who make no claims of material assets, are "within the range" of Krishna's blessing (see also Chapter 2, footnote 30).

To better grasp how a bhagavata-dharma-based communitarian political approach would work brings us to the notion of "anticipatory community."[47] An anticipatory community must be sufficiently well defined through consensus regarding its values of animal care. Then a bhagavata-dharma-based communitarian approach to political practice can serve such a community's purpose of standing for its values (in this case of animal care and more specifically cow care as we have envisioned it in its best form). On such a basis, the community would also be enabled to *promote* these values in the wider society (Cochrane 2010, pp. 74–78). A ready example of this approach may be seen in M. K. Gandhi's efforts to establish ashrams (hermitages) with such practices and ideals. As a current example, we have the Govardhan Eco Village, introduced in the previous chapter, and in Chapter 6, we will look at two similar communities, one in Bengal, India, and one in Hungary. In these cases, the "communitarian" spirit of governance have been based on similar bhagavata-dharma principles, such that all community members have chosen to abide by regulations that are supportive of the respective communities' values, particularly regarding animal care.

In the case of Govardhan Eco Village, one can discern a strong emphasis on pursuit of the four virtue-nourishing practices that we considered earlier, namely compassion, austerity, purity, and truthfulness. More specifically, these values are secured by explicit disavowal of all meat-eating, intake of any form of intoxicants (including tea and coffee), illicit sexual activity, and gambling. These disavowals are taken as the basis for the positive activities of care that constitute the community's vision of

---

[47] In Larry Rasmussen's (Christian-inflected) portrayal of "anticipatory community," such projects must be "intimate communities of moral nurture" in which the "seeds of an Earth ethic" must be planted and nurtured, to meet "adaptive challenges." He defines his term thusly: "'Anticipatory communities' are home places where it is possible to reimagine worlds and reorder possibilities, places where new or renewed practices give focus to an ecological and postindustrial way of life. Such communities have the qualities of a haven, a set-apart and safe place yet a place open to creative risk. Here basic moral formation happens by conscious choice and not by default (simply conforming to the ethos and unwritten ethic of the surrounding culture). Here eco-social virtues are consciously cultivated and embodied in community practices. Here the fault lines of modernity are exposed" (Rasmussen 2013, pp. 223, 226–227).

bhakti-centered life—the way of devoted service to the supreme person, Bhagavan, revered in this community especially in the form of Krishna.[48]

We thus come back to a key principle of the bhakti paradigm, namely discernment and response to divine preference. This principle is particularly highlighted and celebrated at Govardhan Eco Village in the practice of *seva*—attentive service to Krishna, situated in several shrines on the GEV land. Ever celebrating Krishna's identity as divine cowherd, GEV residents are keen to prepare a wide variety of vegetarian—including dairy-based—delicacies for his pleasure. The dairy-based food preparations—mainly sweet preparations—use exclusively milk from GEV's own hand-milked cows, and these are ritually offered to Krishna at designated times each day. Following the offerings, the sanctified food is received and "honored" by the community members in community meals. This culinary practice encompasses the entire range of processes from farming and husbandry to cooking, ritually offering, and receiving the offering "remnants" (*prasada*), creating a cycle of engagement in which food becomes a central vehicle for spiritual as well as physical nourishment. This nourishment then translates into the performance of varied bhakti practices for self-cultivation and outreach, both of which are seen in the context of the dharma paradigm as enactment of nonviolent sacrifice, which takes the specific form of *samkirtana*—collective or congregational celebration of participation in divine activity (*lila*).

Concluding Reflections

I began this chapter with a survey of three Hindu paradigms of thought and practice in relation to animal ethics, namely the dharma paradigm,

---

[48] In considering this community's standard of four strict disavowals, Roy Perrett offers an interesting and relevant discussion on "moral saints." Noting a distinction in Western "commonsense morality" between ordinary and extraordinary morality, morality, narrowly conceived, is concerned with those rules that make human society possible. In contrast, "[t]he extraordinary ideals are concerned with what in ethics lies beyond morality so conceived: the *supramoral*. No one can be morally blamed for not realizing supramoral ideals. "In other words, an ideal like sainthood may be praiseworthy but not obligatory." The point to note here is that the four "regulative principles" (as the community's disavowals are called) constitute in this, and its affiliated communities, as basic morality, even if many would consider them supramoral ideals (Perrett 1998, pp. 31–42).

the yoga paradigm, and the bhakti paradigm. The dharma and bhakti paradigms form a value polarity, with yoga as the linking element between the two. Dharma as normativity emphasizes values of duty, honoring obligation, and observance of regulation, thus locating it largely in deontic and consequentialist normative ethics that is sensitive to the recognition of rights and the observance of duties. Normative dharma includes a sense of duty with respect to all living beings, all of whom have rights by virtue of their non-material identities being qualitatively equal to all other beings, possessing sentience and the potential to realize personhood.

On the opposite end of this value polarity is the bhakti paradigm, which emphasizes contextualized responsiveness and responsibility to individual beings, rooted in reverence that acknowledges a divine reality as the source of all life and that therefore makes all life sacred. I suggest that, while cultivated within a moral space circumscribed by dharma (both descriptive and normative), bhakti particularly resonates with the ethics of care approach to human–nonhuman animal relations. Further, because bhakti that is directed to the divinity Krishna is especially concerned with the care of bovines (*go-seva*), this particular inflection of the bhakti paradigm is an especially important locus for comprehending Hindu animal ethics both as ideal and as an often-challenging practice.

We also briefly considered abolitionist objections to animal—particularly bovine—care as practiced in Hindu traditions. These objections give important cause to reassess current practices and to do all that is possible to eliminate abuse. However, with few exceptions, Hindus will not accept the idea that humans should have no involvement with bovines whatsoever. Rather, they regard human–bovine engagement as a major example of how human–nonhuman animal symbiosis functions in the greater context of a world order of interdependence. Such engagement, if practiced conscientiously (according to principles of dharma, yoga, and bhakti), offers a viable, potentially transformative alternative to the essentially parasitic way of life based on an extractive economy that human society has come to regard as the norm (Ranganathan 2017b, pp. 177–178).

Together, value orientations of dharma and bhakti, linked with practices of yoga, may offer a comprehensive basis for recognizing certain nonhuman animals as citizens—in at least an analogical sense—within communities that are committed to these values. These values are rooted in the vision that all creatures, being of divine origin, have their own trajectories of spiritual progress that may involve enriching interaction with humans. Further, such interactions can occur by conscious cultivation of habits that are liberative for both humans and nonhumans. Through such devotional practice, full personhood in relationship with the primordial supreme person can be realized. Finally, commitment to these values comes with recognition that they afford self-transformation as well as world-transformation, leading toward the full affirmation and protection of all sentient beings' value and dignity.

References

Alexander, Larry, and Michael Moore. 2016. Deontological Ethics. In *The Stanford Encyclopedia of Philosophy*, ed. Edward N. Zalta. https://plato.stanford.edu/archives/win2016/entries/ethics-deontological/. Accessed 26 December 2018.

Babaji, Ananta Das, and Advaita dāsa (trans.). 2010. *Śrī-Śrī Prema Bhakti Candrikā [of] Śrīla Narottama Dāsa Ṭhākura Mahāśaya*. Mathura: Sri Krishna Chaitanya Shastra Mandir.

Bryant, Edwin F. 2009. *The Yoga Sūtras of Patañjali*. New York: North Point Press.

Bryant, Edwin F. 2017. *Bhakti Yoga: Tales and Teachings from the Bhāgavata Purāṇa*. New York: North Point Press.

Clark, Stephen R.L. 2011. Animals in Classical and Late Antique Philosophy. In *The Oxford Handbook of Animal Ethics*, ed. Tom L. Beauchamp and R.G. Frey, 35–60. Oxford: Oxford University Press.

Cochrane, Alasdair. 2010. *An Introduction to Animals and Political Theory*. London: Palgrave Macmillan.

Cochrane, Alasdair. 2012. *Animal Rights Without Liberation: Applied Ethics and Human Obligations*. New York: Columbia University Press.

Dalmiya, Vrinda. 2016. *Caring to Know: Comparative Care Ethics, Feminist Epistemology, and the Mahābhārata*. Delhi: Oxford University Press.

Davis, Donald R., Jr. 2010. *The Spirit of Hindu Law*. Cambridge: Cambridge University Press.

Debroy, Bibek (trans.). 2015. *The Mahabharata*, 10 vols. Gurgaon: Penguin.

Donaldson, Sue, and Will Kymlicka. 2013. *Zoopolis: A Political Theory of Animal Rights*. Oxford: Oxford University Press.

Donovan, Josephine, and Carol J. Adams (eds.). 2007. *The Feminist Care Tradition in Animal Ethics: A Reader*. New York: Columbia University Press.

Ellis, Thomas B. 2013. *On the Death of the Pilgrim: The Postcolonial Hermeneutics of Jarava Lal Mehta*. Dordrecht: Springer.

Fink, Charles K. 2013. The Cultivation of Virtue in Buddhist Ethics. *Journal of Buddhist Ethics* 20. http://blogs.dickenson.edu/buddhistethics/. Accessed 18 October 2018.

Francione, Gary L. 2004. Animals: Property or Persons? In *Animal Rights: Current Debates and New Directions*, ed. Cass R. Sunstein and Marth C. Nussbaum, 108–144. Oxford: Oxford University Press. Available at http://law.bepress.com/rutgersnewarklwps/art21.

Frazier, Jessica. 2017. *Hindu Worldviews: Theories of Self, Ritual and Reality*. London: Bloomsbury.

Freeman, Carrie Packwood. 2010. Embracing Humanimality: Deconstructing the Human/Animal Dichotomy. In *Arguments About Animal Ethics*, ed. Greg Goodale and Jason Edward Black. Lanham, MD: Lexington Books.

Ganguli, Kisari Mohan (trans.). 1991 [1970]. *The Mahabharata of Krishna-Dwaipayana Vyasa*. New Delhi: Motilal Banarsidass.

Glucklich, Arial. 1994. *The Sense of Adharma*. New York: Oxford University Press.

Goswami, H.D. 2015. *A Comprehensive Guide to Bhagavad-Gītā with Literal Translation*. Gainesville, FL.: Krishna West.

Govindrajan, Radhika. 2018. *Animal Intimacies: Interspecies Relatedness in India's Central Himalayas*. Chicago: University of Chicago Press.

Haberman, David L. 2006. *River of Love in an Age of Pollution: The Yamuna River of North India*. Berkeley: University of California Press.

Holdrege, Barbara A. 2013. Vraja-*Dhāman*: Krishna Embodied in Geographic Place and Transcendent Space. In *The Bhāgavata Purāṇa: Sacred Text and Living Tradition*, ed. Ravi M. Gupta and Kenneth R. Valpey, 91–116. New York: Columbia University Press.

Howard, Veena Rani. 2018. Lessons from 'The Hawk and the Dove': Reflections on the *Mahābhārata's* Animal Parables and Ethical Predicaments. *Sophia* 57: 119–131.

Kansal, Vishrut. 2016. The Curious Case of *Nagaraja* in India: Are Animals Still Regarded as 'Property' With No Claim Rights? *Journal of International Wildlife Law and Policy* 19 (3): 256–267. https://doi.org/10.1080/13880292.2016.1204885.

Korsgaard, Christine M. 2011. Interacting with Animals: A Kantian Account. In *The Oxford Handbook of Animal Ethics*, ed. Tom L. Beauchamp and R.G. Frey, 91–118. Oxford: Oxford University Press.

Long, Jeffery D. 2013. The Dharma Paradigm and Ethos: Some Insights from Jainism and Vedānta. *International Journal of Dharma Studies* 1: 2. https://doi.org/10.1186/2196-8802-1-2.

Monier-Williams, Monier. [1899] 1995. Dharma. In *A Sanskrit-English Dictionary*. Delhi: Motilal Banarsidass.

Neiman, Susan. 2008. *Moral Clarity: A Guide for Grown-Up Idealists*. Orlando: Harcourt.

Nussbaum, Martha. 2011. The Capabilities Approach and Animal Entitlements. In *The Oxford Handbook of Animal Ethics*, ed. Beauchamp and Frey. Oxford: Oxford University Press.

Perrett, Roy W. 1998. *Hindu Ethics: A Philosophical Study*. Honolulu: University of Hawai'i Press.

Prentiss, Karen Pechilis. 1999. *The Embodiment of Bhakti*. New York: Oxford University Press.

Ranganathan, Shyam (ed.). 2017a. *The Bloomsbury Research Handbook of Indian Ethics*. London: Bloomsbury.

Ranganathan, Shyam. 2017b. Patañjali's Yoga: Universal Ethics as the Formal Cause of Autonomy. In *The Bloomsbury Research Handbook of Indian Ethics*, ed. Shyam Ranganathan, 177–202. London: Bloomsbury.

Rasmussen, Larry L. 2013. *Earth-Honoring Faith: Religious Ethics in a New Key*. Oxford: Oxford University Press.

Schuster, Joshua. 2016. The Vegan and the Sovereign. In *Critical Perspectives on Veganism*, ed. Jodey Castricano and Rasmus R. Simonsen, 203–223. London: Palgrave Macmillan.

Schweig, Graham M. 2013. The Rāsa Līlā of Krishna and the Gopīs: On the Bhāgavata's Vision of Boundless Love. In *The Bhāgavata Purāna: Sacred Text and Living Tradition*, ed. Ravi M. Gupta and Kenneth R. Valpey, 117–141. New York: Columbia University Press.

Sinha, Jadunath. 1983. *Jivagosvami's Religion of Devotion and Love*. Varanasi: Chowkhamba Vidyabhavan.

Stamm, Katrin. 2015. On the Moral and Spiritual Implications of the Fivefold Sacrifice: Metaphysical Obligations to the Divine in Nature According to Vaishnava Texts and in Contrast with Immanuel Kant. *Journal of Vaishnava Studies* 24 (1) (Fall): 91–120.

Steiner, Gary. 2013. *Animals and the Limits of Postmodernism*. New York: Columbia University Press.

Stewart, James. 2017. Dharma Dogs: Can Animals Understand the Dharma? Textual and Ethnographic Considerations. *Journal of Buddhist Ethics*, vol. 24. Retrieved on January 10, 2019 from http://blogs.dickinson.edu/buddhistethics/?s=dharma+dogs.

Sukthankar, Vishnu S. (ed.). 1942. *The Mahābhārata*, Critical ed. Poona: Bhandarkar Oriental Research Institute.

Sutton, Nicholas. 2000. *Religious Doctrines in the Mahābhārata*. Delhi: Motilal Banarsidass.

Swāmī, Bhānu (trans.). 2006. *Īśopaniṣad Commentary by Madhvācārya, Vedānta Deśika, Baladeva Vidyābhūṣaṇa, Bhaktivinoda Ṭhākura*. Chennai: Sri Vaikuntha Enterprises.

Törzsök, Judit. 2007. *Friendly Advice by Narayana & King Vikrama's Adventures*. The Clay Sanskrit Library. New York: New York University Press.

Whicher, Ian. 1998. *The Integrity of the Yoga Darśana: A Reconsideration of Classical Yoga*. Albany, NY: State University of New York Press.

Wise, Steven M. 2011. Animal Rights, One Step at a Time. In *Animal Rights: Current Debates and New Directions*, ed. Cass R. Sunstein and Marth C. Nussbaum, 16–50. Oxford: Oxford University Press.

Young, Rosamund. 2003. *The Secret Life of Cows: Animal Sentience at Work*. Preston: Farming Books.

Zagzebski, Linda Trinkaus. 2004. *Divine Motivation Theory*. Cambridge: Cambridge University Press.

6

"These Cows Will Not Be Lost": Envisioning a Care-Full Future for Cows

An early seventeenth-century account of what might today be called an interreligious dialogue includes a brief discussion on scriptural justifications—or lack of justifications—for cow slaughter. Krishnadasa Kaviraja, the author of the hagiographic Bengali language Chaitanya Charitamrita (The Ambrosial Exploits of Sri Chaitanya), tells of an encounter between his hero, the young ecstatic saint Vishvambara (later to become known as Shri Krishna Caitanya), and the local Muslim magistrate (*Qazi*). In the course of their conversation, according to Krishnadasa, after Chaitanya challenges the Qazi about Muslim bovine killing practices, the Qazi concedes that Muslims are ill-justified in slaughtering bovines, considering the many benefits they bestow on humans.[1]

---

[1] Prabhupada (2005 [1974], pp. 630–686); *Caitanya-caritamṛta* Adi-lila 17.124–226. In the course of the conversation, Chaitanya provocatively, though politely, asks (in Swami Prabhupada's translation), "You drink cows' milk; therefore the cow is your mother. And the bull produces grains for your maintenance; therefore he is your father. Since the bull and cow are your father and mother, how can you kill and eat them? What kind of religious principle is this? On what strength are you so daring that you commit such sinful activities?" (vv. 153–154).

© The Author(s) 2020
K. R. Valpey, *Cow Care in Hindu Animal Ethics*,
The Palgrave Macmillan Animal Ethics Series,
https://doi.org/10.1007/978-3-030-28408-4_6

Whatever the historical accuracy of this account might be, for us to note is that the story was part of an early vision of possibility, one of tolerance and coexistence between the two communities, Hindu and Muslim. What begins as a sharp confrontation between Chaitanya's followers and the magistrate over the latter's banning of the former's public religious demonstrations concludes amicably: The Qazi safeguards what he had previously banned. There is no suggestion that the Qazi resolves to change his own dietary habits, but neither is this represented as a problem for the Hindus, who are now assured freedom to openly perform their demonstrations of *nagara-hari-kirtan*—singing divine names in the town streets. Krishnadasa here describes what might be called a "moderate heart change," whereby no dramatic conversions or transformations occur, but through dialogue a "live and let live" agreement is reached.[2] And embedded in this agreement is an implied agreement of mutual tolerance of the other community's dietary practices and consequent dealings with animals, specifically cows.

As we have seen, there are competing narratives about bovines in India, narratives that either look toward the past or, alternatively, ignore the past and imagine a future of ever-expanding economic growth afforded by ever-increasing technical efficiency in colonization of bovine bodies. In this chapter, the aim is to sketch, even if only in rough outline, an alternative future for bovines. At the core of this alternative future is the sense that the root of any outward change must be a change of heart—to be sure, a gradual and generally moderate change of heart—of individuals and expanding communities. Yet practical action is equally necessary, action that is energized by vision, inspiration, and knowledge. As a first step in developing vision, we here look at two out of several existing intentional communities in which cow care is an important feature. As "anticipatory communities," one in northeast India and one in southwest Hungary, we look at them as models-in-the-making of a possible future for cow care.

We then examine the issue of care and natural death for bovines, with two cases of conflict with officials in the UK over demands for euthanasia. This points to one area of challenge for cow care expanding outside India,

---

[2]In Krishnadas' Chaitanya Charitamrita account (Adi-lila 17.178–217), in fact the Qazi does show what we could call a change of heart. To be noted is that this episode follows a key "conversion" story, namely, that of Vishvambara/Chaitanya, who had recently returned home from pilgrimage as a changed man, having met and received mantra initiation from his guru, Ishvara Puri.

where differing conceptions of animal welfare (and in one case public health concerns) collide. Returning to India, an account of a "glorious death" of a much-beloved ox calls our attention to the notion of bovines' afterlife futures.

Since we may think of a positive cow care future as calling for public activism, we then examine how certain types of activism may be causing more harm than good. Why this is so needs to be understood in order to avoid such mistakes and develop a broad-based culture of genuine care. I suggest that this aim can be served by awareness of an important teaching of the Bhagavad Gita, namely a threefold typology of action in terms of the three "qualities" of Samkhya (mentioned briefly in Chapter 4). Finally, I offer six positive *affirmations* based on action predominated by *sattva-guna*—the quality of goodness and illumination. These affirmations respond to and embrace six "moral foundations of political life" as a way of exploring how cow care would be able to find place and expand in the wider world. This may be seen as a thought experiment rooted in a notion of dharma as an ongoing process of balancing for the purpose of sustaining cosmic well-being and a moral landscape in which bhakti can thrive. It is one way of affirming for the future the phrase from the ancient Rigveda that we encountered in Chapter 2, "These cows will not be lost."

Anticipatory Communities

As intentional communities, it will be appropriate to regard Mayapur Chandrodaya Mandir (MCM) and New Vraja Dhama (NVD) as "anticipatory communities" in three ways. First, they function as extensive, long-term, multifaceted experiments, *anticipating* specific sorts of outcome while learning from mistakes and building on successes. Cow care is considered integral to these experiments because, as noted earlier, Swami Prabhupada, ISKCON's founder, put so much emphasis on the practice. This engenders a sense of resolve: Somehow or other it must be possible to demonstrate that, with cow care properly practiced, the ideal of sustainable country living is both possible and preferable to modern ways of life that depend on an industrial economy. This is not to say that one day these communities expect to "breathe easily" in confidence that the goal of fully sustainable self-sufficiency has been reached. Rather, the anticipation is for increasing experience and skill in facing the countless challenges that come up in such communities.

Second, MCM and NVD aspire to function as models that can be, at least theoretically and in certain ways, replicated, and thus they *anticipate* a broad application of their principles in the development of more such communities. Larry Rasmussen, from whom I borrow the phrase "anticipatory community," notes that clearly the global environmental destruction and climate change trends call for systematic changes (large scale—national, regional, international). But such changes "usually don't materialize if they are not already present in anticipatory communities, even if those communities are modest in size and number" (Rasmussen 2013, p. 121).

Third, MCM and NVD may be regarded as anticipatory specifically with respect to their cow care programs, in that they show a viable direction of practice conducive to imagining bovines as both "family members" and "citizens," in meaningful, even if figurative, ways. After looking briefly at these two communities, we will discuss this further, in relation to five "basic rules" of cow care rooted in animal rights and care ethics (Meyer-Glitza 2018, pp. 193–194).

Mayapur Chandrodaya Mandir, West Bengal

130 kilometers north of Kolkata along the Bhagirathi-Hooghly River (a tributary of the Ganges) is Shri Mayapur Dhama, an area that Chaitanyaite, or Gaudiya, Vaishnavas celebrate as the birthplace of their founding figure, Sri Krishna Chaitanya (1486–1533). Just south of the temple commemorating Chaitanya's birth is the Shri Mayapur Chandrodaya Mandir, a large and increasingly bustling development with more than 4000 residents, some 30% of whom are foreigners (Fahy 2018, p. 2). In recent years, there has been an explosion of construction, inspired by the community's main project, the massive under-construction Temple of the Vedic Planetarium (TOVP). Initially established in the early 1970s by Swami Prabhupada, as the community expanded, he designated Mayapur as the world headquarters for his mission, the International Society for Krishna Consciousness (ISKCON, which we first encountered

in Chapter 3). The complex includes a goshala with some 360 bovines, mainly of mixed breed, and further breeding is strictly controlled under pressure of limited land—some 12 acres for the goshala proper, plus 80 acres for grazing and growing of fodder, out of some 700 acres in total held by the Mayapur Chandrodaya Mandir.

There are two points to note regarding the future of cow care in connection with Mayapur. The first concerns the present numbers of visitors to the project, hundreds of whom on any given day make the extra effort to seek out the goshala, several hundred meters back from the main areas of attraction (the present temple, gardens, guesthouses, and restaurant). Present visitor numbers are expected to multiply many-fold when the TOVP is anticipated to open, in 2022. On the positive side, for many visitors the goshala serves an awareness and educational purpose, exposing people to the alternative to cow slaughter. Mayapur is in the State of West Bengal, where bovine slaughter restriction or prohibition laws are minimal.[3] As a showcase of cow care, Mayapur Chandrodaya Mandir can have a significant impact on people to simply recognize that there is such an alternative. But while this is the hope, one may wonder if the goshala will serve more as a simulacrum of cow care than as a place of genuine care: It might be argued that the cows are subjected to too much contact with humans, as in a zoo. Being "on exhibit" several hours each day could be seen as compromising their quality of life while instrumentalizing and objectifying them.[4]

---

[3]There are no slaughter prohibition laws in seven of the eight northeastern Union Territories. Of the twenty-nine States and Union Territories, eleven prohibit slaughter of all bovines, including cows, calves, bulls, and buffaloes (Jammu and Kashmir, Punjab, Haryana, Rajasthan, Gujarat, Chhattisgarh, Uttarakhand, Himachal Pradesh, New Delhi, Goa, and Daman and Diu). Another ten states prohibit only slaughter of cows and calves; and one (Madhya Pradesh) prohibits slaughter of cows, calves, and buffaloes, but not bulls. Further details, including various exceptions and punishments for offenses, can be found here: http://www.dahd.nic.in/dahd/reports/report-of-the-national-commission-on-cattle/chapter-ii-executive-summary/annex-ii-8.aspx.

[4]Concerns were recently expressed by some MCM residents about neglect of aging and dying cows. Clearly an institution of this size must guard against the tendency to allow its missionizing priorities to prevail at the cost of its principles of care rooted in bhakti, meant to be the very foundation of the mission. Mayapur Chandrodaya Mandir's 13-point mission statement includes (as the fifth statement), "The cows and bulls are kept happy, protected, worshiped, and fully engaged, setting a standard for cow protection all over the world" (Unpublished document, "Sri Mayapur Project—Articulating Srila Prabhupada's Vision: References, version 4.2").

Reinforcing this concern would appear to be Mayapur Chandrodaya's current managerial priorities. As Mayapur Chandrodaya Mandir anticipates a major influx of visitors, the main source of attraction for them will be the massive TOVP. As a multi-million-dollar construction project, understandably, almost all fund-raising attention goes toward temple construction, leaving the goshala as a lesser priority for the MCM management team. Despite the reasonable justification that the end result will be much greater attention to the goshala, there lurks—for this observer—a sense of irony in the juxtaposition of this globalizing construction project, dubbed by another observer as "a colossal monument to hybridity" (Fahy 2018, p. 15) with the project's goshala (see Fig. 6.1). Practically in the temple structure's massive shadow, the cows may appear like mere tokens of the world of "plain living and high thinking" that Prabhupada so much emphasized as the aim of the project to showcase.

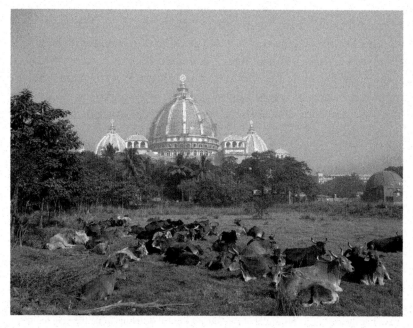

Fig. 6.1 Mayapur goshala cows ruminate in a field before the (under construction) Temple of the Vedic Planetarium

In a sense, the second noteworthy feature of Mayapur Chandrodaya Mandir regarding cow care similarly highlights the contrast between village life and cosmopolitan globalized mission. This feature is a nascent effort to establish a community-supported agriculture (CSA) program with local village dairy farmers.[5] At present, following the pattern of the Indian dairy industry as we have seen, when the greater Mayapur (Nadia District) farmers' cows reduce or no longer give milk, they are typically sold. In this locale, it means that the cows are either slaughtered locally or, more typically, smuggled to the neighboring country, Bangladesh, for slaughter. To create an alternative to this scenario, Pancharatna Das, an American resident of ISKCON Mayapur for 28 years, prepares to launch a CSA program that would attract local Hindu farmers (and possibly even Muslim farmers),[6] to arrange for the retired cows' upkeep through subscriptions. The idea is that since the Western population of Mayapur is growing, it can support an "ahimsa added value" dairy system.[7]

A first step in such a scheme is to convince the local dairy farmers to cooperate by not selling their retired cows or young bulls for slaughter. They would be rewarded in various ways for their self-restraint, such as by building for them better cow shelters than they presently have.[8] The retired bovines would then, ideally, be cared for by the same villagers, motivated by their culturally, and religiously ingrained understanding that human beings should be protecting, not killing, cows.[9] But, says Pancharatna, their capacity to care for these cows, even if subsidized, may be limited:

---

[5]For an explanation of community-supported agriculture, see, for example, Lamb (1994).

[6]The majority of dairy farmers in this area are Hindus, although there is a high Muslim population. Those dairy farmers who are Muslim may, Pancharatna hopes, also take part in the scheme if they see that it is economically viable.

[7]Many westerners (including several hundred Russians, but also an increasing number of Chinese) settle in Mayapur, staying for a few months, alternating with a few months in the West where they earn sufficient funds to live comfortably in Mayapur, where they may have also regular *seva* (service) in one of several departments where their skills are well engaged.

[8]Other benefits that could be offered to the farmers are help in improving yields, help in getting loans, medical support for their cows, help with making biogas facilities, and guidance in growing organic food for which a market would be guaranteed at higher prices.

[9]Again, as mentioned in Chapter 4, because grazing land has become so scarce, even if dairy farmers want to, economically they cannot sustain nonproductive bovines. The village dairy farmers generally own very little, if any, land for grazing.

The fallback plan is that our Vaishnava community would have a place for the cows. We envision a (Indian) nationwide system of regional cow shelters [connected to the several other ISKCON projects around India], in places where land is less expensive, and ideally where there are forests nearby, so that the cows can get at least some of their needs from the forest, national forest … I'm in dialogue with government officers, about possible available land that the government is willing to offer. And those places would be able to accept our retired cows. That is the long-term plan.

With all the financial and other managerial requirements for such a scheme, we can see that it would function within an essentially modern framework of rational organization, and it would function because of its positioning as an added-value dairy that has, as its appeal to a wider (especially, but not exclusively Western) public, the assurance that, in addition to milk quality monitoring (presently completely absent), the bovines in the system are all under lifetime care and the farmers' lives are benefited. Of course, it remains to be seen if this scheme will work, and questions arise whether and how it will be properly managed in the face of the inertia of current local village practices. The question will be whether Western presence, money, influence, and organizational style will bring about the desired standards of cow care.[10] Will such a program serve to realize the aims of "familization" and "citizenship" for bovines that are hoped?

New Vraja Dhama, Hungary

A striking example of a farm community outside India with a strong emphasis on cow care which is sustained with little or no support of an Indian diaspora is the New Vraja Dhama (NVD) community in Hungary, central Europe, some 150 kilometers southwest of Budapest. Residents of NVD engage their oxen in farmwork on its 280 hectares of rolling hills, and a few cows supply milk to the temple for making dairy-based food

---

[10]Pancharatna Das notes that the scheme has many details yet to be worked out, such as whether farmers would continue caring for old bovines supported by the scheme, or whether the old bovines would be bought by the scheme and taken to its (ISKCON's) own regional shelters set up for the purpose. In any case, monitoring—with its additional costs—would be required in all aspects of the scheme.

preparations for the elaborately served temple images of Krishna and his consort Radha (see Fig. 6.2).

New Vraja Dhama is also affiliated with ISKCON, about which we have already discussed in Chapter 3 with respect to the mission's founder, Bhaktivedanta Swami Prabhupada. NVD is a highly structured community, with some fifty organizational departments, each closely monitored for numerical sustainability indexes.[11] The cows and agriculture departments in particular watch very closely their productivity, as the aim is to eventually come to the point where sustainability and self-sufficiency

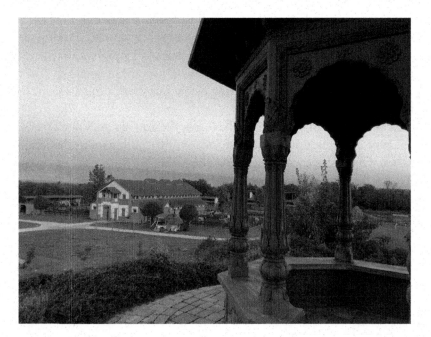

Fig. 6.2 The New Vraja Dhama goshala aims to showcase cow care for increasing numbers of visitors

[11] As currently calculated (by its own managers), based on a detailed set of factors, NVD as a whole is rated at 33% self-sustaining. The cow department has been rated at 50% self-sustaining (Interview with Radha Krishna Das, 27 January 2019). These are considered relatively high percentages compared with other departments and previous years, but of course the aim is to continue to increase the percentages as far as possible, where "possible" is taken to be 80%. Yet managers contend that "when push comes to shove" (if the general surrounding economy would collapse), NVD can run completely self-sufficiently in terms of basic necessities.

become substantial realities.[12] And yet, even though there is concern for rational efficiency and "productivity" in daily cow care, there appears to be a strong sense that the cows are Krishna's (mainly Brown Swiss breed) cows, and hence they must not be regarded or treated in instrumental terms.

An essential principle of sustainable cow care in NVD is maintaining the herd at a sustainable number of bovines. Of course, this is *not* done by "culling"; rather, it is done by paced breeding, the pace being determined by the amount of land available for maintaining each animal. Reckoning one hectare per cow or bull—young or aging—as required for full maintenance, including pasture and winter fodder growing, the current herd number of 44 bovines is expected to be increased to 60. Having seen that the average natural lifespan of these cows is 15 years, the cow care program's managers are allowing four cows to become pregnant each year. In rotation, this means that any single cow may bear a calf twice in her life.

Lactating cows at NVD are milked, but the goshala does not function as a dairy. All milking is done by hand, and the milk goes to the temple kitchen. Ghanashyam, a Hungarian Krishna-bhakta who has been tending the cows at New Vraja Dhama since the project's beginning twenty-two years ago, describes his experience in milking the cows:

> I try to always remember that Krishna says [in the Bhagavad-gita] that we should always remember him. I try to milk with Radhe Shyam (the temple images of Radha and Krishna) in my mind. When I teach someone to milk, I never speak about this, but I teach only such devotees who have the same mood. The cows enjoy it very much: We usually milk outside, where the

---

[12]The main expense for maintaining the bovines would normally be the cost of fodder, but at NVD, this cost is entirely eliminated by having sufficient land for both grazing and fodder for the full year. At this writing, there are 20 cows, 24 oxen, and one bull, and two cows are pregnant. 10 of the animals, mainly oxen, are "retired"; three sets of two oxen are trained and able to do traction work. The milk quantity, presently from four cows, may be some 40 liters per day, most of which goes to the farm's temple kitchen, where the milk is used in various preparations offered to Radha and Krishna. Some milk is used for making ghee, some small amount of which is sold in the temple shop. So essentially there is no income from the cow products. There is, however, regular income from donors who "adopt" a cow. There is a waiting list of people wanting to sponsor cows. The main expense in maintaining the cow care program for NVD is the cost of maintaining the cowherds—the resident community members who oversee and care for the cows, of which there are currently 12.

cows are free. They actually line up to be milked, and some, even after being milked, come back in the line as if wanting to be milked again.[13]

As already noted in Chapter 4, for Vaishnava Hindu cowherds, seeing Krishna as the owner of the cows is conducive for them to feel that by serving the cows, they are serving Krishna.[14]

Ultimately both the devotional mood and good productivity are seen as important by the NVD residents. Both principles are seen to complement each other in such a way that community members feel satisfaction in their work, so that they also experience a sense that they are appropriately honoring principles of dharma. Importantly, here dharma is strongly bhakti-inflected, such that the other three human aims previously mentioned (*purusha arthas*), namely satisfaction of desire (*kama*); pursuit of wealth (*artha*); and pursuit of freedom (*moksha*), are regarded as becoming fulfilled through devotional (bhakti) activity or work. What Christopher Fici (2018, p. 7) calls "embodied and transembodied flourishing" is what is sought. It is such flourishing that frames the sense of satisfaction in residents' devotional activity.[15] Integral to such satisfaction is confidence in being able to show to the wider world progress toward becoming a viable

---

[13]When I visited NVD in summer 2018, Ghanashyam told me that one cow, Radhika, gives 6 liters of milk per day, although her last calving was three years ago. Antardvip also told me of one unusual, no longer living cow, Rati. Rati was a heifer (a cow that has not had any calves), yet she gave milk every day for several years, up to 11 liters per day in one summer (she was kept from becoming a mother due to having a birth defect in one leg that was also present in her mother).

[14]Narayanan (2018a, p. 10) calls attention to the danger of "objectification" as a result of sacralization, citing Martha Nussbaum's theory with seven indicators of objectification among humans, namely instrumentality; (denial of) autonomy; inertness; fungibility; violability; ownership; and denial of subjectivity. Narayanan writes that "In the case of bovines, instrumentality is triply applied through their designation as economic, political and sacred resources." In New Vraja Dhama, one point to be made indicating that this tendency does not apply is the strong sense that, in terms of ownership, it is Krishna who is the owner of the bovines. Thus, all sense of their being "resources" accrues to the divinity. This heightens the sense of responsibility among the cowherds (and administrators of the community) for the bovines to be well cared for. Indeed, regarding Krishna as the supreme *subject* reminds carers of the bovines' subjectivity, for they understand that Krishna is present as *paramatman*, as the supreme sentient self, in the core of each bovine's self.

[15]The biggest challenge to sustainability at NVD, Shivarama Swami (Interview, 13 February 2019) explains, is in the social dimension. Residents here accept considerable physical inconvenience (such as hand-pumping water and having to make wood fires to heat the water for bathing, etc., and living almost entirely without the use of electricity). The present second and third-generation residents do not feel the same fervor to accept the austerities and make the project succeed as the more missionary-spirited first generation. Moreover, Hungary's continental European climate, with its

model of cow-based farming. Thus, my observation was that community members here see themselves as being well positioned to draw a wider public to appreciate cow care practice.[16]

Although not explicitly stated up to now, it should be clear that cow care practice, as we are presenting it, assumes the carers to be at least vegetarian, if not vegan. In NVD, to be vegetarian is an absolute prerequisite for community membership and residency. While not required as yet, members are strongly encouraged to follow the example of the project's founder and main spiritual guide, Shivarama Swami, in keeping an "ahimsa vegetarian" diet. "Ahimsa vegetarian" as defined in this community means abstaining from all dairy products unless they come from lifelong cared for cows. Following a vegetarian diet at the very least is regarded as a crucial step toward understanding the importance of cow care, a key step toward ahimsa vegetarian life, which is regarded as a necessity for what might be called "ethical sustainability," or moral consistency, with the aim of caring for cows in the best possible way.

And yet, conscientious Vaishnava Hindus will say that ultimately no kind of diet restriction frees one from responsibility for suffering, for any food consumption, including non-animal foods of any kind, involves the killing of living beings. As the Bhagavata Purana observes, *jivo jivasya jivanam*, "a living being is the life of (another) living being" (BhP 1.13.47). Far from being a justification for eating anything and everything, the point is to reduce suffering as far as possible. The bhakti principle is to restrict one's diet to only those foods that have been offered in a prescribed devotional manner to the source of all life. Such food is regarded as "remnants" (*prasada*—literally "graciousness" or "kindness") of the divine, sanctified food that is experienced as strengthening and illuminating for the spirit as well as purifying for the body and mind.[17]

---

single annual crop cycle and heavy winters, means that NVD faces numerous challenges that, for example, ISKCON Mayapur in India does not face.

[16]NVD currently receives some 25,000 visitors per year, up 15% from five years previous.

[17]Ideally, all food that is offered to Krishna (through a formal ritual procedure in Krishna's temple) would be grown and harvested or gathered either directly by Vaishnavas or under their direction, avoiding chemical fertilizer, pesticides, and machines such as tractors. More strictly, food offerings for Krishna are to be cooked, especially in temple worship, only by Krishna-bhaktas who have received formal initiation as brahmins. In NVD, this latter standard is strictly maintained, and

For NVD community members, *prasada* sharing is of crucial importance in their outreach efforts. The idea is that if people are to give serious consideration to accepting the radical change in diet that is being proposed, with all the implications for their social lives, and so on, they need to experience directly a "higher taste."[18] They have to literally taste such sanctified food, and by experiencing its rich flavorful quality, they can be more easily open to the ethical reasoning that includes, of course, the care of cows. Therefore, NVD community members will say that admonishments to forgo meat and industrial dairy are, by themselves, usually ineffective. Any call to change must be accompanied by a palatable alternative.

New Vraja Dhama is not an insular community. Quite the contrary, it actively invites visitors, and it has been the object of study for postgraduate students from various universities, with interests from ecology to sociology. The public interface with the community has also meant interaction of various kinds in the political sphere, from the small scale of the adjacent village to the national level. As scholars of religion are fond of saying, "religion and politics are two sides of the same coin." So, it has been unavoidable that the Hungarian Society for Krishna Consciousness (HSKCON) has had to face challenges in the political arena, particularly in 2011–2012, when its status as a legal religion was revoked. For us to note is one occasion, in December 2011, in the course of protesting their religious status denial, when members brought cows from New Vraja Dhama to accompany them in a protest before the Hungarian Parliament building in central Budapest. As it happened, along with seventeen other religious groups in Hungary, HSKCON's religious status was soon reinstated (Dasi 2012).

What this situation in relation to the Hungarian state highlights is the dependency of the NVD project on favorable state recognition, with the

---

many, though not all, foods have been grown on the NVD land. Of course, the only dairy products used are those from NVD cows, making sure the calves are fully nourished first.

[18] A Bhagavad-gita stanza often quoted to underline this point: "The embodied soul may be restricted from sense enjoyment, though the taste for sense objects remains. But, ceasing such engagements by experiencing a higher taste, he is fixed in consciousness" (Prabhupāda 1972, p. 147; Bg. 2.59).

financial benefits such recognition affords.[19] Indirectly, cow care in NVD benefits from its being legally recognized as part of a religious institution. In turn, this relationship with the state points us back to our discussion of animal "citizenship" in Chapter 5, where I drew from Donaldson and Kymlicka's invitation to imagine such a possibility.

Very briefly, in the context of NVD we can revisit the four areas of pre-supposition for citizenship we selected (from nine altogether proposed by these authors). First, mobility and sharing of public space: NVD bovines have ample freedom of movement, especially throughout the warmer months, with daily grazing in generously open areas; and when indoors, they are not tied. Second, the cows' milk is used, not for business, but rather for sanctified food that is shared in the community and with visitors. No attempt is made to artificially increase the milk quantity, nor to deprive calves of their needs. Third, yes, the oxen are trained and engaged in traction work, but they are always carefully worked and not overworked. And lastly, yes, sex and reproduction are controlled, in such a way as to ensure that the already present bovines are not threatened by over-reproduction. Also, artificial insemination is rejected, and motherhood for cows neither denied nor over-frequently imposed.

It can be argued that these practices fall short of indicating that bovines are being regarded as citizens. However, the analogous sense in which the term is used serves to point the community toward honoring the cows as fellow members of the community. It also serves human community members to be reminded that the cows are, as atemporal beings with bovine bodies, ontologically equal to all other community members. However, this is not to minimize or obscure the fact that these are indeed bovines— vulnerable animals with their own specific needs and inclinations.

New Vraja Dhama is not the first or only agricultural community of ISKCON. As mentioned in Chapter 3, Prabhupada inspired followers to develop farm communities in America, and since then, with varied scales and degrees of success, several more have been established in various

---

[19]A significant source of monetary income for HSKCON, including New Vraja Dhama, is a one-percent apportionment of tax money to the religious organization one designates or to which one belongs. Currently there are some 40,000 Hungarian taxpayer citizens who benefit HSKCON, a number that the government multiplies by four, yielding a significant annual supplement to other sources (Shivarama Swami interview, 13 February 2019).

countries of the world.[20] Nor is ISKCON alone in having cow care projects outside India. As we take up our next topic in relation to cow care futures, I will introduce one more ISKCON project outside London and another Hindu project in Wales. One principle these two communities have in common is that bovines should be allowed to live out their natural lives. As we will see, each of the two communities came into conflict with local civic authorities on this point. As we look to bovine futures, we must also reflect on the implications of caring for them through to their natural expiry. In particular, in a Hindu theological context, it is understood that death is the end of the body but not of the self (*atman*) within the body. Thus, animals as much as humans have a post-mortem future. But rather than canceling moral concern for animals' bodies, this understanding of non-temporal selfhood heightens moral concern for temporal bodies, as we will see in the next section.

Departing Bovine Souls

To better appreciate implications of the following events, let us first recall Vrinda Dalmiya's five metaethical themes that frame the ethics of care (introduced in Chapter 5): *relationality* (acknowledgment of the embodied condition of all subjects of moral action); recognition of *needs* (addressing often conflicting needs of corporeal and hence vulnerable, selves); *affectivity* (the recognition that emotions have an important place in moral decision-making); *contextualism* (the awareness that moral judgments always take place in specific relational contexts); and, finally, *responsibility* (the recognition of "moral remainders"—of feelings such as guilt and uncertainty regarding inevitable limits to one's capacity to respond). As broad metaethical understandings, these themes are necessarily abstract, yet paradoxically they emphasize particularity: Care is for particular beings

---

[20] At this writing, ISKCON proper has some 84 projects in which cows are kept. Of these, 47 are in India, 9 in North America, 14 in Europe, 3 in Latin America, 3 in Southeast Asia, 2 in Russia, 2 in Africa, and 4 in Australia. Most projects have very small numbers of bovines—as few as 5–10, a few, such as Gita Nagari in Pennsylvania, have up to 100, and the largest number is currently in Tirupati, with 500 cows and bulls. Additionally, there are several ISKCON members with private projects that include cow care on varying scales.

in particular circumstances. "Particular beings" can, of course, be nonhuman animals, and here we are specifically concerned with possible futures for the care of bovines. How is the gap filled between these very general, though essential, metaethical themes, and the specific aspirations in cow care?

To enlist the ethics of care paradigm specifically for care of bovines, Patrick Meyer-Glitza offers five overlapping "basic rules of the care system."[21] First, care is *universally applied* to all cattle, including both sexes, in all ages and conditions of health. Second, care is *unconditional* in that productivity is no precondition for the animals' right of life, with equal benefits for all animals, whether or not they are "productive." As Meyer-Glitza pointedly notes, "The life of the cattle, their being alive, is the main product." Furthermore, all other farmed animals have the same right of life and care. Third, and elaborating on the previous two rules, *lifetime of care* ensures that during old age, illness and dying, the bovines will be cared for in ways resembling old age homes and other institutions for disabled or vulnerable human beings.[22] Fourth, bovines are *familized*, which is to say the cared-for animals "are looked at as distinct individualities and treated as part of the enlarged family." Although, he notes, the term "family" is used metaphorically, it highlights feelings of bonding between human and animal (the degree and nature depending on several factors) that may resemble feelings of relationship in the family. Finally, *prevention* is a rule of care for animals that embraces farmers' work toward having their farms be models of how to live with farmed animals in such ways as to prevent their slaughter. In the face of state powers, the two following examples point to potential or real difficulties in upholding these rules.

---

[21] Meyer-Glitza (2018, p. 193) refers to two combined systems—the care system, summarized by the five basic rules and characterized by a sanctuary function, and the agri-system of husbandry and animal products. Combined, "these two worlds make up the agri-care-system."

[22] Meyer-Glitza notes that bovines will not, due to disability, be "(re-) commodified." An example of re-commodification would be use of a naturally dead bovine's hide for processing as a leather product. M. K. Gandhi apparently favored re-commodification of dead bovines, specifically their hides, as an income source for goshalas (Burgat 2004, p. 224). In contrast, Swami Datta Sharanananda at Pathmeda rejects re-commodification, arguing that it would have the effect of reducing—even if unconsciously—care for diseased and dying bovines.

Contested Lives at Bhaktivedanta Manor and Skanda Vale

The practice of lifelong cow care in the West is quite new and rare, and it is not being done in a cultural vacuum. While some Westerners appreciate this effort and have some sense of its value, others—especially non-vegetarians, but also persons who may be vegetarian or vegan—may have ethical concerns, in particular regarding end-of-life care and rejection of euthanasia for terminally ill bovines. Two episodes in the UK involving confrontation of cow care practicing Hindu communities with local civic authorities are relevant although, strictly speaking, it is precisely that they need *not* have been terminal cases that they are noteworthy.

In the northwest part of London's Green Belt zone is Bhaktivedanta Manor, a very active and expanding community of Vaishnava Hindus established in 1973.[23] The main property of some 77 acres includes a *goshala*, presently with 50 bovines (mainly Meuse Rhine Issel breed), cared for as an integral feature of the Manor's missionary work to show people an alternative way of life and to share the tenets and practices of "Krishna consciousness." In 2007, one thirteen-year-old cow named Gangotri suffered a fall and a damaged leg when one of the goshala's bulls tried to mount her. With attentive nursing by the Manor's cowherds, Gangotri was slowly recovering, and although she still could not walk, she was helped to stand twice a day. Despite the improvement and her general good health aside from her condition of lameness, and despite positive indications from the Manor's two regular veterinarians that she was steadily improving, word got to the local animal welfare agency, the Royal Society for the Prevention of Cruelty to Animals (RSPCA) that a sick cow was being neglected. Through what the Manor managers regarded as blatantly deceptive means, the RSPCA arranged to have Gangotri euthanized.

The news of this act soon went public in the local Asian press in which, to a published response to accusations against the RSPCA by a representative thereof, the Manor countered (in part),

---

[23]Bhaktivedanta Manor was purchased and gifted by "Beatle"-musician George Harrison to the International Society for Krishna Consciousness (ISKCON). Swami Prabhupada, ISKCON's founder, visited here in 1973 and expressed his wish that cows be acquired and cared for on the property. For a detailed discussion of cow care at Bhaktivedanta Manor, see Prime (2009).

The Manor runs a Cow Protection Project and as such animal welfare is its first consideration. The position of the RSPCA is that nursing animals beyond a certain level is not animal welfare and in this position they are judging the practice of the Hindu faith where animals are cared for until their natural end. They say to allow Gangotri to continue to live would have been wrong; in other words, they are condemning the beliefs of the Hindu tradition as being wrong.

By framing the RSPCA's action as an affront and repudiation of "the beliefs of the Hindu tradition," the Manor challenged the agency's understanding of animal welfare as being deficient if not wrong-headed. Noteworthy is that, in this case, the conflict was eventually resolved amicably: The RSPCA issued a public apology to the Manor and the UK Hindu community, and it donated a cow to the Manor goshala (Aditi who, in early 2009, gave birth to a female calf, receiving the name Gangotri).[24]

A positive result of this incident was that the Manor's goshala manager, Shyamasundara Das, became a temporary consultant for the UK Department for Environment, Food and Rural Affairs (DEFRA) in the drafting of its "Protocol for handling welfare cases in cooperation with the Hindu Community" (DEFRA 2009).[25] Yet this document also reaffirms governmental authority to determine if "unnecessary suffering" of an animal is occurring, such that it may decide that euthanasia is to be done, despite

---

[24] ISKCON News Weekly Staff (2009). https://iskconnews.org/rspca-donated-cow-gives-birth-at-bhaktivedanta-manor,1027 (accessed 8 June 2018).

[25] In its favor, this protocol explicitly "acknowledges that the manner in which the Hindu community cares for bovine animals is governed by strict ethical and religious beliefs. It also acknowledges that financial or such other considerations will not limit the efforts of the Hindu community to provide palliative care as they might in a situation where commercial farming practices are involved" (DEFRA Protocol 2009, para. 3). However, authority remains with government agencies to decide if an animal is to be euthanized, according to British animal welfare legislation (see especially paras. 17 and 19).

disapproval of (in this case) cow carers.[26] The protocol also states (para. 5) that it "does not apply to any action required for disease control purposes."

Disease control was considered to be the issue in the case of the bull Shambo at Skanda Vale Ashram in West Wales, in 2007. Skanda Vale ashram, officially the Community of the Many Names of God (CMNG), is a quite small "multifaith, multispecies community" with a prominent Hindu orientation, with currently some twenty-eight human members, two of whom are lay members, the others being monks, nuns, or novices (Hurn 2018, p. 264). Nonhumans of the community include cows, as well as water buffalo, a variety of smaller species, and one Asian elephant. Although the community is small, it receives some 90,000 pilgrims annually, mostly Hindu South Asians of Britain with Tamil backgrounds. Founded in 1973 by the Sri Lankan Tamil Guru Sri Subramanium, the central principles of the ashram are ahimsa and *sanatana-dharma*, defined here as "timeless consciousness of God, manifest in practice at Skanda Vale through the recognition and preservation of the sanctity of life of all living beings" (Hurn 2018, p. 264; Warrier 2010, p. 262).

As already mentioned, in 2007 Shambo, Skanda Vale's resident black Friesian bull, was tested positive for bovine tuberculosis (bTB). Maya Warrier (2010) describes in detail the government's determination that the bull must be slaughtered for disease control, leading to a multi-layered battle, ending with the government's power prevailing, bringing death to Shambo. An important feature of this battle narrative is CMNG's shift from an eclectic multifaith identity to an explicitly Hindu identity. This served well to martial widespread Hindu support (mainly British, but also from other countries). A point for us to note is that the plea of Hindu religious tradition and its ahimsa principle failed to carry sufficient weight to reverse the government's decision on the plea of disease control.

---

[26] More recently, in March 2019, Bhaktivedanta Manor's cow named Shyama Gauri suffered a broken leg which, when she rolled over on it, broke further and protruded through the skin. Her state of obvious agony could not be mitigated despite injections of painkillers. In this case, the managers decided they had no choice but to allow her to be euthanized, following government regulations. In a letter addressed to the Manor community, senior manager Gauri Das explained the situation, concluding with a comparison to the case of Gangotri, twelve years previous: "However, this [present] incident proved too extreme. Shyama Gauri was in sustained and helpless agony despite all efforts. We turn in prayers to Lord Krishna now, for the soul of Shyama Gauri, and for the wisdom to know how to best serve His cows."

We might step back to view this incident in terms of late modern cultural theory about how knowledge and power are interwoven. This episode at CMNG serves as an example of how contemporary discourse about animals functions in a delimited scope, within a "discourse of law" and a "discourse of lines" (Johnson 2012, pp. 39–62).[27] From this perspective, within certain "conditions of truth" recognized by the state, Skanda Vale's "transmigration of souls discourse" was one of *subordinated knowledge*, a way of understanding reality that carried no weight with the government. In this context, ironically, the discourse of law, in which animal ownership is decisive, was in a sense inverted, so that the CMNG's ownership of Shambo was, in effect, superseded by state ownership. This quasi-transfer of ownership meant that fungibility replaced uniqueness: Sambho, suspected of carrying a contagious disease, was regarded by the state as disposable because replaceable. Whatever the degree of threat to public health there might have been by his condition,[28] the CMNG's offer to quarantine and treat the apparently curable Shambo had no leverage against the inertial legal system. Still, as we are here considering bovine futures, what may prove to be significant about this episode is that it became a platform on which the subordinated knowledge of transmigration of souls came more into public awareness. It would be possible, in course of time, for the subordinated knowledge of transmigration to become a prominent, and perhaps even a dominant, knowledge. The hope would be that then the "discourse of animals as *beings*," which is, as Johnson puts it, currently "buried in plain sight," could come to the public surface, for the substantial, life-preserving benefit of animals (Johnson 2012, p. 100) and hence, for the benefit of all human society.

---

[27] Michel Foucault (1926–1984), well known for his analyses of the relationship between power and knowledge, is the key thinker behind Lisa Johnson's analysis of these two components in relation to animals. The expression "discourse of lines" refers to the way language "works to shape the form of our knowledge about things. Specifically, the discourse of lines requires us to see parts, rather than wholes" (Johnson 2012, p. 22). Although not using this expression directly Carol Adams (2010) elaborates extensively on how this discourse works with respect to animals and the meat industry.

[28] Compounding the ironies and adding an element of pathos to this episode, apparently Shambo's post-mortem examination showed him to be tuberculosis free (Prime 2009, p. 29. No source for this information is given).

Krishna the Ox Breathes His Last in Vrindavan

It would be reasonable to assume that such a recognition of animals as beings is necessary to appreciate the Hindu conviction that bovines should be cared for to their natural end. One account of the life, final days, and funerary honoring of a particular ox in India can give us a sense of how such "beingness" of a bovine was experienced by his carers.

In 2008, at the Care For Cows goshala in Vrindavan, the ox (of Kankrej breed) named Krishna died. It had been seven years since Krishna had twice walked a circuit around the entire coast of India and across the north, from east to west, over a period of ten years, together with his counterpart ox, Balaram. These journeys were with a *padayatra*—a walking procession, enacted as part of the Chaitanyaite Vaishnava mission to bring Krishna-bhakti (the message of devotion to Lord Krishna) to villages throughout the country.

On being suddenly retired from his service of pulling the *padayatra* cart "[Krishna, the ox] protested by being irritated and unruly for almost a year. We brushed him for hours, took him for long walks and built him a cart, but nothing seemed to pacify him" (NA, "Tribute" 2008). Eventually he became again calm (possibly because of "bonding" with a goshala co-resident cow, Vanamali). Eventually the ox contracted horn cancer, gradually lost interest in eating, and lost his ability to stand. After a peaceful death, several friends of Care For Cows gathered to help bury him.[29] The newsletter report continues,

> After being placed in the grave, about twenty-five devotees [Krishna-bhaktas] offered Ganges water, flowers and incense and began to circum-ambulate him in *kirtan* [singing divine names]. With moist eyes we all filled our hands with Vrindavan dust and showered it all over his body.

---

[29] Sanak-Sanatan Das, from Germany, recalled with wonder the ox's death, and the fact that he happened to be present at that moment, feeling that the ox had "called" him "[After I arrived, Krishna] started stirring as if wanting to stand, lifted his head to the sky, opened his mouth, and expired....We [Krishna, the ox, and myself] had been really, really good friends. I had purchased him [and Balaram], I had donated him [to the *padayatra* project], I grew up with him for almost ten years." Regarding his experience of friendship with the ox, Das goes on to tell of the ox's remarkable friendship with his counterpart, Balaram. "They were more like lovers, Krishna taking the feminine role and Balaram the masculine role. We used to call them Mr. and Mrs. Patel."

This strikingly handsome ox, with the very large horns of the Kankrej breed and his ten years of *padayatra* cart-pulling service, made him much admired—so much so that letters of condolence were received from around the world. Further, the family sponsoring his maintenance after retirement also sponsored the construction of a permanent memorial structure, a *samadhi*, in his honor. The final paragraph of the newsletter article speaks of him as a devotee of Lord Krishna, rather than as an animal:

> [Krishna] is an inspiring example of one who served selflessly to spread the Holy Name to every town and village. His passing in Vrindavan at an auspicious moment, in the company of well-wishers and without excessive suffering attests to his greatness. May he remember us favorably as we continue to struggle in this material world. (NA, "Tribute" 2008)

"May he remember us favorably" is a telling reminder of the pan-Indic notion that, as we have discussed in relation to Jada Bharata in Chapter 5, the atemporal self continues after the body dies. There is also an indication of the conviction that this particular being, temporarily in a bovine body, had attained after death the much coveted destination of Goloka Vrindavan, by virtue of having died in the earthly land of Vrindavan.

I call attention to this account because it articulates a Vaishnava Hindu understanding of what the perfect future for an individual being—bovine or otherwise—would be, following death. Another way of putting it, I suggest, is that this particular bovine was regarded as having attained what we might call "full citizenship," in the only realm where it is possible, namely beyond the realm of temporality. In the temporal realm, any citizenship status for any beings, including humans, can at best be an approximation, for it is contingent upon changing factors. Also to be noted is the sense of satisfaction that the human carers for this particular ox had, that they had properly done their parts in facilitating the best possible conditions for the remainder of his life.[30] In this case, a sense of perfect human–animal

---

[30] In the CFC newsletter, it is also mentioned that after Kṛṣṇa's second tour of India, three senior persons who felt responsible for him discussed at length whether he should be allowed to go on a third tour. Knowing that he was getting older, they decided not to risk that his life might end outside Vrindavan, instead having him remain where they saw he would be best cared for.

cooperation reached a summit secured by bhakti—dedication in sharing lives across the species boundary to please the supreme person.

Finally, this is an example of what was seen as an ideal case of species boundary-crossing as human/nonhuman animal cooperation. As such, it is seen as a demonstration that it is possible to transcend the "discourse of lines," the discourse that permits humans to see nonhuman animal bodies as parsable, or divisible, to serve human ends (in a doomed attempt of humans to make themselves whole, de-alienated) (Johnson 2012, pp. 61–62). This, then, becomes dharma in the deeper sense suggested in Chapter 5: The dharmic sensibility is a recognition of agency and choice that enables us humans to "access hidden possibilities and bring them under our control" (Frazier 2017, pp. 195–198). In this case, the "hidden possibility" is the potential to transcend the species boundary as well as the boundary of death by caring for a being in a dying bovine body in hopes of ushering him toward a permanent life beyond suffering.

When Cow Protection Activism Becomes Counterproductive

In thinking of futures for cows with the aid of a dharmic sensibility, we do well to reconsider efforts for cows in the public sphere, specifically activism in its various forms. The Cow Protection movement in India that initially took formal shape in the 1880s has continued in various ways and forms up to the present day. As we discussed in Chapter 3, in its early form it served to shape and galvanize a nationalist identity as essentially Hindu, arguably accelerating the process that led to India's independence from British rule in 1947. Since independence, cow protection activists are known to cite M. K. Gandhi for his setting cow protection as a priority equal to if not higher than independence.[31] Sadly, however, the long and continuing history of Indian bovine protection legislation is, as mentioned in Chapter 3, a narrative largely of persistent failure to protect bovines from slaughter. It

---

[31] Lodha (2002, Chapter 1, paragraph 39) quotes Gandhi, from December 1927: "As for me, not even to win Swaraj [independence], will I renounce my principle of cow protection." I was not able to verify this quote from the CWMG. In any case, it is clear from his numerous references to "cow-protection" that he considered it a high priority.

is also a story of ignoring the manifold abuses to bovines *during* their lives. Ironically, much of this failure may be attributed to insistence on cows' sacrality. How this is so has been explained in detail by Yamini Narayanan (2018a), based on her interviews with several cow protectionists of three different types, namely religious protectionists, political protectionists, and "secular" animal welfare organization members. Here, as we look to possible cow care futures, I want to consider her findings to show the need for deeper understanding of how persons may best serve cows in the political sphere. More constructive than abandoning affirmations of cows' sacrality, I suggest, is to extend the category of sacrality, aiming toward inclusion of all sentient beings. But this requires replacing the tendency to objectify the sacred with the essential meaning and purpose of sacrality, namely to *subjectify*—to acknowledge and affirm the subjective reality and being of all creatures.

The notion that cows in general or specific breeds of bovines are sacred is often represented by cow protectionists in a way that, unfortunately, amplifies cows' objectification. This means that a cow's being, as a creature with vulnerabilities, becomes obscured by her *function* as a symbol.[32] As a symbol, she becomes an abstraction, because what she symbolizes are abstractions: *The* cow is a symbol *of* "Hinduism," "purity," "the Indian nation," "*sanatana-dharma*," and so on. Further, all these meanings are one side of binary oppositions. What is *not* "Hinduism," and so forth, are opposed to these concepts, and being in opposition, they are seen as a threat to them. Although these terms are abstractions, they are rhetorically very powerful, such that persons identify themselves either with them or in opposition to them. Then, with further rhetorical moves, the divisions become sharpened, intensifying from difference to antagonism to hatred and to violence.[33]

---

[32]Further to n. 14 in this chapter, "objectification" is a term used in feminist discourse to critique how women are objectified and thereby exploited by men. The term has been extended by some animal ethicists to call attention to a similar dynamic in human treatment of animals. Ironically, the effort to protect the cow by identifying her as "mother" can have the effect of affirming her as an object of exploitation, thus inverting the whole purpose of highlighting her identity as "mother."

[33]Purushottama Bilimoria (2018, p. 57) aptly asks, "Is modern Hinduism even as it becomes more secular …, McDonalized [sic], and globalized, after the Gandhian interlude, far behind in abrogating the moral inclusiveness of animals in a reformed Hindu ethos? Or is the evangelism and self-righteousness of Hindutva with its almost absolute embracing or 'revivification' of vegetarianism

Such antagonism can be further aggravated by what Narayanan (2018a, p. 5) calls "casteised speciesism," whereby certain animal species are associated with specific human castes or *varnas*. This association echoes the Samkhya system of metaphysics (briefly introduced in Chapter 4): Nature's (*prakriti's*) quality of luminosity (*sattva-guna*) is said to be prominent in brahmins as well as cows; the quality of passion (*rajo-guna*) is prominent among *kshatriyas* and horses; and the quality of inertia and darkness (*tamo-guna*) is thought to characterize *shudras* and dogs. This association can easily be misconstrued as imputations of superiority and inferiority such that one type of animal (the cow) is privileged in such a way that other animals are neglected or condemned. Such is typically the case with buffaloes, whereby they are associated with lower castes or even with demonic beings. As a result, with little or no stigma against the slaughter of buffaloes, farmers often prefer owning them to owning cows. As a result, it is buffalo milk that constitutes most of the Indian dairy industry product, and it is buffaloes that are first to be slaughtered when they become no longer productive. The sharp distinction and hierarchizing of cows and buffaloes are mirrored in a widespread distinction between indigenous (*deshi*) cow breeds, "Jersey" (nonindigenous, Western) breeds, and mixed (*deshi* and Western) breeds. As the latter two types are considered inferior to any of the some thirty-nine officially recognized indigenous breeds, this distinction also serves to reinforce the sacrality of indigenous bovines. Again, the problem is that such sacralization leads to objectification, which can undermine the aim of protection by ignoring bovines' animality and hence their vulnerability (Narayanan 2018a, pp. 12–17).

One practical result of such objectification is that cow protectionists tend to regard cow slaughter as the only issue to be addressed. There are two possible negative effects from cow protectionist activism's focus on the single issue of protecting cows from slaughter. First, there is no attention given to the main cause of cow slaughter in India today, which is, arguably, the dairy industry. For dairies to maintain their profit margins, they engage their cows to produce as much milk as possible, and when their milk yield reduces or when they are no longer productive, the cows

---

likely [to] alienate secular Indian animalists, by underscoring more the orthodoxly religious rather than the moral grounds?"

are sent for slaughter, along with the male calves and bulls. Second (tied to B. R. Ambedkar's analysis of untouchability, discussed in Chapter 3), the focus on protection exclusively of cows translates into persecution of the marginal classes of people accustomed to eating meat. This provokes reactions, often resulting in defiant increase of cow slaughter where it had otherwise been minimal. In a similar vein, agitation against cow slaughter has fueled defiant demonstrations in the form of "beef festivals," in which people—not necessarily from marginal castes—demonstrate their solidarity with the marginal castes by public displays of beef eating (Narayanan 2018b; Sunder 2018).[34]

Surely all who are involved in cow protectionism have the best of intentions to bring an end to the abuse of bovines, and to this end since decades they have been making immense efforts on numerous fronts. And yet, as Gandhi lamented already in 1921 (see Chapter 3), it must be asked to what extent these efforts are effective or indeed counterproductive. Since our concern here is specifically with Hindu animal ethics and cow care, I suggest that a valuable guide for analyzing actions aimed to aid and protect bovines may be the sacred text so broadly revered by Hindus, the Bhagavad Gita. More specifically we shall look at the Gita's quality-analysis (*guna-bhedana*) which we have already referred to as the Samkhya system of metaphysics.

Cow Protection in Three Qualities

In the Bhagavad Gita, Krishna sets out the classical threefold typology of cosmic dynamics in terms of "qualities" (*gunas*, literally "threads"

---

[34] Sunder offers a striking analysis of the complexities involved in the issue of cow protection versus slaughter, through samples of recent Dalit ("Untouchable") literature, noting, for example (p. 15) that "[t]he Indian Left's deployment of meat as a signifier of progressive politics presents an ethical dilemma for those with a stake in animal welfare or rights … Calls for animal justice in India that do not take into account such complexities risk imposing upon Muslims, Dalits, and untouchable communities an ethics of privilege propagated by First Worlders and caste Hindus who, intentionally or not, 'do no harm' to animals as a matter of luxury, class mobility, and the violent oppression of the poor. Questions of animal rights or welfare paradigms cannot easily apply to Indian meat politics, but nor can we efface the lives of animals as we struggle to grant liberation and dignity to South Asia's most marginalized and vulnerable people."

or "strands," but also "qualities" or "constituents").[35] We have already encountered this typology briefly: *sattva*—illumination or "goodness," *rajas*—passion, and *tamas*—darkness can be compared to three primary colors—yellow, red, and blue, respectively—from which all color mixtures are derived and which thereby "color" experience. The Gita's eighteenth and final chapter, which is largely concerned with effective practices of world renunciation, takes the analysis of action (*karma*) as a key theme. Since action invariably binds human beings to its results, and it is impossible to refrain from action even for a moment, the question becomes how to upgrade or refine the *quality* of action such that its binding effect is reduced and ultimately eliminated in realization of one's spiritual identity. Here is how Krishna characterizes action in terms of these three qualities:

> Prescribed action, free of attachment, done without passion or aversion by one not seeking the fruit, is said to be in goodness. But action done by one seeking selfish pleasure, or done with egotism and much trouble, is declared to be in passion. Action undertaken in illusion, disregarding consequences, waste, harm and human limits, is said to be in darkness. (Bg. 18.23–25, transl. Goswami 2015, p. 208)

In this clearly hierarchical typology of moral values, it is the attitude of the actor that is crucial. Beginning at the low end, *tamo-guna*, darkness characterizes action under this quality because it is counterproductive, harmful, and wasteful. In the context of bovine protection and advocacy, illusion predominates where differences are considered essential—differences among human communities and differences among species and breeds. It may happen that activists locate their own identity in the designation "Hindu," defining themselves in contradistinction to "Muslim" or "Christian" identities. In like manner, they may identify with a particular political party over against another political party, claiming that it is their party that champions the cow, not the other party. As we have discussed, when this attitude predominates, it leads to antagonism, hatred, and violence. Such action is therefore bound to be counterproductive, typically aggravating rather than alleviating conflict.

---

[35] For further explanation of the *guṇas*, see Rusza, "Sankhya" in the Internet Encyclopedia of Philosophy, Section 4b: *Prakṛti* and the Three *guṇa-s*. https://www.iep.utm.edu/sankhya/#SH4b.

Similarly, action in which *rajo-guna*—passion—predominates is characterized by egotism (*ahamkara*), whereby one thinks oneself to be of crucial importance in making positive changes for cow care, or one seeks recognition and praise for one's cow care activism. The passionate quality also predominates in expectations of quick results, such as getting a law passed or winning a legal case expected to favor bovines. *Rajo-guna* is likely to be exhibited by politicians who make promises and schemes for cow protection to win votes—promises and schemes that may never materialize. Similarly, it can be exhibited in the making of laws meant to protect cows that are unenforceable, or in making state-led schemes for cow protection that prove to be unsustainable or abusive of cows, or both.

If cow protectionists were to pursue their purposes in ways characterized by *sattva-guna*, how would this look? Gandhi once gave an indication of this when he wrote: "Cow slaughter can never be stopped by law. Knowledge, education, and the spirit of kindliness towards [cows] alone can put an end to it" (Gandhi 1999, CWMG 92, p. 119).[36] I would modify Gandhi's assertion slightly, shifting the word "alone" to the first sentence, to read "Cow slaughter can never be stopped by law *alone*...." Law has its place (Cochrane 2012, pp. 13–14), and it can only be supported and sustained by a broad-based culture of what I am repeatedly calling "cow care." Such cow care needs to be practiced in a spirit of *sattva-guna*, characterized by valuing and pursuing worldly detachment and, more specifically in the present context, detachment from expectation of quick favorable results for cow care in the wider public sphere.[37]

To further reflect on cow care in which *sattva-guna* predominates, the second half of Gandhi's above statement (regarding knowledge, education, and a spirit of kindliness) bears further attention in terms of this conception of qualities, especially the quality of illumination and goodness.

---

[36]Earlier, in 1942, Gandhi wrote, "[Regulation of cow slaughter] cannot be achieved by legislation. In the first instance people ought to be trained. Hindus have got to put up with cow-slaughter. Killing Muslims will not stop them from slaughtering the cow....What will the law do in this?" (Gandhi 1999, CWMG 82, p. 95).

[37]Despite numerous good reasons for skepticism about the efficacy of legal regulation for care and protection of bovines, there are occasionally hopeful signs. As I write, the central Government of India has "approved a proposal for the setting up of 'Rashtriya Kamdhenu Aayog' (National Commission for Cows) for conservation, protection and development of cows and their progeny" (Times News Network, *Times Nation*, 7 February 2019, p. 14).

However, before doing so, a further aspect of Samkhya's threefold quality typology must be considered: In terms of cosmic order and change, the Bhagavata Purana associates passion (*rajo-guna*) with creation; goodness and illumination (*sattva-guna*) with sustenance, regulation, and preservation; and darkness or inertia (*tamo-guna*) with entropy and destruction. The association of sustenance, regulation, and preservation with *sattva-guna* is particularly relevant in considering how cow protectionism in *sattva-guna* might look, because it recalls the essential meaning of the term *dharma*—to hold, uphold, or sustain. Therefore, to elaborate a vision of future cow care, for the remainder of this chapter I will suggest, through six *affirmations on the dharma of cow care*, what we can characterize as cow protectionism predominated by the quality of goodness and illumination.

Six Affirmations on the Dharma of Cow Care

Keeping within a Hindu vocabulary, I return to the notion of dharma, albeit an expanded understanding that includes what we have discussed about dharma in Chapter 5. In addition, dharma will be used here as a *balancing sensibility*, giving priority to practices of cow care that foster balance among the conflicting interests that surround bovines. To this end, I draw on a non-Hindu, contemporary Western typology of six "moral foundations of political life" developed by social psychologist Jonathan Haidt and his colleagues (Haidt 2012). Drawn from his extensive empirical research, Haidt identifies five positive foundational moral themes underlying and energizing political discourse. Each positive theme has a negative counterpart—conditions or principles sought to be avoided or suppressed. These five positive/negative moral theme pairs are: *care* versus *harm, fairness* versus *cheating, loyalty* versus *betrayal, authority* versus *subversion*, and *sanctity* versus *degradation*. A sixth moral foundation awaiting more empirical confirmation is *liberty* versus *oppression*. Haidt and his colleagues have found definite correlations between one's political leanings and which of these five or six moral foundations one will value or, negatively, abhor, above other foundations. Here, our aim is to see how, in the practice of cow care, all six positive moral foundations can be honored, such that the interests of bovines are upheld and cow care becomes an important means by which the expanding moral community is fostered and sustained.

Taking each positive moral foundation in turn, what follows will be in the form of affirmations—present-tense positive as-if statements that aid in sparking the imagination to envision a possible better future that is rooted in the pursuit of self-integrity (Cohen and Sherman 2014).

1. *Cow Care and Care.* The first of Haidt's six moral foundations is *care*, the opposite of which is *harm.* We frame our care practices in the general terms identified by Dalmiya (see Chapter 5) in relation to bovines. More specifically, we have instituted a certification system (through a network similar to that of worldwide organic farmers) to monitor and ensure that all institutions and individuals who care for cows and wish to have the monitoring agency's seal of approval must follow minimum standards summarized in the five "basic rules of the care-system" for lifelong care of animals (Meyer-Glitza 2018, pp. 193–194; see above, in the section "Departing bovine souls"). Further, and as an integral aspect of this monitoring system, we observe standards of care for all humans serving as cow carers, in terms of appropriate remuneration and medical care. In caring for cows, we further strive to realize, as far as feasible, the nine aspects of citizenship for bovines (see Chapter 5). We do not discriminate types of bovines with respect to care, either by breed or by species, but we do have programs to preserve indigenous breeds of various regions and countries. We pursue the ideal of *go-seva*—service to cows in a spirit of selfless dedication that characterizes the bhakti ethical paradigm. By all these practices, we seek to minimize *harm* to bovines and to the planet's biosphere and, rather, to foster regenerative practice that sustains bovines, humans, and the earth.

2. *Cow Care and Fairness.* A comprehensive monitoring system ensures that any physical products or byproducts from bovines are obtained only under strict conditions of respectful and caring treatment: Milk in particular is never denied to a dam's calf; cows are preferably milked by hand; and no artificial means of increasing milk are used. Under similar strict monitoring, working oxen are engaged in traction services such that they are never overworked. In the interest of fairness

to all recipients of goods received from our bovines, we label all products accurately, including indication of the type or breed of cow (and whether cow or buffalo) from which the products originate. Further, our accounting of cow care expenses is transparent: All donors can know how their donations are being used, and they can be informed of any challenges the cow care organizations face. On a deeper level, we pursue social justice and environmental justice by showing how cows deserve to be protected, thus approaching the ideal of proper respect and dignity for domestic and farm animals, in a way analogous and pursuing the ideal of citizenship. Further in the interest of fairness to persons suspected of breaking any laws related to bovines—in matters of welfare or protection from slaughter—we respect and uphold the rule of law and we condemn any illegal and violent acts of "cow vigilantism"; rather, "neighborhood watches" are trained to inform authorities of improper activity involving cows.

3. *Cow Care and Liberty.* Cow care activists recognize that all people are at liberty to follow the diet of their choice, within various sorts of constraints. If they are accustomed to eating meat, we encourage them and explain reasons for, reducing meat consumption, and we appreciate and applaud the work of any environmental activism that explicitly confronts the environmental cost of carnism. We also urge anyone consuming dairy to source their dairy products from cow care families and institutions that are authorized (as described in # 1 above). Persons unable to source ahimsa dairy are encouraged to move toward this goal in a progressive manner.[38] To persons accustomed to eat meat, we explain traditions of animal sacrifice, and where this is legal, we

---

[38] Madhava Candra Das (Seattle and Bangalore) suggests a five-stage progression to "liquid dharma": (1) One continues to buy commercially produced milk while becoming aware of the hidden "karmic cost"—the consequences of one's action (karma); (2) one buys organic commercial milk, and sets aside the equivalent amount spent as "cow credit" to be donated in support of an "ahimsa" dairy; (3) one makes arrangement with a local dairy farmer to keep one's own cow(s), to be protected for life, whatever the cost; (4) one creates a community "ahimsa" dairy together with local like-minded persons, pooling resources and hiring the necessary management and labor; and (5) one has one's own cows, caring for them at or very near one's home.

encourage them to restrict meat to animals thus immolated (by quali-fied priests), preferably having been personally present at the event.[39] To dairy farmers in particular, we offer free workshops on methods of converting their operations into nonviolent, cow care-based establish-ments. Similar workshops and information events, as well as media, are available for the public for learning to adopt a nonviolent vegetarian or vegan diet. Anticipatory communities have well-organized outreach programs, especially to schools and colleges, explaining how cow care is vital to a culture of human liberty that is not anthropocentric and speciesist. On a deeper level, the moral foundation of liberty is served by education in the principles and processes of yoga, the aim of which is final liberation from the bondage of temporal life. We show how cow care can be integral to realizing this aim.

4. *Cow Care and Loyalty.* Loyalty of cow carers to their own nations is encouraged, as is loyalty to their particular communities. Dharma-based cow carer culture is such that these loyalties are not energized by antagonism against other nations or communities. Rather, by car-ing for cows, these persons make a deep connection with the earth and their environment in such ways that they cultivate knowledge in the quality of goodness and illumination, as described in the Bha-gavad Gita: "Knowledge in goodness is that by which one sees a single unchanging reality in all beings, undivided in the divided" (Bg. 18.20; transl. Goswami 2015). In turn, this knowledge nurtures cow carers' dedication to the bovines in their charge, such that they do all that is necessary for the bovines to be cared for properly for life, thus never to have their trust in their carers *betrayed.* Such knowledge also protects carers from the tendency to commodify bovines and their products against their own interests, which would also be a form of betrayal.[40] Thus, cow carers, who are well trained and practiced in their duties, are

---

[39]This suggestion is bound to be controversial, as most modern states prohibit ritual slaughter of animals—ironically so, since they strongly allow and support the non-ritual, factory slaughter of animals. Numerous questions arise regarding how such ritual slaughter would be done in practice. In this positive affirmation exercise, suffice to mention that in a Hindu context it would be done according to the appropriate ritual texts; it would be regulated by an appropriate agency; and it would surely involve a system of state taxation.

[40]Thomas Berry wrote, "To reduce any mode of being simply to that of a commodity as its primary status or relation within the community of existence is a betrayal" (Berry 2006, p. 9).

dedicated to the cause of cow care as a key means of bringing well-being to the world. In their dedication to this cause, however, they do not make the mistake of holding abstract cause above interpersonal duties. The possible danger of tribalism being fostered in the name of loyalty associated with cow care is avoided by eschewing the quality of passion with its tendency to sharpen tribal identities.

5. *Cow Care and Authority.* Authority in relation to cow care is specifically located first and foremost in persons with extensive experience in all aspects of cow care, including cow-based organic agriculture. Indeed, these persons are recognized and accredited as teachers of cow care, in learning institutions connected with cow care centers and cow-based organic farms and village communities throughout the world. At a few larger such centers research projects related to cow care and cow-based organic farming are undertaken, with results published in peer-reviewed journals and disseminated to other educators, farmers, and cow carers.[41] Such educational and research facilities serve the purpose of bringing knowledge and education forward as requirements for protection of cows, as expressed by M. K. Gandhi. Cow care organizational entities network extensively with a variety of organizations dedicated to deep reform of human-environment relationships, sharing knowledge and experience.[42] All levels of practical knowledge related to cow care are, in turn, supported by the spiritual knowledge in goodness mentioned previously, namely the recognition of a "single unchanging reality in all beings." As farmers realize practically the advantages of cow care for sustainable farming (possibly supported by various schemes in connection with goshalas and community agriculture organizations), the *subversive* activities involving cow smuggling or other illegal or abusive practices are replaced with effective local communities of cow protection. For persons and communities who do not understand the importance of cow care and therefore allow or take part in bovine

---

[41] A dedicated, multi-disciplinary, peer-reviewed journal, *Cow Care*, is also planned.

[42] For example, they could network with IFOAM—Organics International (including Good Food for All); the Global Ecological Integrity Group (see Westra et al. 2017; the Bhumi Project—http://www.bhumiproject.org/; the Vegetarian Resource Group—https://www.vrg.org/).

abuse, there are substantial dedicated staff of "animal police" with special training in all relevant skills.[43] At the same time, the cow care community is deeply challenging to and subversive of self-destructive lifestyles centered in the consumption of animal bodies.

6. *Cow Care and Sanctity.* Those who care for cows regard them as bearers of sanctity in that they are unique in their ways of creaturely being in the world such that humans can care for them. For many Hindus, cows are special because they are regarded as especially dear to the supreme divinity Krishna. Therefore, they are practiced to give cows' special attention. Such special attention is not at the cost of other creatures (indeed, in the bovine family, Krishna is said to have a pet buffalo); rather, to again quote M. K. Gandhi, "We can realize our duty towards the animal world and discharge it by wisely pursuing our dharma of service to the cow. At the root of cow-protection is the realization of our dharma towards the sub-human species" (Gandhi 1999, vol. 81, pp. 139–140). Cow care practitioners "wisely pursue" such dharma by balancing sanctity with care, the first of these six moral foundations of political life in which cow care is practiced. In this way, they realize the true sanctity of all life, and thus they contribute significantly to protection of the biosphere from *degradation*—the direct result of the absence of a sense of sanctity.

These six affirmations serve to point us in a positive, and not implausible, direction toward a bright future for cows and thereby for other creatures and for human beings on this planet. Again, these affirmations are nourished by a sense of dharma as a cosmic principle of balance, which in turn supports action characterized by the mode of goodness and illumination. Conscientious Hindus pursuing such a dharma culture would claim that the aim of sustainability (which is also a feature of this mode) on all levels, including environmental and political, is achievable. Anticipatory communities in which these ideals are pursued need to be supported and their

---

[43] Maneka Gandhi reports the institution of "animal police" in Holland, with an initial 500 officers dedicated to overseeing observance of animal protection laws in the country. Gandhi laments that in India, far from such services existing, the existing police generally take *hafta*—bribes—from cow smugglers and other animal law offenders. https://www.peopleforanimalsindia.org, "Animal Police" (accessed 9 February 2019).

examples followed to spread the awareness that an alternative way of living is available, and we have much to learn from well-cared-for cows about how to realize this alternative.

With the six cow care affirmations, we arrive at what may seem a utopian vision located in dharma culture upheld by *sattva-guna* practices. But, one might well ask, even if such a culture would become established and even widespread, what is to keep it from degenerating back down to *rajo-guna* and even *tamo-guna*? According to the Bhagavad Gita, the three modes of phenomenal nature tend to transmute from one into another. Therefore, Krishna urges Arjuna to rise above these modes and be situated in transcendence, constituted of bhakti, the culture of devotion, and practice of care. Thus, the negative tendency that *sattva-guna* carries in relation to cow care, namely the tendency for one to become preoccupied with "correctness" at the expense of genuine care, is overcome. Such transcendent cow care assumes and includes correct action in relation to cows and other beings, from a position of joyful heightened relational awareness that sees all life in connection with divine being.

References

Adams, Carol J. 2010 [1990]. *The Sexual Politics of Meat: A Feminist-Vegetarian Critical Theory*. New York: Continuum.

Berry, Thomas. 2006. Preface. In *A Communion of Subjects: Animals in Religion, Science and Ethics*, ed. Paul Waldau and Kimberly Patton, 5–10. New York: Columbia University Press.

Bilimoria, Purushottama. 2018. Animal Justice and Moral Mendacity. *Sophia* 57: 53–67. https://doi.org/10.1007/s11841-018-0652-y.

Burgat, Florence. 2004. Non-violence Toward Animals in the Thinking of Gandhi: The Problem of Animal Husbandry. *Journal of Agricultural and Environmental Ethics* 14: 223–248.

Carlson, Laurie Winn. 2001. *Cattle: An Informal Social History*. Chicago: Ivan R. Dee.

Cochrane, Alasdair. 2012. *Animal Rights Without Liberation: Applied Ethics and Human Obligations*. New York: Columbia University Press.

Cohen, Geoffrey L., and David K. Sherman. 2014. The Psychology of Change: Self-Affirmation and Social Psychological Intervention. *Annual Review of Psychology* 65: 333–371.

Dasi, Krishna-lila (Krisztina Danka). 2012. ISKCON Retains Its Religious Status in Hungary. Retrieved December 10, 2018 from https://iskconnews.org/iskcon-retains-its-religious-status-in-hungary,3148/.

DEFRA. 2009. *Protocol for Handling Welfare Cases in Cooperation with the Hindu Community*, 2nd ed. London: Department of Environment, Food and Rural Affairs.

Dharampal and T.M. Mukundan. 2002. *The British Origin of Cow Slaughter in India—With Some British Documents on the Anti-Kine-Killing-Movement of 1880–1894*. Mussoorie: Society for Integrated Development of Himalayas.

Fahy, John. 2018. The Constructive Ambiguity of Vedic Culture in ISKCON Mayapur. *Journal of Hindu Studies* 11 (3): 1–26. https://doi.org/10.1093/jhs/hiy008.

Fici, Christopher. 2015. The Spiritual Ecology of Gaudiya Vaishnavism in Praxis: The Govardhan Eco-Village (GEV). *Journal of Vaishnava Studies* 24 (1) (Fall): 205–226.

Fici, Christopher. 2018. Ahimsa for Vaishnava Earth Ethics. *Journal of Vaishnava Studies* 26 (2) (Spring): 5–16.

Frazier, Jessica. 2017. *Hindu Worldviews: Theories of Self, Ritual and Reality*. London: Bloomsbury.

Gandhi, Mohandas K. 1999. *The Collected Works of Mahatma Gandhi (CWMG)* (Electronic Book). New Delhi: Publications Division Government of India.

Ganeri, Jonardon. 2003. Hinduism and the Proper Work of Reason. In *The Blackwell Companion to Hinduism*, ed. Gavin Flood. Oxford: Routledge.

Goswami, H.D. 2015. *A Comprehensive Guide to Bhagavad-gītā with Literal Translation*. Gainesville, FL: Krishna West.

Haidt, Jonathan. 2012. *The Religious Mind: Why Good People Are Divided by Politics and Religion*. New York: Pantheon Books.

Hurn, Samantha. 2018. Exposing the Harm in Euthanasia: Ahimsa and an Alternative View on Animal Welfare as Expressed in the Beliefs and Practices of the Skanda Vale Ashram, West Wales. In *Routledge Handbook of Religion and Animal Ethics*, ed. Andrew Linzey and Clair Linzey, 264–274. London: Routledge.

Johnson, Lisa. 2012. *Power, Knowledge, Animals*. New York: Palgrave Macmillan.

Klostermaier, Klaus K. 1988. A Universe of Feelings. In *Shri Krishna Caitanya and the Bhakti Religion*, Studia Irenica 33, ed. Edmund Weber and Tilak Raj Chopra, 113–133. Frankfurt am Main: Peter Lang.

Lamb, Gary. 1994. Community Supported Agriculture: Can It Become the Basis for a New Associative Economy? *The Threefold Review* (Summer/Fall), Issue 11. The Margaret Fuller Corporation. https://plantbiology.rutgers.edu/faculty/robson/AGECOLOCT28-6.pdf. Accessed 11 May 2018.

Lodha, G.M. (ed.). 2002. *Report of the National Commission on Cattle* (Chapter I Introduction). New Delhi: Department of Animal Husbandry, Ministry of Agriculture and Farmers' Welfare, Government of India. http://dahd.nic.in/related-links/chapter-i-introduction. Accessed 25 September 2017.

Lokhit Pashu-Palak Sansthan and Ilse Köhler-Rollefson. 2005. *Indigenous Breeds, Local Communities: Documenting Animal Breeds and Breeding from a Community Perspective*. Sadri, Rajasthan, India: Lokhit Pashu-Palak Sansthan (LPPS).

Long, Jeffery D. 2013. The Dharma Paradigm and Ethos: Some Insights from Jainism and Vedānta. *International Journal of Dharma Studies* 1: 2. https://doi.org/10.1186/2196-8802-1-2.

Meyer-Glitza, Patrick. 2018. Cattle Husbandry Without Slaughtering: A Lifetime of Care Is Fair. In *Ethical Vegetarianism and Veganism*, ed. Andrew Linzey and Clair Linzey, 192–200. Abingdon: Routledge.

NA. 2008. Tribute to Krsna the Padayatra Ox. *Care for Cows Newletter*, February. http://www.careforcows.org/cfc/download/newsletters/CFCNewsFeb2008.pdf. Accessed 11 December 2018.

NA. 2013. *Symbiotic Development: 9 Case Studies in Service of Mother Earth*. Thane, Maharashtra, India: Govardhan Eco Village.

Narayanan, Yamini. 2018a. Cow Protection as 'Casteised Speciesism': Sacralisation, Commercialisation and Politicisation. *South Asia: Journal of South Asian Studies* 41 (2): 331–351. https://doi.org/10.1080/00856401.2018.1419794.

Narayanan, Yamini. 2018b. Cow Protectionism and Indian Animal Advocacy: the Fracturing and Fusing of Social Movements. Lecture, Institute for Critical Animal Studies Oceania Conference, 14 July 2017, Melbourne. Retrieved December 6, 2018 from https://archive.org/details/YaminiN.

Prabhupāda, A.C. Bhaktivedanta Swami. 1983 [1972]. *Bhagavad-gītā as It Is*. Los Angeles: Bhaktivedanta Book Trust.

Prabhupāda, A.C. Bhaktivedanta Swami. 2005 [1974]. *Śrī Caitanya-Caritāmṛta of Kṛṣṇadāsa Kavirāja Gosvāmī* (Nine Volume Edition), Ādi-līlā, vol. 2 (Chapters 8–17). Los Angeles: Bhaktivedanta Book Trust.

Prabhupāda, A.C. Bhaktivedanta Swami, and Hridayananda Das Goswami, trans. 1993. *Śrīmad Bhāgavatam*. Cantos 1–12 in 18 Vols. Sanskrit text, translation and commentary. Los Angeles: Bhaktivedanta Book Trust.

Prime, Ranchor. 2009. *Cows and the Earth: A Story of Kinder Dairy Farming*. London: Fitzrovia Press.

Rasmussen, Larry L. 2013. *Earth-Honoring Faith: Religious Ethics in a New Key.* Oxford: Oxford University Press.

Rusza, Ferenc. n.d. Sankhya. Internet Encyclopedia of Philosophy, 4b: *Prakṛti* and the Three *guṇa-s.* https://www.iep.utm.edu/sankhya/#SH4b. Accessed 7 July 2019.

Sunder, Jason. 2018. Religious Beef: Dalit Literature, Bare Life, and Cow Protection in India. *Interventions: International Journal of Postcolonial Studies,* 1–17. https://doi.org/10.1080/1369801X.2018.1558097. Accessed 10 March 2019.

Warrier, Maya. 2010. The Temple Bull Controversy at Skanda Vale and the Construction of Hindu Identity in Britain. *International Journal of Hindu Studies* 13 (3): 261–278.

Westra, Laura, Janice Gray, and Franz-Theo Gottwald (eds.). 2017. *The Role of Integrity in the Governance of the Commons: Governance, Ecology, Law, Ethics.* Cham, Switzerland: Springer.

7

Concluding Ruminations

The previous chapter sketched a vision for cow care in the late modern world, in the form of anticipatory communities and affirmations regarding cow care's ethos and practices. As a vision, it is a proximate echo to the temporally distant vision portrayed in Chapter 2: There, we glimpsed the Rigveda's mysterious world in which cows and words for "cow" converge and diverge, the words sometimes seeming to take lives of their own in poetic flights that stretch linguistic parameters of meaning. As we traversed through later Sanskrit and eventually non-Sanskrit Indic literature in search of "bovinity," we found it to be ever in proximity to divinity. This is most apparent in the world of the Bhagavata Purana, where he who is seen as *purna-bhagavan*—the supreme divinity-in-full, Krishna—makes cowherding his daily, playfully pleasing vocation.

Between these two visions are two fields of modern discourse. The first (discussed in Chapter 3) is a debate on how to regard ancient Indian tradition with respect to cows and, more broadly, what should be understood from textual accounts of animal (including cow) sacrifice and the apparent opposite, namely textual exhortations to nonviolence. The second field of

© The Author(s) 2020
K. R. Valpey, *Cow Care in Hindu Animal Ethics*,
The Palgrave Macmillan Animal Ethics Series,
https://doi.org/10.1007/978-3-030-28408-4_7

discourse (discussed in Chapter 5) is how traditional Hindu ethical ideals may be brought into conversation with contemporary animal ethics thought. In the middle of this sandwich, in Chapter 4, we viewed the varied and complicated present-day situation in India regarding cow care and, sadly, the widespread *lack* of care for cows as a consequence of changing economic, social, cultural, and political pressures.

As we step back to reflect on the terrain thus traversed, I see a broad conceptual binary emerge, one of a "utopian/dystopian" character. The two visions that open and close this account may strike us as utopian, in the sense of being imaginary, nostalgic, and wishful thinking. Yet within the ancient idyllic vision lurks always the threat of dystopian chaos, embodied in the demon serpent Vritra (disruptor of environmental balance), in the Panis (disruptors of the Vedic ritual order), and in the threat of cattle rustlers (disruptors of social well-being). Further, toward the end of the Bhagavata Purana there is a detailed anticipation of a pervasive cultural breakdown in the progression of the present age, *kali-yuga*. We recall that Kali personified senselessly tortures the earth-cow and the dharma-bull, but is nevertheless given shelter in places of impiety by King Parikshit, enabling Kali to insidiously spread his debilitating influence throughout the world. This account near the Bhagavata's beginning prepares readers for the much more detailed description of the Kali age near the text's conclusion.

Sage Shuka begins this latter account (BhP 12.2) by listing characteristics of human life that diminish day by day. Dharma, truthfulness, cleanliness, tolerance, mercy, life duration, and physical strength all dwindle by the force of time. As good qualities diminish, dark qualities become prominent, such that truth gives way to hypocrisy and audacity, dharma yields to the desire for fame, and justice is cloaked in greed for power. In this state of affairs, Shuka asks rhetorically, "What can a person who injures other living beings for the sake of his body know about his own self-interest, since his activities are simply leading him to hell?" (BhP 12.2.41; translation: Goswami et al., in Prabhupada 2017). But then, following his description of the Kali age, Shuka recites the Bhumi-gita—the Song of the Earth (BhP 12.3). In this song, Earth (as a feminine personage) laughs at the folly of countless kings in their futile efforts to conquer her. In seeking control of her, they fail to control their own sensory urges and become oblivious to their own impending death (BhP 12.3.4–5). The upshot of such ignorance is misuse of the earth's gifts, leading to scarcity. Swami Prabhupada discussed this dynamic on numerous occasions, for example in a lecture he gave in Los Angeles:

> As soon as you make misuse, the supply will be stopped. After all, the supply is not in your control. You cannot manufacture all these things. You can kill thousands of cows daily, but you cannot generate even one ant. And you are very much proud of your science. You see. Just produce one ant in the laboratory, moving, with independence. And you are killing so many animals? Why? So how long this will go on? Everything will be stopped. (Prabhupada 2017; Lecture, Bhagavad Gita 3.11–19, Los Angeles, 27 December 1968)

Again, mistreatment of cows is linked to mistreatment of the earth, and these are seen as products of human arrogance. Such arrogance is epitomized in scientists who make brash, unfounded claims to the effect that humans' well-being will always be secured by their (scientists') inexhaustible powers to create. Therefore—so the arrogant reasoning goes—the killing of animals can continue without restriction. And so, as the slaughter continues, it is such "reasoning" that drives the dystopia that humans are making of this planet today.

We wonder, what is the trajectory of our collective human behavior toward our planet earth? A related question concerns the possibility, or impossibility, of changing our habits, perhaps our very "nature." From one perspective of early Sanskrit literature, one should not hope for such change. The well-known guidebook of prudent conduct (*niti*), the Panchatantra, consists of several talking animal fables. Among these, a dominant theme is that one cannot expect persons to change their nature (*svabhava*), and in particular, predators will always remain predators, no matter their apparently "reformed" behavior (Taylor 2007, pp. 47–50). By this understanding, as long as humans see themselves as meat-eating predators, all our philosophies can only serve to perpetuate this identity and our *wild*—unrestrained—behavior. As G.K. Chesterton (1909, p. 265) aptly put it,

> We talk of wild animals; but man is the only wild animal. It is man that
> has broken out. All other animals are tame animals; following the rugged
> respectability of the tribe or type all other animals are domestic animals;
> man alone is ever undomestic, either as a profligate or a monk.

Further, if the present age is characterized by diminishing observance of
normative precepts—dharma—what can be expected to motivate persons
to "tame" themselves in their eating habits? For clearly, this is the crucial
point. Humans have allowed themselves to be conditioned to regard the
taste of animal flesh as greatly pleasurable, and any amount of ethical
or even medical argumentation for avoiding meat—however compelling
to reason this might be—fails to change our hearts. To give up meat is
regarded as an unwanted austerity, maybe good for saints but not for
"normal" people. Habit persists, justified simply by virtue of being habit,
which we can at least label as "carnism" (Joy 2010, p. 29).

And yet, our human inquisitiveness impels us to ask, can human wildness be tamed? Could it be that what makes us human is quintessentially
our capacity for inner reform and transformation, a capacity facilitated
and nourished by spiritual wisdom, ethical reasoning, reflection, and conscious choice? This, I would argue, is particularly the view represented
in the Bhagavad Gita and in the entire bhakti stream of Hindu tradition. Further, this view is of critical importance for understanding and
changing taste, which is so foundational to the existence and changing of
eating habits. More on this in a moment, but first some background by
way of a short look at general principles espoused in the Bhagavad Gita,
linking these to the story of King Yudhishthira and the dog, discussed in
Chapter 5.

We have already considered one key theme of the Bhagavad Gita, namely
equal vision (*sama-darshana*): "A learned brahmin, a cow, an elephant, a
dog, or a 'dog-eater'—a wise person sees [them all] with equal vision"
(Gita 5.18). It was such equal vision that enabled King Yudhishthira to
insist that his companion dog be admitted with him into heaven; and
by this insistence, he exercised his power of *choice* (*iccha*). With these
two foundational capacities—seeing with equal vision and making a conscious choice based on that vision, the king was empowered to practice
nonviolence (*ahimsa*) and, in the process of doing so, to *teach by example*
(*acharya*) to the world. To hold fast to this teaching despite all resistance

from the world required and enabled him to realize *humility* (*amanitva*), which he could experience blossoming into true *affection* (*priti*) for fellow beings.[1]

Changing Taste

A key stanza early in the Bhagavad Gita (2.59) gives a clue about how all six of these themes are realized, through a subtle but decisive shift in "taste" (*rasa*):

> Sense objects fade away for the embodied who does not partake of them, except for the taste; for one who has seen the Supreme, even this taste fades. (translation based on Schweig 2007, p. 52)[2]

The word *rasa*, here translated as "taste," has a rich constellation of meanings, bringing the physical, sensory experience of tasting into direct application in the sphere of classical Sanskrit aesthetic theory. For us to note here is the link indicated in this stanza between two sorts of perception, namely perception of sense objects, on the one hand, and, on the other, perception of divinity (the latter referred to in this stanza as "seeing"—from the Sanskrit verbal root *drish*). Bhakti is the means by which the sensate self (*atman*), ordinarily absorbed in matter, is enabled to experience its counterpart—the trans-temporal higher self (*paramatman*) in an aesthetically pleasing, or "relishable" relationship (Valpey 2019). Such a relationship is the culmination of realizing the six above-mentioned themes, with reciprocal affection experienced as an ever-dynamic *sharing* (a basic translation of the word *bhakti*). Such affectionate relationship becomes the basis for molding action according to *divine preference*, as we discussed in Chapter 5.

---

[1] I am grateful to Shaunaka Rishi Das for calling attention to this sixfold thematic understanding of the Bhagavad-gita.

[2] H.D. Goswami's alternative translation (Goswami 2015, p. 159) replaces "who has seen the Supreme" with "on seeing something better." The Sanskrit term in question is *param*, which can have both senses. Arguably, the entire Bhagavad-gita makes the case that the "something better" that one aspires to see is none other than the supreme person. See also Swami Prabhupada's translation of the stanza in n. 18 of the previous chapter.

Bhakti, as presented in authoritative Hindu texts, has both an individual, private dimension and a social, public dimension. Reciprocal affection with the divine cowherd Krishna has practical implications that extend outward into the world to include a positive, care-full (caring) engagement with the environment to the furthest extent of human influence on the environment. Naturally, such care-full engagement impacts human political and economic behavior, whereby fresh, feasible ideas for bringing about the good for all can be welcomed and implemented. From "good taste" in spiritual matters, good choices for long-term well-being are made.[3] Good choices include wise—restrained—uses of technology based on a clear sense that human life becomes humane only when there is self-restraint.

For Vaishnava Hindus, in its most aesthetically refined and perfected form, wise engagement inspired by the bhakti paradigm brings about the realization of Vraja-Vrindavan, the land in which bovinity and divinity find their perfection. Krishnadasa Kaviraja offers a striking vision of such realization in his Chaitanya Charitamrita account of the Vaishnava bhakti saint, Sri Chaitanya. According to Krishnadasa, to fully appreciate the potential of this vision, we best regard Chaitanya as none other than Krishna incarnate.[4] But although he is Krishna, he covers his divine identity for the duration of his earthly manifest life (during the late fifteenth and early sixteenth centuries), preferring to be absorbed in the identity and mood of Krishna's devotee. It is in this mood (*bhava*) that Chaitanya, after having taken the vows of a renunciant (*sannyasin*), had set out from Puri, on India's eastern coast, journeying by foot with a single companion, Balabhadra, toward far-away Vrindavan. For our discussion, it is an episode said to have occurred along the way to Vrindavan that is significant.

As Chaitanya and Balabhadra were passing through the Jharikhanda forest (present-day Jharkhand, central India), they encountered many animals, including elephants, tigers, rhinoceros, boars, deer, and assorted bird

---

[3] With consideration of economics, I am thinking of Alf Hornborg's radical proposal for "redesigning money for sustainability, justice, and resilience" as a viable means for consequential transformation of human–environmental relations that would have immediate and far-reaching benefits for the planet as a whole and for individual animals. See Hornborg (2017).

[4] Krishnadas elaborates a detailed theological treatise to justify this claim in the opening four chapters of his Chaitanya Charitamrita. Here, suffice to say that he refers extensively to scriptural proof-texts, but he also offers his own theological reasoning and, through the entire work, an account of Chaitanya's life by way of confirming his claim.

varieties. These creatures, attracted by Chaitanya and his joyous singing of divine names, would follow him along the path, prompting Chaitanya to feel that he was already in Vrindavan and to recite a certain Bhagavata Purana stanza:

> Vṛndāvana is the transcendental abode of the Lord. There is no hunger, anger or thirst there. Though naturally inimical, human beings and fierce animals live together there in transcendental friendship. (CC Madhya 17.39, quoting BhP 10.13.60; translation Prabhupada 2005, Madhya-Lila vol. 4, pp. 20–21)

Krishnadasa tells his readers that Balabhadra, initially fearful of the jungle animals, became shocked and amazed to witness how Chaitanya would induce them not only to "sing" the name "Krishna," but to also "dance." Indeed, "the tigers and deer began to embrace one another, and touching mouths, they began to kiss. When Śrī Caitanya Mahāprabhu saw all this fun, He began to smile. Finally He left the animals and continued on His way" (CC Madhya 17.40–43; translation Prabhupada 2005, Madhya vol. 4, pp. 21–22).

This is a vision that may be said to go beyond the two visions presented in the second and sixth chapters of this study. As fantastical as it sounds, this vision of divine-human–animal celebratory interaction awakens our imagination to a state where our most fundamental presuppositions about the workings of nature and the necessity of biotic violence are, at least momentarily, suspended. It also points to a particular notion prominent in Hindu aesthetic tradition, namely the experience of *wonder* (*adbhuta-rasa*). Wonder can be seen as the seed of humility—the acknowledgment of our smallness, vulnerability, and limited reasoning power, that can open us to the sort of inner transformation—the change of heart—necessary for a truly ethical way of life in relation to all living beings in this world. Out of such humility may come the sort of understanding that could allow us to embrace and live by the implications of Chaitanya's assertion (which he is said to have spoken to his student Sanatan Goswami, on his return journey to Puri from Vrindavan): "All creatures (*jivas*) are eternal servants of the supreme person, Krishna" (CC Madhya 20.108). The simple shift in consciousness from trying to be masters to accepting that we are servants can, according to Vaishnava Hindu understanding, make all the difference for realizing our proper relationship to all beings.

Throughout this book, I have attempted to bring Hindu thought and practice regarding nonhuman animals—especially cows—into view for consideration in the broader area of animal ethics. The fact that we specify as a "branch" of ethical reflection our approach to nonhuman animals already indicates a major distinction we make, between humans and nonhumans (and it seems to imply that this branch is at best peripheral to what are regarded as the central issues of ethics, confined within human society). Here, I have made a further distinction, namely between humans who regard themselves or are regarded as Hindus and other humans (many of whom may have never heard the term "Hindu"). With this distinction and a further distinction—between cows (a type of *bovinae*) and other nonhuman animals—I have added complexity to the discussion about desirable behavior of humans in relation to nonhuman animals. I have also attempted to show how, by looking closely at how Hindus regard cows in the context of a worldview that fundamentally questions the nature of selfhood—human or otherwise—we can, despite our wildness, open ourselves to broader and better ways of thinking about and acting within our—non-nonhuman—relationships with nonhuman animals (Figs. 7.1 and 7.2).

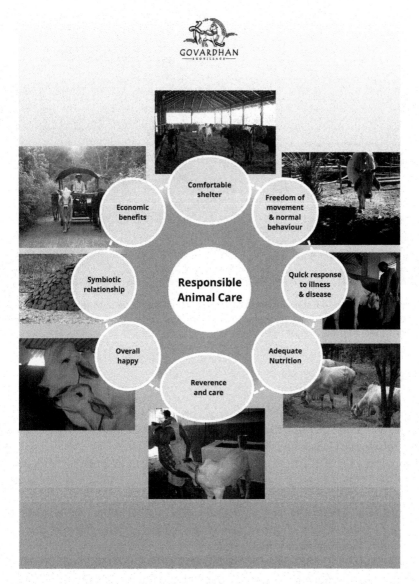

Fig. 7.1 Govardhan Eco Village Responsible Animal Care brochure indicates cow care as care affirmation (Used with permission of Govardhan Eco Village [Thane, Maharashtra, India], all rights reserved)

258 K. R. Valpey

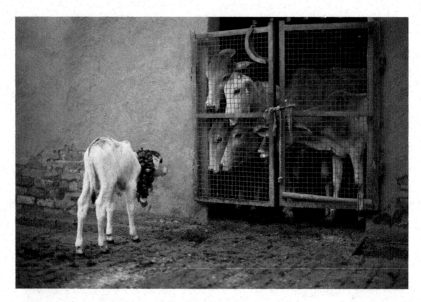

Fig. 7.2 Week-old Balaram (same calf as on front cover) is examined by his bovine seniors at Care For Cows goshala, Vrindavan (*Source* Image courtesy of the photographer, Filip Cargonja)

References

Chesterton, Gilbert K. 1909. *Orthodoxy*. London: John Lane.

Goswami, H.D. 2015. *A Comprehensive Guide to the Bhagavad-gītā with Literal Translation*. Gainesville, FL: Krishna West.

Hornborg, Alf. 2017. How to Turn an Ocean Liner: A Proposal for Voluntary Degrowth by Redesigning Money for Sustainability, Justice, and Resilience. *Journal of Political Ecology* 24: 623–632.

Joy, Melanie. 2010. *Why We Love Dogs, Eat Pigs, and Wear Cows: An Introduction to Carnism, the Belief System That Allows Us to Eat Some Animals and Not Others*. San Francisco: Conari Press.

Prabhupāda, A.C. Bhaktivedanta Swami. [1974] 2005. *Śrī Caitanya-Caritāmṛta of Kṛṣṇadāsa Kavirāja Gosvāmī* (Nine Volume Edition), Madhya-līlā, vol. 4 (Chapters 17–20). Los Angeles: Bhaktivedanta Book Trust.

Prabhupāda, A.C. Bhaktivedanta Swami. 2017. *The Complete Teachings of His Divine Grace A.C. Bhaktivedanta Swami Prabhupāda*. Vedabase CD-ROM Version 2017.2. Sandy Ridge, NC: Bhaktivedanta Archives.

Schweig, Graham M. 2007. *Bhagavad Gītā: The Beloved Lord's Secret Love Song.* New York: HarperSanFrancisco.

Taylor, McComas. 2007. *The Fall of the Indigo Jackal: The Discourse of Division and Pūrṇabhadra's Pañcatantra.* Albany, NY: State University of New York.

Valpey, Kenneth. 2019. From Devouring to Honouring: A Vaishnava-Hindu Therapeutic Perspective on Human Culinary Choice. In *Ethical Vegetarianism and Veganism,* ed. Andrew Linzey and Clair Linzey, 222–231. London: Routledge.

Index

© The Editor(s) (if applicable) and The Author(s) 2020
K. R. Valpey, *Cow Care in Hindu Animal Ethics*,
The Palgrave Macmillan Animal Ethics Series,
https://doi.org/10.1007/978-3-030-28408-4

Printed by Printforce, United Kingdom